Dictionary of

Communication Disorders

Third edition

Dictionary of Communication Disorders

Third edition

David W. H. Morris

M.A., B.Ling., Dip.C.C.S., MRCSLT (reg)

Consultant Speech and Language Therapist,
VOCA*tion* Partnership, Monifieth, Dundee, Scotland.

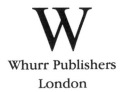

Whurr Publishers
London

First published by Taylor and Francis in 1988
All right reserved by Whurr Publishers Ltd 1990
Reprinted 1990
Second edition published by Whurr Publishers Ltd 1993
Reprinted 1994
Third edition 1997
Published by Whurr Publishers Ltd
19b Compton Terrace London
N1 2UN, England

British Library Cataloguing in Publication Data
A catalogue record for this book is available from the
British Library.

ISBN 1-897635-83 4

Printed and bound in the UK by Athenaeum Press Ltd,
Gateshead, Tyne & Wear

Contents

Dedication
To my parents

Preface to third edition

This third edition of *Dictionary of Communication Disorders* marks the tenth anniversary of the author's conception of a dictionary to clarify terminology for students and practitioners.

As with most new editions, it has been updated to include new terminology in the field of communication disorders including terms which may have been omitted in previous editions.

As many of the references as possible have been updated including the latest editions of the main texts. The references range from the 1950s to the 1990s with literature from each of the intervening decades. There are 285 references in all, and the number of references and percentage for each of the decades are: 1950s (3; 1%), 1960s (16; 5.6%), 1970s (63; 22%), 1980s (106; 37%) and 1990s (97; 34%).

Various comments made about the second edition have proved to be invaluable in the writing of the third edition. In general, technology changes very rapidly and no less so than in the field of communication disorders. A dictionary of communication disorders should include descriptions of all relevant terminology, including the different types of high-tech communication aids and appropriate computer software, especially when these are not extensively covered in a Speech and Language Therapy course. This follows the original aim of the dictionary to be a useful guide to the essential terms used in Speech and Language Therapy and its allied subjects.

This third edition has also been made as politically correct as possible. Thus, all references to 'mental handicap' have been changed to 'learning disability' and the word 'suffer' has been replaced with the verb 'have'.

The cross-references within definitions have been made more consistent and many cross-referenced terms within the text have been removed to provide for easier reading.

It is unfortunate in the changing world of communication disorders with new assessments, rehabilitation packages and technology, that a dictionary can become out of date quickly. I hope that, with regular updating of terminology and references, this dictionary can keep pace with the changes and maintain my original aim of clarifying the terminology which may mystify many entering or already working in the field of communication disorders.

David W. H. Morris

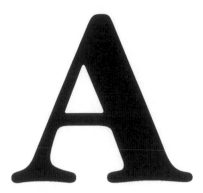

AAC *see* ALTERNATIVE AUGMENTATIVE COMMUNICATION.

abdomen the lower part of the trunk which contains within its cavity the gut, liver, kidneys and urogenital system. The walls comprise muscles and bones. The roof of the abdomen is formed by the diaphragm which separates the thoracic and abdominal organs. This structure produces abdominal–diaphragmatic respiration. The anterior wall is wholly muscle while the back wall is made up of muscles. *See* Tortora and Grabowski (1993).

abdominal–diaphragmatic respiration breathing produced by the movement of the diaphragm. In inspiration, the diaphragm decreases in size and pushes out the abdominal wall. In expiration, the opposite happens. This form of breathing is most common in men. It is opposed to THORACIC RESPIRATION (*see* CLAVICULAR). *See* Tortora and Grabowski (1993).

abducens nerve (cranial nerves vi) *see* CRANIAL NERVES.

abduction a description of movement away from the midline. It is opposed to adduction. *See* Tortora and Grabowski (1993).

aberrant a psychological description of behaviour which is found to be abnormal.

ability tests *see* INTELLIGENCE TESTS.

ABLB *see* ALTERNATE BINAURAL LOUDNESS BALANCE TEST.

abnormal behaviour behaviour that departs from the norm. Such behaviour can be found in those with conditions such as SCHIZOPHRENIA, AFFECTIVE DISORDERS, ANXIETY DISORDERS, personality disorders and drug-dependency. Treatment can include BEHAVIOUR THERAPY and PSYCHOANALYSIS although some disorders may be improved through drug therapy. *See* Atkinson et al (1993).

ABR *see* AUDITORY BRAIN-STEM RESPONSE.

abreaction *see* PSYCHOANALYSIS.

abrupt release during the production of plosives, there is a sudden release of built-up pressure in the mouth. It is opposed to DELAYED RELEASE. *See* Cruttenden (1994).

AC an abbreviation for air conduction (*see* PURE-TONE AUDIOMETRY).

acalculia an arithmetic disorder which can present as a person's inability to cope with arithmetic processes or as difficulty in the spoken or written production of symbols used in calculation. It can be associated with APHASIA, especially if the client has a lesion in the right hemisphere producing problems of spatial orientation. *See* Eisenson (1984).

accent

1. The part of a word, phrase or sentence which is given increased loudness as well as a change to the intonation pattern. In English, the

accent is regular in that the main accent is always on a specific syllable of each word. See Cruttenden (1994).

2. The regional variations of pronunciation of a language. These variations are caused by differences in the type of vowel and consonant used as well as in the phonological and prosodic patterns produced by the speaker. It is differentiated from a DIALECT. See Wells (1982).

acceptability an acceptable utterance made by one native speaker to another native speaker is one which follows the syntactic rules of that language. See Lyons (1968).

acceptable stammer the criterion of success used by speech therapists using the STAMMER MORE FLUENTLY approach.

access

1. The process by which the computer obtains data or other information from a disk in a disk drive or instructions from a memory so that they can be carried out (e.g. from a program in the computer's memory). See Brookshear (1991).

2. In ALTERNATIVE AUGMENTATIVE COMMUNICATION, access refers to the means by which a person uses a communication aid. This may be by direct manual selection, headpointing or by using switches. See Beukelman and Mirenda (1992).

accessory nerve (cranial nerve XI) see CRANIAL NERVES.

Acorn computers Acorn produced the BBC series of microcomputers. They began by producing the BBC A, BBC B and BBC B+ models. Since that time, there have been further additions: the Master 128, the Master compact and the Archimedes ranges and RISC Personal Computers.

acoupedics see EDUCATION OF HEARING-IMPAIRED CHILDREN.

acoustic method see EDUCATION OF HEARING-IMPAIRED CHILDREN.

acoustic neurinoma this is a retrocochlear problem producing a unilateral hearing loss, TINNITUS and forms of imbalance. The audiologist can determine the presence or otherwise of an acoustic neurinoma. If it is found that the client has a unilateral sensorineural hearing loss, this should be taken as possible evidence of an acoustic neurinoma. If some of the following are found from carrying out a battery of audiometric tests – absence of RECRUITMENT, positive TONE DECAY, a poor word discrimination ability – a retrocochlear pathology is suggested. CT (COMPUTED TOMOGRAPHY) scans and MRI (MAGNETIC RESONANCE IMAGING) scans can also be used to determine this lesion site. See Ginsberg and White (1985).

acoustic phonetics the physiological study of the ways in which sounds are produced. Acoustic phonetics is the procedure used to carry out such a study. The three main acoustic features which describe the ways in which sounds are produced are frequency, intensity and time. Frequency is the number of times in which the vocal cords open and close when a sound is produced. The unit used to measure frequency is the hertz (Hz). A hertz is the number of cycles per second used in producing a sound (i.e. the number of times the cords open and close). So, if a sound causes the cords to vibrate 550 times per second, then the frequency of the sound will be 550 Hz or 550 cps. The higher frequencies of the sound, which are whole multiples of the fundamental frequency, are known as harmonics. To work out the harmonic series of a sound, the fundamental frequency is multiplied by successive whole numbers. For example, if a sound has a fundamental frequency (i.e. 100 cycles per second) and a frequency of 300 cycles per second, this is the third harmonic of the sound. Intensity is the measure of how loud the sound is which a person produces. The unit used to measure intensity is the decibel (dB). Quality of a sound changes in relation to the change in frequencies between sounds. Thus, there is a difference in the quality of any two vowels that are held to be different. *See* Ladefoged (1993).

acquired agnosia *see* AGNOSIA.

acquired aphasia *see* APHASIA.

acquired apraxia a disorder caused by trauma to the brain after birth affecting the person's coordination. As a speech disorder, it is characterised by the person groping for the correct order of sounds which produces trial and error realisations of the required sounds. In the most severe forms of acquired apraxia, people may not even be able to start off a word with the correct sound. The programming of the movements required to make sounds in a particular order becomes disordered, particularly, though not exclusively, with polysyllabic words. There is also disruption to PROSODY, articulatory inconsistency and difficulties in initiating utterances. *See* Miller (1986).

acquired disorders any disorder not caused at birth (i.e. congenital disorders) in the PRENATAL or PERINATAL stages. Acquired disorders usually have an organic cause (e.g. CEREBROVASCULAR ACCIDENT, HEAD INJURY, etc.). The most common acquired disorders of communication are APHASIA, DYSARTHRIA and DYSPRAXIA. They can occur at any time in the person's life. *See* Crystal (1993).

acquired dyslexia occurs following damage to the brain caused by such conditions as CEREBROVASCULAR ACCIDENT, HEAD INJURY or brain tumour (*see* TUMOURS OF THE CENTRAL NERVOUS SYSTEM). There are four types:

1. Phonological dyslexia: the inability to read non-words (*see* NONSENSE WORDS) aloud, e.g. 'dup', 'getuld' etc., while the ability to read everyday words aloud remains intact. Other symptoms such as 'visual errors' in reading aloud non-words e.g. [dek] for /desk/ can appear. Derivational errors are also present when reading words aloud, especially when they contain bound morphemes (*see* MORPHOLOGY).

2. Deep dyslexia: semantic errors are present when reading. Other symptoms can also be present e.g. visual impairment, function word substitution and derivational errors. Low-imageability words are harder to read aloud than high-imageability words; verbs are harder to read than adjectives, which are harder to read than nouns. However, deep dyslexia can only be diagnosed if a semantic error is present in reading aloud, even if there are none of the other symptoms.

3. Letter-by-letter reader (word-form dyslexia): what is being read aloud can only be understood by reading one letter at a time. This is the only acquired dyslexia that is produced by a focal lesion, the link between the ANGULAR GYRUS in the left cerebral hemisphere (*see* CEREBRAL HEMISPHERES) and the visual input system in both hemispheres being broken. Since the angular gyrus is unaffected per se, writing is relatively unimpaired. It is also known as Déjérine's syndrome after the neurologist who discovered the disconnection.

4. Surface dyslexia: a disturbance between the visual word recognition system and the semantic system. However, the word can still be spoken since the visual recognition system and phonemic system are still intact. *See* Patterson and Kay (1982); Ellis (1993); Nickels (1995).

acquired dysphasia *see* APHASIA.

acquired hearing loss a hearing loss produced by disease, tumours, natural ageing, excessive noise, otoxic drugs and trauma at any time during a person's life after birth.

acquisition a learning process opposed to INNATENESS. The phrase language

3

acquisition is used to describe the stages of language development in children between the ages of 9 months and 5 years. It can also be used to describe how children with specific learning difficulties, or adults with speech and language disorders, develop communication skills which they have hitherto lacked. *See* Clark and Clark (1977); Fromkin and Rodman (1993).

acrocephalosyndactyly *see* APERT'S SYNDROME.

Action Picture Test devised by Renfrew in 1966 (2nd edn, 1971; 3rd edn, 1989) it is a quick means of finding out if a child has a LANGUAGE DELAY or SPECIFIC DEVELOPMENTAL LANGUAGE DISORDER. Answers are sought to simple questions regarding what is being enacted in each of the ten coloured pictures of everyday events. Responses are analysed for (1) amount of correct information given and (2) the grammatical forms used, which should include some irregular forms of verbs and nouns as well as complex and compound sentences. The test is standardised in the UK and can be applied to children from 3;6 to 8;6 years. *See* Renfrew (1989) in Appendix I.

active voice usually contrasted with passive, it refers to a grammatical construction in which the grammatical subject is typically the actor as in:

1. The dog bit the man.

In earlier versions of transformational generative grammar (*see* TRANSFORMATIONAL GRAMMAR), active sentences and their passive equivalents were related by a transformational rule. *See* Clark and Clark (1977); Fromkin and Rodman (1993).

acuity the sounds which the ear can pick up. These can vary depending on how near the sound source the person is. *See* Denes and Pinson (1973).

acute

1. A description of the sudden onset of

an illness or disease. It is opposed to chronic.

2. A distinctive feature used by Jakobson and Halle to distinguish sounds made towards the front of the mouth and produced using the high frequencies such as alveolar, dental and palatal consonants (*see* ARTICULATION) from vowels made in a similar position. These are denoted as [+ACUTE].

See Hyman (1975).

acute laryngitis inflammation of laryngeal mucosa and of VOCAL FOLDS. The symptoms are hoarseness leading to DYSPHONIA, malaise, pain when speaking, redness and swelling of the LARYNX. Vocal rest is usually recommended and possibly a period of speech and language therapy. *See* Pracy et al (1974); Greene and Mathieson (1989).

adaptation *see* ASSIMILATION (1).

address in computer terms, a number which identifies one memory location in the computer's memory, or one peripheral device or unit. Each part of the computer's memory has an address, so the information which goes into the memory always goes to a specific location. *See* Bishop (1985); Brookshear (1991).

adduction a description of movement towards the midline. It is opposed to abduction. *See* Tortora and Grabowski (1993).

adenoidal facies *see* MOUTH BREATHING.

adenoids lymphatic tissue found in the posterior wall of the nasopharynx (*see* PHARYNX). At birth, the adenoids are small and as the child grows older, the adenoids grow until puberty when they atrophy. If they become large, they may block the eustachian tube (*see* EAR) causing hearing problems and/or nasal obstruction. Such obstruction results in mouth breathing and snoring. There is a particular facial appearance known as 'adenoidal facies' associated with the condition.

The obstruction may become so significant that an adenoidectomy, in which the adenoids are removed, is necessary. *See* Pracy et al (1974).

adiadochokinesis an inability to produce rapid sequences of movement. In speech, this relates to rapid alternating movements of the articulators. It occurs as a feature of DYSPRAXIA and DYSARTHRIA. *See* Darley et al (1975); Robertson and Thomson (1986).

adjective adjectives appear in NOUN PHRASES and are also used as predicates. This is exemplified by the following sentences:.

1. An interesting question.
2. The question is interesting.

In noun phrases, the adjective comes between the determiner and the noun, as will be found in the discussion concerning CONSTITUENT ANALYSIS. However, when two or more adjectives are used in a noun phrase, they are placed in a particular order. Following analysis of sentences in which the noun is premodified by one or more adjectives, the following order can be found:
determiner – general – age – colour – participle – provenance – noun – denominal – head noun.
This order takes account of sentences such as those shown in the box below.
In all cases, the noun phrase will make sense by using any or none of these adjectives. *See* Strang (1968); Fromkin and Rodman (1993).

adverb an adverb is usually an adjunct to the verb. The most common and most recognisable form of adverb is an adjective with '-ly' attached to it, e.g. quickly, slowly, etc. These adverbs are found in sentences such as:.

1. He ran quickly.
2. The tortoise moves slowly.

However, adverbs can take other forms. They can mark time and place, e.g. here, now, there, perhaps, seldom, etc. These can only be used as adverbs. Other words such as 'yesterday, downstairs, first, etc.' can be used as adverbs although they can function in other ways. Adverbs, like adjectives, can be used in the positive, comparative and superlative forms. They can be differentiated from adjectives by the use of 'than' which requires a comparative and 'of all' which requires a superlative. Consider, for example, the following sentences:

1. The world cup is the greatest football competition of all [football competitions].
2. Stephen Hendry played better than Jimmy White.

See Strang (1968); Fromkin and Rodman (1993).

affect an emotional response to a thought. If there is no emotion shown, such as in SCHIZOPHRENIA, there is FLATTENING OF AFFECT. *See* Atkinson et al (1993).

affective disorders a group of disorders which produce abnormal moods in a person, e.g. DEPRESSION and MANIC-DEPRESSION. *See* Atkinson et al (1993).

afferent a description of how sensory nerve impulses reach the CENTRAL NERVOUS SYSTEM. Afferent neurons are those which carry nerve impulses from the body tissue into the central nervous system. It is opposed to efferent or motor neurons. *See* Taverner (1983); Tortora and Grabowski (1993).

det.	gen.	age	colour	partic.	proven.	noun	head noun
The	large	old	grey	crumbling	English	country	house
A	small		blue				ball
The	great	young		battling	French	rugby	team.

(based on Quirk and Greenbaum, 1979)

afferent (motor) aphasia an APHASIA described by Aleksandr Luria in the 1960s. It is similar to ACQUIRED DYSPRAXIA. The person is unable to predict where or how to position the articulators for sound production. A severe afferent aphasia results in a global problem; in a mild form, only similar sounds may be confused, e.g. bilabials /p,b,m/, alveolars /t,d,n/, etc. There may also be a disorder in the person's writing ability by confusing what Luria calls articulemes, i.e. sounds. The lesion causing such a disorder occurs in the secondary zones of the postcentral kinaesthetic cortex. *See* Eisenson (1984).

affix a general term used in MORPHOLOGY to refer to the adding of morphemes (prefixes and suffixes) to the base form. *See* Allerton (1979); Fromkin and Rodman (1993).

affricate *see* ARTICULATION.

AFP an abbreviation for alpha-fetoprotein. *See* AMNIOCENTESIS.

age-equivalent scores scores that are obtained after working out the results of assessments by looking up tables in the manuals of the assessments concerned. Such tests have undergone standardisation and so these scores can be compared to the chronological age of the assessed person.

ageing the process of becoming older. During this process a person undergoes physical changes, e.g. anatomical, physiological and skeletal changes, increasing problems with vision and hearing; psychological changes, e.g. possible changes in intellectual levels; memory changes, e.g. memory loss in senile dementia or, more generally, memory problems that occur with retaining material requiring full attention and ability to organise it. Neugarten et al (1963) (*see* Bromley, 1988) showed that, as they grow older, people have different reactions to their old age. These reactions can be positive where a person substitutes other activities for lost activities, becoming less positive where a person gradually withdraws from the world to one who is deeply pessimistic and no longer takes part in life. In a study of 87-year-old men, Reichard (1962) (*see* Bromley, 1988) found similar reactions to the ageing process. Davison and Neale summed up growing old as: '...the greatest challenge of old people is to cope with reality, the gradual loss of loved ones and friends, the deterioration of physical and psychological capacities, the low regard in which they are held by the culture at large' (Davison and Neale, 1994, ch. 17). *See* Bromley (1988); Davison and Neale (1994).

Agenda a high-tech communication aid which is a portable word processor and can be used also as a diary, address book, alarm and calculator. It has a 4-line, 20-character display screen and can be attached to computers or printers, etc. It has a 32K memory with two slots for additional memory packs. Agenda has two keypads – an alphanumeric keypad and a microwriter-type keyboard allowing a quick entry of messages using different finger/thumb combinations.

aglossia *see* GLOSSECTOMY.

agnosia a disorder of understanding speech or knowing what objects are although speech can still be heard and objects touched. There are five main types which may be congenital or acquired:

1. Acoustic – difficulty in sound discrimination.
2. Pure word deafness – a specific difficulty in recognising speech sounds resulting in an inability to repeat what has been said but, with difficulty, can use some spontaneous speech, read or write. At times, by watching the therapist's face intently, lip-reading may be possible for auditory comprehension.
3. Visual – inability to understand various situations by failing to recognise visual stimuli.

4. Tactile – inability to recognise objects by feel or touch.
5. Auditory verbal – the inability to understand spoken language.

See Eisenson (1984); Byers Brown and Edwards (1989).

agonist muscle a description of the contraction of one muscle against another that acts as an antagonist muscle. This muscle contraction is also known as a prime mover. *See* Tortora and Grabowski (1993).

agrammatism restricted use of grammar, often associated with aphasia. *See* APHASIA (1).

agraphia disorders of writing which may be neurological in origin. There are three types:.

1. Phonological dysgraphia: impaired ability to write and spell non-words (*see* NONSENSE WORDS) while the ability to write real words is preserved.
2. Surface dysgraphia: inability to write and spell real words.
3. Deep dysgraphia: semantic errors occur in writing.

See Rosenbek et al (1989).

AI *see* ARTIFICIAL INTELLIGENCE.

air bone gap *see* PURE-TONE AUDIOMETRY.

air conduction *see* PURE-TONE AUDIOMETRY.

air-conduction hearing aid the main type of hearing aid given to those who have a hearing loss. There are also BONE-CONDUCTION HEARING AIDS. *See* Miller (1972).

airstreams the source of power for the production of most sounds is made by air from the lungs. There are four types of airstream:.

1. Pulmonic egressive airstream: the normal airstream used by all speakers using all varieties of English. The speaker uses ABDOMINAL-DIAPHRAGMATIC RESPIRATION or clavicular breathing (*see* CLAVICULAR) although the length of message which can be produced in the former will be more than that pro-

duced in the latter. Thus, if a deep breath is taken in and let out from the lungs producing a fricative (*see* ARTICULATION), e.g. /s/, a very long uninterrupted sound will be produced until the breath runs out. No other type of airstream allows the speaker such a long uninterrupted flow for producing speech.
2. Pulmonic ingressive airstream: this airstream works in the opposite way to the egressive airstream. The lungs are emptied of air followed by the speaker producing speech while drawing air into the lungs. If a similar fricative is produced as in (1), the sound will not be sustained for very long. Speech can become very distorted.
3. Glottalic airstream: an airstream produced by a movement of the larynx with glottal closure. An upward movement of the larynx produces a glottalic egressive airstream which produces an ejective, while a downward movement of the larynx produces a glottalic ingressive airstream which produces an implosive.
4. Velaric airstream: an airstream which produces velaric ingressive stops or clicks.

See Ladefoged (1993).

akinetic seizures a type of seizure that usually affects only children. It produces a loss of tone that may be generalised throughout the body or specific to the neck. In the former, the child collapses to the ground while in the latter, the head falls forward onto the chest. It can be controlled by clonazepam or sodium valproate. Children may have other types of seizure. *See* Gilroy and Holliday (1982).

alexia *see* ACQUIRED DYSLEXIA and DEVELOPMENTAL DYSLEXIA.

alexia with agraphia a disorder of both reading and writing but EXPRESSIVE LANGUAGE and auditory comprehension are intact. *See* Ellis (1993); Rosenbek et al (1989).

alexia without agraphia also known as pure alexia, it is a rare condition in which the person cannot read but can write. Oral expression, auditory comprehension and repetition are intact. Benson and Geschwind (1969) suggested the following specific symptoms: right homonymous hemianopia, inability to identify colours, an impairment in calculation, occasional problems with naming objects, severely impaired reading and relatively intact writing. *See* Rosenbek et al (1989).

allomorph *see* MORPHOLOGY.

allophone *see* PHONOLOGY.

AllTalk a high-tech communication aid with digitised speech unit. An overlay of 128 cells can be used with each programmed with individual messages. Alternatively, groups of cells can be programmed with the one message or even all 128 can be programmed with one message. The messages can be customised for each individual user. The memory has a standard capacity of 600 words but can be expanded to 1200 words. Different levels can be programmed so that the levels can be entered by operating the 'level keys' and accessed by the 'talk key' in the correct order. It is operated by rechargeable batteries.

alpha-fetoprotein *see* AMNIOCENTESIS.

Alpha Talker a high-tech communication aid with digitised speech output. It uses MINSPEAK to organise vocabulary to store into the device. It has a memory of three minutes for standard speech and five minutes for extended speech. With an extra memory card this can be increased to 15 minutes standard and 25 minutes extended. It can be accessed using direct manual selection, optical headpointing, single, dual or two switch scanning. Overlays of 4, 8 and 32 locations can be used. Other features include icon prediction, which shows by illuminating a light on a symbol which symbols have messages stored under them and shows the others in the sequence; and pre-dictive selection, which makes symbols with nothing stored under them inoperative when using with direct manual selection or optical headpointing, while with scanning, the scanning light jumps the unused symbols. The Alpha Talker also allows for auditory prompts to be stored. This allows for a user to hear the names of the symbols before they are activated. This feature can be used either with direct manual selection, optical headpointing or using a switch for scanning. The device's memory can be backed up on computer, and basic computer emulation is possible as well as attaching the DIRECTOR, an environmental control system. The Flash Eprom system means the device should never lose its memory. *See* Appendix IV.

alternate binaural loudness balance (ABLB) test a test for recruitment used with those who have a unilateral hearing loss. It attempts to match the loudness level of two tones. It requires a two-channel audiometer to send a signal to each ear. The tester presents a tone of 20 dB SL (SENSATION LEVEL) to the better ear and the same tone to the poorer ear. The tone is increased until it is heard at the same loudness in each ear.

alternate hypothesis the hypothesis must be proved by statistical analysis. This hypothesis states that a significant difference between scores does exist if it is proven by carrying out either a parametric or a non-parametric test (*see* PARAMETRIC TESTS). The alternate hypothesis must be set out before the results of the experiment are known and be based on what is known about the subject under investigation from other experiments, surveys etc. It will be proved if the null hypothesis is rejected. Both hypotheses are used in inferential statistics. The alternate hypothesis is also known as the experimental hypothesis. *See* Miller (1975); Porkess (1988); Clarke and Cooke (1992).

alternative augmentative communication (AAC) the forms of communication offered to those who cannot speak or whose communication attempts are unintelligible and to those who require help to overcome word-finding difficulties. Systems which are described as being high-tech are operated by mechanical, electronic or computerised means. Low-tech systems comprise sign languages, such as MAKATON, BRITISH SIGN LANGUAGE or PAGET-GORMAN SIGN SYSTEM, gesture systems and communication books or boards. The International Society of Alternative Augmentative Communication (ISAAC) promotes the use of AAC techniques throughout the world. *See* Enderby (1987); Beukelman and Mirenda (1992); Jones (1995a) (training in the use of AAC systems).

Alzheimer's disease a type of dementia. The cause is unknown but there is an increasing rate of loss of neurons in the brain. Atrophy occurs in both the white and grey matter of the BRAIN while the sulci widen and the gyri atrophy. A person with this disease will have a gradual loss of short-term memory which becomes worse while long-term memory (*see* MEMORY) is retained intact until the later stages of the disease. A change in personality occurs as well, e.g. a quiet person can become aggressive, and transient hemiplegias may also occur. Women are affected twice as frequently as men and death may occur 2–5 years after the original onset. The language impairment of someone with Alzheimer's disease reflects quite closely the disorders found in Wernicke's aphasia (*see* APHASIA (2)), especially in the later stages of the disease. However, in the early stages, there may be language problems such as the use of circumlocution in naming tasks and verbal paraphasias which may be self-corrected. In conversation, the patient in the early stages of the disease will digress quite frequently and will find difficulty returning to the subject and will often fail to answer a specific question but not a related one. This latter problem, as with others, gets worse as the disease progresses. The person will respond better to specific comprehension tests than in conversation and will succeed in repetition tasks when asked to repeat high probability phrases, e.g. near the table in the dining room, while they become confused and make paraphasic errors with low probability phrases, e.g. the Chinese fan had a rare emerald. As the disease progresses, all these problems become worse with an increase in verbal and literal PARAPHASIAS and circumlocution. Cueing strategies such as phonemic or semantic cueing have little effect. In conversation, the digression from the subject is much more marked. In the later stages, PRAGMATICS become a problem with the person becoming mute or using palilalia or ECHOLALIA. Jargon (*see* JARGON APHASIA) becomes more evident and discourse becomes empty. During a naming task, the correct label may be produced amongst other language but the person will be unaware of producing the correct word. *See* Obler and Albert (1981); Gilroy and Holliday (1982) (medical); Stafford-Clark and Smith (1983) (psychological); Stevens (1992) (communication); Patel and Satz (1994).

American Speech-Language Hearing Association (ASHA) the governing body for those who work with speech/language and hearing disorders in the United States. Its equivalent in the United Kingdom is the ROYAL COLLEGE OF SPEECH AND LANGUAGE THERAPISTS.

Amerind a sign language originally used by the American Indians. It is used more often with those people who have some degree of word-finding difficulty in APHASIA. It can be used as a means of augmenting the person's communication. The use of sign language can help the person to think of the word they are wanting to produce.

Many of the signs can be produced by one hand which can be useful with patients who have an accompanying hemiplegia. *See* Skelly (1979).

amitriptyline the most commonly used antidepressant drug (*see* ANTIDEPRESSANT DRUGS). Its side effects can be dry mouth, palpitation, tachycardia, postural hypotension, dizziness, constipation, vomiting, glaucoma, loss of accommodation, i.e. eye problem with focusing, and urinary problems. The person may not have any of these side effects or may have only some of them. *See* Stafford-Clark and Smith (1983); Atkinson et al (1993); Davison and Neale (1994).

amniocentesis an invasive technique to monitor the development of the fetus *in utero* at 14 weeks into the pregnancy. A quantity of amniotic fluid, which surrounds the fetus, is drawn off so that its protein content and cells can be examined. A chromosomal analysis will show if there are the correct number of chromosomes, if they have the correct structure and if the sex chromosomes are present or damaged. Alpha-fetoprotein is also measured. This is a protein which can leak out of the fetal circulation. *See* Hosking (1982); Tortora and Grabowski (1993).

Amsterdam-Nijmegen Everyday Language Test an assessment devised by Blomert and colleagues for those with APHASIA. It is designed to measure the level of communicative abilities of aphasic individuals and the changes in their abilities over time. Communicative effectiveness is measured by the adequacy of getting a message across while verbal communication is measured by the understandability of the message and the intelligibility of the utterance. The assessment uses real-life scenarios found in everyday situations. There are two parallel versions each comprising 10 items. The responses for every item are scored on two five-point scales. *See* Blomert et al (1994) in Appendix I.

Amstrad Amstrad was founded in 1968 by Alan Sugar. AMSTRAD itself is an acronym for Alan Michael Sugar Trading. Locoscript is the software designed for use with Amstrad's word processing systems. Amstrad was one of the first companies to market low price clones of the IBM PC. As with IBM compatible computers, these machines use MS-DOS as their operating system. Amstrad have also produced small compact word processors which can have an address book, database and spreadsheet programs.

anacoluthon an utterance during which the speaker changes from one syntactic structure to another without finishing the first.

once upon a time there was a – are you listening to me?

The speaker has shown that he has the intention of making an utterance but has broken off without finishing it to make another utterance. *See* Huddleston (1976).

anal stage *see* PSYCHOSEXUAL STAGES OF DEVELOPMENT.

anaphora a process which allows for one linguistic unit to refer back to one previously given. This is usually with a pronoun:

George wrote that himself.

'Himself' is the reflexive pronoun which anaphorically relates to George. *See* Huddleston (1976).

anarthria the severest form of DYSARTHRIA wherein articulate speech is grossly affected. It arises from impairment of the CENTRAL NERVOUS SYSTEM or of peripheral cranial nerves controlling movement of the articulators. As a result, the person may need to use some form of AAC (ALTERNATIVE AUGMENTATIVE COMMUNICATION) to allow communication to take place. *See* Darley et al (1975).

anatomy a study of the structures that exist in the human body. Some of these are visible to the eye, such as the mouth, face, arms and legs, while others cannot be seen until the body is dissected or 'cut-up' (the word 'anatomy' means 'cutting-up'). *See* Tortora and Grabowski (1993).

angiography a method of examining the blood vessels proposed by Egas Moniz in 1927. A radio-opaque solution is injected into an artery, followed by serial X-ray photographs being taken every second or so. It is a useful technique for pinpointing vascular malformations and aneurysms. Information is also provided of occlusive vascular disease and space-occupying lesions. A safer and improved technique for carrying out angiography is DIGITAL SUBTRACTION ANGIOGRAPHY. *See* Barr (1979).

angioma a tumour composed of blood or lymphatic vessels. Usually benign, it may be found in any tissue of the body. *See also* TUMOURS OF THE CENTRAL NERVOUS SYSTEM. *See* Gilroy and Holliday (1982).

angular gyrus a structure found in the parietal lobe of the brain. There are two parts which form the inferior parietal lobule: the angular gyrus is one and the supramarginal gyrus is the other. The angular gyrus is considered to be important in the acts of reading and writing. A disorder can produce letter-by-letter reading or Déjérine's syndrome (*see* ACQUIRED DYSLEXIA (3)). *See* Barr (1979).

ankyloglossus more commonly called a tongue-tie, it is produced by the lingual frenulum being attached all the way along the underside of the TONGUE. Tongue movement is restricted which can produce articulation problems. The frenulum can either be snipped surgically or the child can be shown how to compensate to improve his articulation. *See* Tortora and Grabowski (1993).

anomia word-finding difficulties which may be developmental or acquired. *See also* APHASIA (4).

anorexia nervosa an eating disorder characterised by the pathological desire not to gain weight. In the USA, its incidence is 1–2 per cent and is in the ratio of 20:1 in favour of females; it is common in young women in their late teens and twenties. Most people who have anorexia usually think they look overweight although they may lose 25 per cent of their normal body weight which can result in undernourishment and other associated problems. *See* Atkinson et al (1993).

anosognosia failure of a person to recognise the disabled side of the body caused by trauma to one of the cerebral hemispheres. Language may remain intact.

ANS *see* AUTONOMIC NERVOUS SYSTEM.

antagonist a muscle contraction which is opposed to the contraction of the prime mover, i.e. agonist muscle. *See* Tortora and Grabowski (1993).

anterior a distinctive feature proposed by Chomsky and Halle. It is used to produce a distinction of sounds produced towards the front of the mouth. The sounds which are denoted as [+ANTERIOR] are dentals and labials (*see* ARTICULATION). *See* Hyman (1975).

anterograde often referring to a type of amnesia, it refers to the inability to acquire new information or remember what happens in the person's daily routine. *See* Atkinson et al (1993).

antidepressant drugs tricyclic drugs given to treat those who have endogenous DEPRESSION. The most commonly used antidepressant drugs are:

amitriptyline,	protriptyline,
imipramine,	dothiepin,
clomipramine,	trimipramine,
noritriptyline,	doxepin.

For the side effects of these drugs, *see* AMITRIPTYLINE. *See* Stafford-Clark and Smith (1983); Atkinson et al (1993); Davison and Neale (1994).

anxiety a neurotic disorder. Abnormal anxiety is caused by acute fear which is often irrational and produces feelings of panic. Someone with such irrational anxieties may show some of the following features:

11

1. Anxiety may dominate their mental status.
2. Physical symptoms (e.g. tachycardia – abnormal heart rhythms).
3. Restlessness, sleeplessness and sweating, etc.
4. Choking, suffocation, collapse.
5. HYPOCHONDRIASIS.

Not everyone with anxiety has all of these symptoms. It will depend on severity of the anxiety condition. Treatment can be given by PSYCHOTHER-APY, ANXIETY DRUG THERAPY, BEHAVIOUR THERAPY and self-help groups. *See* Stafford-Clark and Smith (1983); Atkinson et al (1993); Davison and Neale (1994).

anxiety disorders a group of disorders which produce abnormal behaviour. The main symptom is anxiety or anxiety-producing PHOBIAS or OBSESSIVE-COMPULSIVE DISORDERS. *See* Atkinson et al (1993); Davison and Neale (1994).

anxiety drug therapy the main drugs used are benzodiazepines. They act partly on the brain and partly by decreasing the activity of the spinal reflex centres. The drugs which take a long time to act are diazepam, chlordiazepoxide medazepam, clorazepate and oxazepam. The main side effect of these drugs is drowsiness. The drugs which take a shorter time to act are lorazepam, temazepam and triazolam. They can produce problems with the kidneys. The drug is taken at night so that the person can be fully aware of what is happening during the day.The only problem with such drugs is a growing dependence on them resulting in the person becoming unreceptive to other non-medication forms of therapy. Other drugs used in the treatment of anxiety are MONOAMINE OXIDASE INHIBITORS and tricyclic ANTIDEPRESSANT DRUGS. Beta-blocking drugs can also be given to reduce an abnormally fast heartbeat and for sedation during the night. *See* Stafford-Clark and Smith (1983); Atkinson et al (1993); Davison and Neale (1994).

apathy a reaction of certain people to various situations (e.g. frustration). They withdraw and become indifferent to certain situations whereas others react with aggression to similar situations. It is uncertain why this should happen but it may be learned behaviour, their in-born personality or due to their surrounding environment. *See* Atkinson et al (1993).

Apert's syndrome a condition which involves an abnormal growth of the cranium and malformed fingers and toes. The face has a particular appearance with wide-set, bulging eyes, abnormally small maxillae, crowded teeth and a protruding mandible. Usually, intelligence is within normal limits although there can be a degree of LEARNING DISABILITY. It is also known as acrocephalosyndactyly. *See* Hosking (1982); Goodman and Gorlin (1983).

apex in articulatory terms, the tip of the tongue which is used, for example, to produce dental and some alveolar sounds, known as apico-alveolar. *See* Catford (1989).

Apgar score devised by Virginia Apgar, it is a test given to new born babies. If the numerical test scores remain low for a considerable time, the prognosis for the baby's life and possible neurological sequelae are poor. It gives a value of 0, 1 or 2 to the baby's heart rate, respiratory effort, reflex irritability, muscle tone and colour. It is repeated at 1 and 5 minutes of life. *See* Illingworth (1987).

aphasia also known as dysphasia. The most common causes are CEREBROVASCULAR ACCIDENT (CVA), HEAD INJURY or brain tumour (*see* TUMOURS OF THE CENTRAL NERVOUS SYSTEM) which have affected part of the BRAIN, usually the left cerebral hemisphere (*see* CEREBRAL HEMISPHERES) which controls the use of language – both comprehension and expressive language. Both can be disordered to a lesser or greater degree. Both children and adults are affected. In most cases, it is more accurately termed acquired dysphasia as language has already been acquired. Those who are diagnosed as having acquired dysphasia can have word-finding difficulties, comprehension problems, both auditory and reading, problems with reading out loud, repetition, serial speech and writing. Those who have word-finding difficulties are said to have a non-fluent aphasia while others who produce fluent speech that is syntactically correct but may be meaningless have a fluent aphasia. Different classifications have been used to describe different kinds of aphasia. They have been produced by the Boston School, Schuell and Aleksandr Luria, among others. Probably the most common classification in use presently is the Boston classification. The following types of aphasia are recognised by this school:

1. Broca's aphasia – speech production is non-fluent. It is marked by phonetic disintegration, by reduced vocabulary, especially of function words, and by restricted grammar (agrammatism). Prosody and written language affected. Auditory verbal comprehension is relatively intact. Luria's terms for this type of aphasia are 'afferent kinaesthetic aphasia' and 'efferent kinaesthetic aphasia'.
2. Wernicke's aphasia – speech is fluent and grammatically and prosodically intact. It is interspersed with neologisms and paraphasias which may be semantic (inappropriate selection of words) or phonemic (deletion, addition, substitution, or mis-sequencing of sounds). Verbal comprehension is severely impaired. Both reading and writing are affected. Luria's term for this type of aphasia is 'acoustic amnesia'. Eisenson described it as being JARGON APHASIA.
3. Conduction aphasia – an inability to repeat words. Short bursts of speech can be fluent though there may be phonemic PARAPHASIAS. Auditory com-

prehension is good relative to the expressive deficit. Luria called this type of aphasia a 'dynamic aphasia'.
4. Anomic aphasia – comprehension is good and speech is fluent and grammatical. There is, however, a marked word retrieval deficit. Recall of proper names and names of objects is most affected. Ideas are expressed through circumlocution. Luria called this type of aphasia 'semantic aphasia'.
5. Transcortical aphasia:
   (a) Motor: a rare condition bearing certain similarities to Broca's aphasia except that there is a disproportionate ability to repeat fluently. Spontaneous speech is dysfluent. Auditory verbal comprehension is good.
   (b) Sensory: also rare. It shares certain features with Wernicke's aphasia. There is good ability to repeat. Propositional speech is empty and echoic. Auditory comprehension is impaired.
6. Global aphasia – a very severe disorder in which all language modalities are affected. Speech is fragmented and reiterative and may be unintelligible. Serial speech may be retained. See Mark et al (1992); van Mourik et al (1992).
7. Pure aphasias – rare conditions in which only one modality is affected leaving the remainder intact.

In a review of the literature concerning thalamic and striato-capsular aphasia, Kennedy and Murdoch (1994) suggest they can be seen as independent aphasic syndromes with the following characteristics:

1. Acute thalamic aphasia (0–3 months post-onset): lack of spontaneous speech (once speech is initiated syntax is intact); naming impairments with semantic and phonemic PARAPHASIAS, neologisms (see JARGON APHASIA), circumlocutions and jargon (see JARGON APHASIA); PERSEVERATION; relatively intact repetitions; some degree of auditory and reading comprehension impairment; impaired writing

13

abilities and fading or lowered voice volume.

2. Chronic thalamic aphasia (more than 3 months post-onset): relatively fluent language; naming deficit, mild auditory and reading comprehension impairment; disorder of writing.

In their review of the literature concerning striato-capsular aphasia, they found that not all lesions in this area of the dominant hemisphere (*see* CEREBRAL HEMISPHERES) result in aphasia and that those who do have an acute form of striatocapsular aphasia exhibit relatively intact abilities to severe impairment in language tasks such as spontaneous speech, naming, repetition, auditory and reading comprehension. There is no uniform type of language disorder; subgroups of aphasia based on lesion site have been proposed. However, at least three distinct patterns of language deficit have been reported to occur:

1. Acute striatocapsular aphasia (0–3 months post-onset):
   (a) anterior lesion: Broca's type aphasia; transcortical motor aphasia; anomic aphasia.
   (b) posterior lesion: Wernicke's type aphasia.
   (c) anterior-posterior lesion: global-type aphasia.
2. Chronic striatocapsular aphasia (more than 3 months post-onset):
   (a) anterior lesion: Broca's type aphasia; transcortical motor-type aphasia.
   (b) posterior lesion: Wernicke's type aphasia; minimal/high level aphasia.
   (c) anterior-posterior lesion: global-type aphasia.

The main assessments used to test for aphasia are the BOSTON DIAGNOSTIC APHASIA EXAMINATION (BDAE), the WESTERN APHASIA BATTERY (WAB), the MINNESOTA TEST FOR THE DIFFERENTIAL DIAGNOSIS OF APHASIA (MTDDA) and various screening tests such as those devised by Whurr (the APHASIA SCREENING TEST) or by Enderby and her colleagues (the FRENCHAY APHASIA SCREENING TEST or the SHEFFIELD SCREENING TEST FOR ACQUIRED LANGUAGE DISORDERS). With the advent of cognitive neuropsychology, Kay and her colleagues have devised the PSYCHOLINGUISTIC ASSESSMENTS OF LANGUAGE PROCESSING IN APHASIA (PALPA). *See* Satz and Bullard-Bates (1981); Eisenson (1984) (adult dysphasia); Rosenbek et al (1989); Sarno (1991); Kay et al (1992) in Appendix I; Basso (1992) (prognostic factors); Martins and Ferro (1992) (recovery in acquired aphasia in children); *Aphasiology* 1993, 7;5 (complete volume on acquired childhood aphasia); Lees (1993); Kennedy and Murdoch (1994); Code and Müller (1995, 1996); Morris (1995a, 1995b) (AAC and Aphasia).

Aphasia Screening Test devised by Whurr in 1974, it is a SCREENING TEST to assess the severity of APHASIA. It covers all modalities of communication in both comprehension (20 tests) and expressive language (30 tests). Each subtest is scored out of 5. The scores are plotted onto a profile chart to give an instant idea of the person's difficulties and where treatment can begin. In some cases, it may be necessary to use a more formal, standardised assessment such as BOSTON DIAGNOSTIC APHASIA EXAMINATION (BDAE), the WESTERN APHASIA BATTERY (WAB), the MINNESOTA TEST FOR THE DIFFERENTIAL DIAGNOSIS OF APHASIA (MTDDA) or the PSYCHOLINGUISTIC ASSESSMENTS OF LANGUAGE PROCESSING IN APHASIA (PALPA). *See* Whurr (1974) in Appendix I; Beech et al (1993).

aphasiology the study of aphasia in all its forms.

aphemia the former (historical) term for APHASIA used by Broca to describe his patient, Leborgne. However, it seems to be thought of more as a term for describing APRAXIA rather than aphasia. *See* Eisenson (1984); Rosenbek et al (1989).

aphonia complete loss of voice. This may be organic in origin, e.g. vocal nodules, or psychogenic, e.g. conversion aphonia. *See* Greene and Mathieson (1989); Fawcus (1991).

Apple Apple was founded in 1981 by Grant Martin and Simon Rowley. Apple can claim to have invented the PC in its business form in the early 1980s with the production of the Apple II. In response to the IBM PC, Apple produced the Macintosh. Apple popularised the concepts of windows, pull-down menus and mice devices although these had originated from Xerox. The original Macintosh, the Mac Classic, was slow and underpowered but as Apple recognised the strengths of the IBM PC, later versions have taken account of limited compatibility with the IBM PC. Since these early computers, Apple have become more commercially orientated and produced the Performa range followed by the latest Power PC Macs which can run IBM PC compatible software without special software. There are also portable Apple computers known as Powerbooks and Power PC Powerbooks. As well as the usual peripherals of printers, CD ROM drives, MODEMS, etc. Apple have produced a Notepad known as the Newton. It can recognise handwriting, which, when sent to the computer, is translated into print.

applied linguistics putting theoretical linguistics into practice. This can happen in speech and language therapy when forming a treatment programme for those who have communication disorders. In such programmes, therapists have to use their knowledge of SYNTAX, SEMANTICS, PRAGMATICS, SOCIOLINGUISTICS and PSYCHOLINGUISTICS to assess the status of the person's linguistic systems. *See* Pit Corder (1973).

applied psychology *see* PSYCHOLOGY.

apposition a linguistic phenomenon which makes an implicit coordination of constituents without the use of a conjunction or pronoun:

1. Fred, the baker's son, went home.
2. Fred who is the baker's son went home.

(1) demonstrates apposition while (2) shows an explicit linkage with a pronoun. *See* Allerton (1979).

appropriateness the type of language people use differs from situation to situation. For example, informal language occurs at parties and among friends while much greater care is taken in the type of language used, for example, in religious services. Variation occurs in both spoken and written forms of English. *See* Crystal and Davy (1969).

apraxia a severe form of dyspraxia. It may be developmental (*see* DEVELOPMENTAL VERBAL APRAXIA and DEVELOPMENTAL VERBAL DYSPRAXIA) or acquired (*see* ACQUIRED APRAXIA) and in the latter case is usually associated with CENTRAL NERVOUS SYSTEM impairment. There is a total inability to programme certain skilled purposeful movements in the absence of loss of motor power, sensation or coordination. It can appear in different forms including constructional, motor, ideo-motor, ideational, verbal and dressing apraxia. Usually, two or more types appear together while it is very rare to find only one type in isolation.

Apraxia Battery for Adults devised by Dabul in 1979, it is an assessment to diagnose the severity of ACQUIRED APRAXIA. There are six subtests:

1. DIADOCHOKINESIS.
2. Increasing word length (e.g. thick – thicken – thickening).
3. Limb and oral apraxia – 10 oral directions for the volitional manipulation of the oral structures and 10 oral commands requiring use of arms and hands.
4. Latency and utterance time for polysyllabic words – 10 polysyllabic words are represented in picture form and the person has to name them immediately after presentation, both latency and utterance times are measured.

15

5. Repeated trials test – the same pictures as used in subtest 4, each word is repeated three times.
6. Inventory of articulation characteristics of apraxia.

See Dabul (1979) in Appendix I.

aprosody absence of appropriate non-segmental parameters of speech, i.e. intonation, stress, rhythm, pause. *See* Crystal (1992).

aptitude tests tests which are designed to predict the client's future performance levels. Unlike achievement tests, which test what the person has already learnt, aptitude tests do not depend on past experience. Thus, intelligence tests can be called aptitude tests as they aim to predict the person's performance over a range of abilities and do not rely on memory recall or practised skills. *See* Atkinson et al (1993).

arcuate fasciculus a band of fibres which links Broca's area to Wernicke's area (*see* CEREBRAL HEMISPHERES). A disturbance in this area of the brain produces conduction aphasia (*see* APHASIA (3)). It is sometimes called the superior longitudinal fasciculus. *See* Barr (1979).

Arnold-Chiari malformation *see* HYDRO-CEPHALUS.

articulation the production of vowels and consonants by the active and passive articulators in the mouth. The active articulators are the moving parts in the mouth which can produce sounds whilst the passive articulators are the non-moving parts of the mouth against which, in the production of many sounds but not all, the active articulators come into contact. There are three ways for describing articulations of sounds:

1. Place of articulation – the different places in the mouth used to produce consonants are:
   a) bilabial – both lips are placed together, e.g. [p, b];
   b) alveolar – the tongue comes either into direct contact with the alveolar ridge, e.g. [t,d] or close to it, e.g. [s, z];.

c) interdental – the only time the tongue is placed between the teeth, e.g. [θ, ð];
d) dental – the tip of the tongue is placed against the top teeth, e.g. [t, d];
e) retroflex – the blade of the tongue is turned back to touch the hard palate, e.g. [ʈ, ɖ,, ʂ, ʐ, ɳ];
f) palatal – the flat of the tongue is placed against the hard palate, e.g. [c, ɟ, ɲ, ç, ʝ j, ʎ].
g) palato-alveolar – the sound is made in two places, both at the alveolar ridge and hard palate, e.g. [tʃ,dʒ];
h) labial-dental – the top teeth are placed over the bottom lip, e.g. [f, v, ɱ, ʋ];
i) labial-velar – the lips approximate to each other and move apart while at the same time there is a slight closure at the velum, e.g. [w];
j) velar – the back of the tongue comes into contact with the soft palate, e.g. [k, g, ŋ, x, ɣ];
k) uvular – the back of the tongue is placed close to the uvula, e.g. [g, ɢ, N, R, χ, ʁ];
l) pharyngeal – the back of tongue is pushed against the wall of the pharynx, e.g. [ħ ʕ];
m) glottal – the vocal folds come together in the glottis producing a break in the production of a word, e.g. [ʔ, h, ɦ].

2. Manner of articulation – the different ways in which the articulators are moved in the mouth:
   a) plosive – the articulators are brought firmly together, pressure is built up behind the closure followed by abrupt release, e.g. [p, b, t, d, ʈ, ɖ, c, ɟ, k, g, q, ɢ, ʔ];
   b) fricatives – the articulators are brought close together without meeting and the airstream is allowed to pass though producing a hissing quality to the sound, e.g. [ɸ, β, f, v, θ, ð, s, z, ʃ, ʒ, ʂ, ʐ, ç, ʝ, x, ɣ, χ, ʁ, ħ, ʕ, h, ɦ];
   c) affricates – a combination of (a) and (b) which occurs in quick sequencing, e.g. [tʃ, dʒ];

d) lateral – the sides of the tongue are lowered while the tongue touches the alveolar ridge in the centre of the mouth, e.g. [l, ɬ, ɭ, ʎ, ʟ];

e) trill/tap – a trill is a series of taps whilst a tap is a very brief, loose contact with the alveolar ridge, e.g. [r, ʀ, ɾ, ɽ];

f) nasal–the soft palate is lowered away from the back wall of the pharynx allowing the airstream to pass into the nasal cavities. There is also an obstruction in the mouth produced by the lips [m], the tongue against the alveolar ridge [n], and the back of the tongue against the soft palate [ŋ];

g) approximant – the articulators are brought close to each other and there is no abrupt release, e.g. [u, ɹ, ɭ, j, ɥ].

3. Voicing sounds can be produced either with the vocal folds vibrating (i.e. voiced), e.g. [b,d,g,v,...] or with them at rest (i.e. voiceless), e.g. [p,t,k,f,...].

Consonants can be described as:
[p] – voiceless bilabial plosive.
[d] – voiced alveolar plosive.
[v] – voiced labiodental fricative.

The CARDINAL VOWEL SYSTEM is used to describe the production of vowels. *See* Ladefoged (1993).

Articulation Attainment Test devised by Catherine Renfrew, it is not meant to be used as a diagnostic test of the child's articulation problem but rather is intended to find out how many consonants a child can produce. The test uses 38 words made up of 100 consonants. The child has to name 38 objects spontaneously as well as produce some serial counting and phrases for repetition. *See* Renfrew (1971) in Appendix I.

articulation delay many children have an articulation difficulty, failing to produce sounds correctly because they cannot place their articulators in the correct position. An articulation delay occurs when a child's articulation development is below the child's chronological age (CA) and fails to acquire the adult articulatory patterns. However, the child will catch up with his CA with regular therapy and/or a home therapy programme. It is also called articulatory immaturity. *See* Grunwell (1987).

articulation disorder the deviant production of speech sounds. It may be structural, e.g. associated with orofacial abnormalities; neurological, e.g. cerebral palsy, or degenerative, e.g. ageing. A child who has this condition requires a very systematic programme to improve his articulation. In other words, unlike an articulation delay, it will not improve with ordinary therapy or in the fullness of time. *See* Grunwell (1987).

articulation tests assessments used by speech and language therapists to find out the severity of the articulation disorder or delay. Two of the most common tests used in the UK are the EDINBURGH ARTICULATION TEST (EAT) and the GOLDMAN-FRISTOE ARTICULATION TEST. *See* Anthony et al (1971) in Appendix I.

articulatory dyspraxia *see* DEVELOPMENTAL VERBAL DYSPRAXIA.

articulatory phonetics a study within phonetics of the way in which articulation of sounds takes place. For this study, introspection and observation of what is going on in people's mouths are carried out as well as the use of such techniques as electromyography, spirometry and palatography. These devices seek to find out how the vocal organs produce speech sounds such as those described under articulation. *See* Catford (1989); Fromkin and Rodman (1993).

artificial intelligence (AI) the attempt to make a computer or other machine make decisions using similar sensory techniques to human beings. The aim is to make the machine 'understand' the input and act upon it using some kind of reasoning processes. The 'intelligence' is written in the computer program and is not contained in the machine itself. *See* Brookshear (1991).

artificial larynx   there are several artificial laryngae available to those who have undergone total laryngectomy. With the larynx removed, to produce voice the person requires artificial techniques such as the Bart's Vibrator, the Medici Speech Vibrator, the Siemen's Servox, the Rexton Laryngophone, the Weston Electronic No. 5A (male) and No. 5B (female). Each works by being placed next to the skin under the chin; a button on the side is pressed, which starts a diaphragm vibrating on top of the device; this produces a voiced sound as the person mouths the sounds. There are facilities to control volume, pitch and tone of voice produced. Most have rechargeable batteries. There are also two pneumatic devices – the Tokyo and Osaka. These consist of a tube which leads from the tracheostoma, passing through a cylindrical unit which contains a rubber membrane. The membrane is vibrated by air from the lungs as a sound source and directs the sound into the mouth by the mouth tube. *See* Edels (1983); Greene and Matheson (1989).

arytenoids   cartilages and muscle found in the LARYNX which control the vocal folds. *See* Tortora and Grabowski (1993).

ASCII   abbreviation for American Standard Code for Information Interchange. The computer uses codes to represent alphabetic, numeric and punctuation characters which are stored in memory or put on the screen. The ASCII characters are those found on the tops of the keys on the keyboard. *See* Brookshear (1991).

asemantic jargon   *see* JARGON APHASIA.

ASHA   *see* AMERICAN SPEECH-LANGUAGE HEARING ASSOCIATION.

aspect   grammatical aspect signals features of the 'temporal contour' of actual states or events. In English, progressive aspect, signalled by a form of the auxiliary 'be + -ing' inflection, conveys a durative timing for the verb to which it is attached as in:

1. The boy went to the factory.
2. The boy is going to the factory.
3. The boy was going to the factory.

See Huddleston (1976).

aspiration   the airflow which follows the release of a plosive sound before the onset of voicing for the following vowel. It is marked with the diacritic [ʰ] placed above the sound with which it is made. *See* Ladefoged (1993).

assertive training   a form of treatment given during social skills training. It exists for those who allow themselves to be dominated either, in the case of children, by younger children, or, in the case of older people, by those with less authority. Such people are placed in situations in which they have to assert themselves either gradually, by giving step-by-step training, or very quickly by placing them in the situation and not allowing them to leave the situation until they show themselves to be sufficiently assertive. *See* Trower et al (1978); Atkinson et al (1993); Argyle (1994); Davison and Neale (1994).

Assessment and Therapy Programme for Dysfluent Children   devised by Rustin in 1987, this programme allows for the assessment of dysfluent children, aged between 2.5 and 11 years of age, and provides a comprehensive therapy and monitoring programme. The initial assessment is carried out using a structured interview with both parents and their child. A two-week intensive therapy programme follows, incorporating parental involvement and follow-up sessions. Workbooks for both parents and children are provided which contain the exercises related to programme modules. Parents fill in a homework sheet regularly during the initial two-week course and each week after the end of the course. *See* Rustin (1987) in Appendix I; Beech et al (1993).

assessment of phonological processes   tests that show the number of phonological processes which a child produces at a particular age.

assessments measures used by various professionals throughout the rehabilitation process. Speech and language therapists use them to find out what communication disorders a person may have and the severity of the disorder. There are assessments for almost all disorders but since some people may have a mixture of problems, e.g. dysphasia with dyspraxia, two or more tests may be required. Most assessments are made up of smaller tests called subtests. The two main types of assessments are formal and informal assessments. The former types have been published like those described in this book. They themselves have been tested to check their reliability and validity. Some assessments also undergo standardisation. These assessments have been administered to a large number of the population covering the age range for which they are intended to be used. In this way, the tester can discover the most frequent and normal responses of the different age groups and, thus, be enabled to compare the scores obtained from those tested with those of the norm for that age range. The informal assessments are tests made up by the therapist to assess certain parts of a particular treatment programme or to assess a communication disorder in a more relaxed environment than that in which a formal assessment takes place. *See* Aiken (1985); Kersner (1992); Beech et al (1993).

assimilation

1. The process whereby one sound is changed because of the influence of another sound next to it. For example, [n] becomes [n̪] because of [ð] in the phrase 'in the' (based on Ladefoged, 1993). There are three type of assimilation:
   (a) anticipatory (or regressive) where the sound is influenced by the next sound; this is the most common form of assimilation in English;
   (b) progressive where the sound is influenced by the preceding sound;
   (c) coalescent where two or more sounds can come together to form one sound. For example, 'got you' becomes [gɔtʃa] where the 't' and 'y' sounds come together to form [tʃ].

   See Fromkin and Rodman (1993); Cruttenden (1994).

2. A phenomenon proposed by Piaget to explain the development of the child's ability to 'understand'. He introduced the notion of schema or schemata which are 'well-defined sequences of actions...their chief characteristic, whatever their nature or complexity, is that they are organised wholes which are frequently repeated and which can be recognised easily among other diverse and varying behaviours' (Beard, 1969). Assimilation occurs when the child brings new experiences into schemata which already exist. Accommodation occurs when a child has to work out a response to a new experience which allows him to modify his schema continually. Eventually the child can organise all this information into a whole and so one schema can be subordinated to another. Piaget called assimilation, accommodation and organisation invariant functions. There are three types of assimilation:
   (a) reproductive – the child assimilates an experience to a schema but cannot fit it into an organisation, so keeps assimilating the experience, getting nowhere;.
   (b) generalisation – the child begins to extend the range of objects or experiences to a schema;.
   (c) recognitory – as the child generalises his range of objects into a schema, he realises he has to accommodate certain actions to the object, e.g. there is only one way to hold a cup.
   See Beard (1969).

astereognosis an inability to recognise shapes by tactile means. Oral stereognosis is the recognition of differing shapes and textures intraorally. *See* Kolb and Whishaw (1990).

Aston Index devised by Newton and Thomson at Aston University in 1976, it is a screening test to assess the use of children's language between the ages of 5 and 14 years. It has two levels of which level 1 is suitable for the screening of 5–6 year olds while level 2 is for use with the older age range. It contains six tests to measure general ability; the results provide age-equivalent scores and ten performance tests which measure the ability necessary for learning to read and write. All the results are plotted onto graphs provided on the score sheets. Thus, the therapist or teacher can discover any delay in development or the most significant difficulties a child may possess. *See* Newton and Thomson (1976) in Appendix I.

astrocytomas *see* TUMOURS OF THE CENTRAL NERVOUS SYSTEM.

ataxia *see* CEREBRAL PALSY.

ataxic dysarthria speech disorders resulting from this type of DYSARTHRIA are caused by a lesion in the CEREBELLUM. It is primarily a disorder of pitch, time and stress. Speech gives the impression of being scanning and monotonous because of disintegration of syllabic structure. Vowels are prolonged and there is lengthening of word segments so that the duration of words is greatly increased. Phonation and articulation are also affected. *See* Darley and Holliday (1975).

athetosis *see* CEREBRAL PALSY.

atrophy the wasting away of structures in any part of the body. It is often used in referring to the wasting of part of the brain, which may produce such communication disorders as DYSARTHRIA or APHASIA. *See* Gilroy and Holliday (1982).

attachment the way in which children bond with their parents, usually their mother or the person who provides the initial care and security. The children tend to explore unknown environments when this person is with them. It has been suggested that a failure to develop such bonding may lead to the failure in making close personal relationships in later life. Ainsworth (1979) set up a laboratory experiment called the 'Strange Situation' in which the child is faced with the mother and a strange female and the researchers tried to find out the type of attachment the child made in different situations. They found three groups: those who were 'securely attached'; those who were 'insecurely attached: avoidant'; and those who were 'insecurely attached: resistant'. From these results, they could conclude all babies become attached to their mothers by 1 year of age but the quality of the attachment depends on the mother's responses to the child. While most babies are securely attached, some form insecure attachments often because the mother will only respond to the baby's cries when she wants to and fails to respond at other times. The avoidant behaviour is related to maternal hostility and rejection while resistant behaviour is related to the unresponsiveness of the mother. (*See* Atkinson et al, 1993, pp. 494-495). Further studies have shown that those children who are securely attached by 2 years of age are better equipped to cope with new experiences and relationships. Erikson (1963) suggested eight stages of psychosexual development which people go through from birth to old age. He believed a person's psychological development depended on the kinds of social relationships made at various times in their lives but each relationship had problems that had to be faced. He produced them as opposites: trust vs mistrust (1 year old); autonomy vs doubt (2 year old); initiative vs guilt (3–5 years); industry vs inferiority (6 years–puberty); identity vs confusion (adolescence); intimacy vs isolation (early adulthood); generativity vs self-absorption (middle adulthood) and integrity vs despair (after 65 years). *See* Atkinson et al (1993).

attention the selection of relevant stimuli from the environment as part of the process of comprehension. The stimuli may be auditory, visual or tactile kinaesthetic. *See* Atkinson et al (1993).

Attention-Deficit Hyperactivity Disorder (ADHD) a disorder in which the child cannot attend for any significant period of time to a particular activity especially when asked to sit still, for example at school or at mealtimes. The diagnosis is reserved for those children who behave in an extreme way, not for those who are just overactive and slightly distractible. There has been a move away from a variety of different symptoms to separating those children with attention-deficit disorder (ADD) only and those with both attention deficit and hyperactivity. The latter group, ADHD children, seem more likely to develop CONDUCT DISORDERS, whilst the fomer group, those with ADD, have more problems with focusing attention or speed of information processing, which can lead to academic problems in such subjects as maths, reading or spelling. Both drug therapy and BEHAVIOUR THERAPY have been used to treat the condition. *See* Davison and Neale (1994).

Attitudes and Strategies towards AAC a training package for AAC users and carers providing a ready-to-use resource for training people who are involved in AAC. It is workshop based and focuses on attitudes to AAC and strategies used in AAC conversations.These priority areas have been highlighted by the many AAC users and their communicative partners whom the authors have known. There is a manual and a video. *See* Murphy and Scott (1995).

audiology a science concerned with the hearing mechanism used by humans. Audiologists study the development, anatomy, physiology, and pathology of the auditory system. This is done mostly by the use of tests, the results of which are analysed by audiologists. They are also concerned with the psychological aspects of hearing loss as well as with treatment strategies used in the rehabilitation of the client's hearing loss. *See* Katz (1985).

audiometric tests tests which are carried out by an audiologist to find out if a person has a hearing loss. The most common test is PURE-TONE AUDIOMETRY. If people are found to have particular problems in the hearing mechanism other tests are used specifically for the problem. When younger children are presented to have their hearing tested, the audiologist may use DISTRACTION TESTS or FREE FIELD AUDIOMETRY. *See* Katz (1985).

audiometric zero the sound pressure level required to make any frequency barely audible to the average person with normal hearing. It is also the hearing threshold level setting on an audiometer marked at 0 dB. *See* Katz (1985).

audiometry the process used by audiologists to test a person's hearing. The most common test is PURE-TONE AUDIOMETRY.

auditory aphasia *see* APHASIA (2).

auditory brain-stem response (ABR) an audiometric test to diagnose the neurological causes of hearing loss and to find the site of lesion. An audiological assessment is made. Electrodes are placed on the earlobes or the mastoids and on the vertex. Testing begins at 60 dB SL or 90 dB sound pressure level. The audiologist compares the results from the testing with normal responses. Disorders of the cranial nerve VIII or brain-stem will show up in the ABR. It is a non-invasive technique, does not affect the state of the client and is regarded as providing a good objective test of the client's hearing threshold level. *See* Josey (1985).

auditory comprehension the processing of incoming auditory stimuli leading to recognition. It involves sound discrimination, perception of sequence and retention and can be a symptom of APHASIA. Auditory comprehension is a subtest of the main tests in aphasia such as the BOSTON DIAGNOSTIC APHASIA EXAMINATION (BDAE), the WESTERN APHASIA BATTERY (WAB) or the MINNESOTA TEST FOR THE DIFFERENTIAL DIAGNOSIS OF APHASIA (MTDDA). When it is found that auditory comprehension is a particular problem, more specific tests can be used to assess this further, for example the TOKEN TEST and the TEST FOR RECEPTION OF GRAMMAR (TROG). *See* Riedel (1981); Rosenbek et al (1989).

Auditory Discrimination and Attention Test devised by Morgan-Barry for children from 3 to 12 years of age with a speech deficit. It assesses the child's ability to discriminate between 17 minimal pairs, i.e., words that are minimally differentiated by a single PHONEME. The minimal feature contrasts are voiced/voiceless, place of articulation, manner of articulation (*see* ARTICULATION) and constituents of CONSONANT CLUSTERS. The child is presented with a page showing two pictures. The child places a counter below the correct picture named by the therapist. Each pair of pictures is presented six times to prevent a random response. Norm tables to convert error scores into percentages and standard scores are provided. The test was standardised on 650 children. The manual reports extensive research studies comparing the results of those with a language disorder, those with a hearing loss and children with a LEARNING DISABILITY, as well as non-handicapped children. It was developed in the UK. *See* Morgan-Barry (1988) in Appendix I. Beech et al (1993).

Auditory Discrimination Screening Test devised by Catherine Renfrew, it assesses the phonological feature contrasts and semantic confusions often found in children with speech and language problems. It can be used with children of 5 years and upwards but if it is to be used with younger children, the therapist must cover up the bottom row of pictures. In scoring, errors in auditory discrimination must be distinguished from vocabulary errors. *See also* ACTION PICTURE TEST.

auditory method *see* EDUCATION OF HEARING-IMPAIRED CHILDREN (1a).

auditory phonetics the study of how people perceive sounds. The two main components of this study are:

1. Pitch: this feature describes the way in which the listener works out the difference between a high and a low pitched sound. Pitch is the equivalent of the acoustic feature of frequency.
2. Loudness: this feature describes the amount of air pressure in the speaker's voice which is required for the listener to hear the message. Loudness is the equivalent of the acoustic feature of intensity.

Sound reaches our ears by the movement of air particles hitting each other. The stage where the particles come together is called compression which is followed by them spreading out, known as rarefaction. Compression and rarefaction can be seen clearly when shown in the form of a sine wave where compression is at the highest positive while rarefaction is at the lowest negative value on the sine curve.

However, compression and rarefaction can be found in a complex wave form as such a wave form is made up from the products of a sine wave. Normal atmospheric pressure is represented by the horizontal axis, known as equilibrium. Sound waves spread around from the sound source. *See* Fromkin and Rodman (1993); Cruttenden (1994).

auditory speech perception a learnt skill for accepting auditory information. The various parts of this skill which have to be learnt by the child are:

1. Awareness of the presence of the sound.
2. Localisation of the sound, so that the child knows where it comes from and so can pick up on linguistic cues as well as seeing the person producing the sound.
3. Cutting out of background noise and focussing his attention solely on the sound he perceives.
4. Extraction of linguistic information from the acoustic phonetic characteristics of the phonemes produced.
5. Use of memory, particularly the short-term memory to retain and process the utterances produced by the speaker.

However, if the child has a hearing loss during this period, these skills are more difficult to acquire:

1. Those who have a conductive loss have a problem of receiving information and so will require a hearing aid or will ask the speaker to speak louder for him to receive such information.
2. Those who have a sensory hearing loss have a problem in receiving information and also in discrimination.
3. Those who have a neural/central hearing loss have a problem in obtaining meaning from the information they receive.
4. Those who have a mixed hearing loss will have elements of (1)–(3).

See Sanders (1977).

augmentative communication aids *see* ALTERNATIVE AUGMENTATIVE COMMUNICATION.

aural rehabilitation *see* EDUCATION OF HEARING-IMPAIRED CHILDREN.

autism a childhood psychosis. It is a syndrome characterised by a severe failure to develop social relationships, language retardation with ECHOLALIA, lack of comprehension and various ritualis-

tic and stereotyped phenomena. Most of these characteristics develop before 2;6 years. It affects 2 in 10 000 children, three-quarters of whom require special education.

1. Poor social relationships: children who have autism do not cling to their mothers in strange situations as unaffected children do; they treat people like objects and other children like toys; they have little warmth and behave in strange ways; they fail to make personal friendships; they spend very little time playing and behave with a lack of social propriety toward their peers.
2. Speech and language problems: these include 'I/you' reversal; robotic voice and flattening of affect; language delay/disorder (only about half the children suffering from autism acquire language normally); lack of imitation; delayed echolalia; use of platitudes; understanding only concrete instructions and extreme idiosyncrasy in their language.
3. Ritualistic and stereotyped phenomena: stereotypical play is found quite commonly, e.g. twirling things around. They are fascinated by what most people find peripheral, and use a facsimile of normal speech while insisting on doing things as they have always done them.

There is uncertainty as to the cause of autism. It may arise from some difficulty in forming a relationship with the natural mother. Young autistic children are more sluggish at sucking, tend not to smile, may not respond to the human voice and are undemanding. While not completely rejecting environmental causes, investigations are being made into organic causes of autism. Researchers are looking for possible brain pathologies such as ENCEPHALITIS in early years, complications of rubella passed to the child by the mother during pregnancy, TUBEROUS SCLEROSIS, untreated PHENYLKE-

TONURIA, infantile spasm (severe epileptic attacks during the first year) and complications in the perinatal stage. These causes have been found in one-third of children who have autism. Site of lesion in the brain is another possible cause, but no conclusive evidence has been provided although proposed sites are in the dominant hemisphere, RETICULAR SYSTEM or BASAL GANGLIA. The different psychological behaviours of the autistic and non-autistic child may lead to a possible cause. However, the most likely outcome of all this research will be to provide a group of interrelated causes and not just one cause for autism. Treatment is aimed at improving the child's socialisation and providing him with socially acceptable behaviour. Such treatment is aimed at removing the child's 'self-encapsulation in an isolated world' (Jaspers, 1963 in Wolff, 1981). *See* Wing, (1980); Wolff, (1981); Ellis, (1990); Fay, (1993).

Autistic Continuum: An Assessment and Intervention Schedule devised by Aarons and Gittens in 1992, the schedule is designed to look at various developmental areas. There is no time limit or complex scoring. The authors' approach looks at autism as a continuum and not as a particular disorder existing within its own boundaries. It is a revision of an earlier publication *Is this Autism? See* Aarons and Gittens (1992) in Appendix I.

autonomic nervous system (ANS) part of the nervous system which innervates smooth muscle. It is divided into two parts:

1. Sympathetic nervous system
2. Parasympathetic nervous system

The ANS supplies the HEART, sweat glands and digestive glands. *See* J.H. Green (1978); Tortora and Grabowski (1993).

autosomal dominant *see* CHROMOSOMES.

autosomal recessive *see* CHROMOSOMES.

autosomes a human has 23 pairs of CHROMOSOMES, of which 22 are autosomes while the twenty-third pair are the sex chromosomes. *See* Hosking (1982); Tortora and Grabowski (1993).

auxiliary verb auxiliary verbs such as 'be', 'have', 'do', 'can', 'shall', etc., subordinate to lexical verbs in English (in declarative sentences), and help to convey distinctions in tense, aspect and modality. They also have an important syntactic role in negation and in forming interrogative structures. For example:

1. John is singing.
2. Mary might arrive soon.
3. Bill didn't finish the job.
4. Can Sophie come out to play?

See Strang (1968); Fromkin and Rodman (1993).

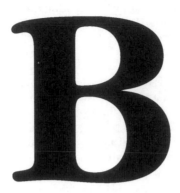

babbling an early stage of language acquisition (*see* ACQUISITION and Appendix II). The child will babble when he is comfortable and this is reflected in the type of sounds the child produces, e.g. velars, sounds made by the tongue against the top of the mouth, and open vowels. By nine months, babbling has become more human. Strings of sounds follow, put together in a CVCVCV structure. The pitch pattern is similar to the one used in normal English, with cooing and vocal play where the child experiments considerably with voice quality, and airstreams are also produced. It is also an indication of the development of motor coordination, of audition and of cognition. Absence of babbling may be associated with subsequent speech disorder though this is not absolutely established. *See* Cruttenden (1970); Byers Brown and Edwards (1989); Fromkin and Rodman (1993).

Babinski reflex a reflex obtained as part of the plantar response during a neurological examination. The reflex takes the form of the great toe being extended with extension of other toes which separate in the shape of a fan. *See* Gilroy and Holliday (1982); Tortora and Grabowski (1993).

baby talk a phenomenon which occurs in language development (*see* ACQUISITION and Appendix II) which refers to

the special use of a simplified language used by a mother to communicate with her child. At first, she may use simple words to refer to objects, animals or people, e.g. [brm, brm] = 'car'; [horsie] = 'horse'; [doggie] = 'dog'; [mama, dada] = 'mummy and daddy', etc. As the child's language develops, he begins to use two-word phrases, e.g. [cake allgone] = 'there is no more cake'; [dada shoe] = 'there are Daddy's shoes'. The mother seems to know intuitively at what level to pitch her language, so that she is always one step ahead, thus encouraging the child to reach another stage in his language development. It is also described as parental speech, motherese or parent talk. *See* Cruttenden (1979).

back-up in computer terms, a copy of one program, document, graphic etc. from an original, in case the original is lost or corrupted. The original may be kept on a hard disk while the back-up copy is kept on a floppy disk. *See* Bishop (1985).

Bangor Dyslexia Test devised by Professor T.R. Miles as a screening test to find out if a child's difficulties in reading and/or writing are those typically found in dyslexia or not. There are ten subtests: (1) Knowledge of left/right body parts; (2) repetition of polysyllabic words; (3) subtraction;

(4) multiplication tables; (5) months forward; (6) months reversed; (7) digits forward; (8) digits reversed; (9) b/d confusion; (10) familial incidence. *See* Miles (1982) in Appendix I.

basal ganglia a mass of grey matter at the base of the BRAIN. The nuclei found in this structure include the corpus striatum (caudate, globus pallidus putamen) and the amygdaloid nucleus. If this structure becomes diseased, tremor and rigidity (*see* PARKINSON'S DISEASE) may occur. *See* Barr (1979).

base 10 devised by LaPointe, it is a therapeutic technique for showing the success of a treatment programme, usually in APHASIA therapy. It comprises a printed form on which the aims of the therapy are entered and baseline scores are recorded. Progress is shown graphically, thus giving positive feedback to the person and providing the therapist with a record of success. The activities can be modified if improvement occurs. It is very useful for intensive therapy. *See* LaPointe (1977) in Appendix I; Code and Müller (1989); Rosenbek et al (1989).

base form the part of a word which remains after all the affixes have been removed. For example, the base form of 'quickly' is 'quick' after the affix '-ly' has been removed. It is also described as the base word. It is used in the morphological study of word formation. *See* Matthews (1974).

BASIC an acronym for Beginner's All Purpose Symbolic Instruction Code. BASIC is one of several languages used for programming computers. It is very versatile and easy to use. Most manufacturers of microcomputers produce computers able to run software written in BASIC. It works on a line-by-line basis, with each line numbered, so that the program can run logically. The lines can be changed as the program is being written. *See* Bishop (1985); Brookshear (1991).

basilar membrane *see* EAR.

baud rate the rate per second at which data move from one processor to another, e.g. from computer to printer. *See* Bishop (1985); Brookshear (1991).

BBC microcomputers *see* ACORN COMPUTERS.

BC bone conduction *see* PURE-TONE AUDIOMETRY.

BDAE *see* BOSTON DIAGNOSTIC APHASIA EXAMINATION.

Beck's cognitive therapy an approach to producing acceptable behaviour by treating thought processes. Beck provided therapy which was aimed at making people aware of their thinking processes, teaching them to recognise maladaptive thoughts in various situations, producing more normal thought patterns for such situations and, having accomplished this, the therapist gives praise and reinforcement to cognitive and behaviour changes during therapy. *See* Rachman and Wilson (1980); Atkinson et al (1993).

behaviour modification *see* BEHAVIOUR THERAPY.

behaviour therapy aims at the modification of abnormal patterns of behaviour which do not have a medical origin. It is sometimes called the two-factor model of learning as it consists of two learning procedures – CLASSICAL CONDITIONING and OPERANT CONDITIONING. In the former, several behaviour therapies have been evolved such as SYSTEMATIC DESENSITISATION, FLOODING, MODELLING, and ASSERTIVE TRAINING, while in the latter the behaviour therapies of individual conditioning paradigms (*see* OPERANT CONDITIONING) and TOKEN ECONOMIES have evolved. Behaviour therapy occurs also in the form of COGNITIVE BEHAVIOUR THERAPIES such as RATIONAL-EMOTIVE THERAPY (RET) (Ellis), SELF-INSTRUCTIONAL TRAINING (SIT) (Meichenbaum) and BECK'S COGNITIVE THERAPY. Sjödé described the most important aspect of behaviour therapy as 'being task-specific rather than based on personality. The therapist has respect for the client as a learning, striving and a coping person who is not sick but will benefit from guided experiences in dealing with particular specified situations'. (Sjödé et al. 1979). *See* Atkinson et al (1993).

Békésy audiometry a procedure used in PURE-TONE AUDIOMETRY. Earphones are placed over the listener's ears and he is given a button to control the intensity of the tones. The button must be pressed in order to make the tone audible and released when it is audible (causing the intensity to decrease again). The whole range of frequencies, from low to high, should be tested. The audiometer does the sweep automatically and different tracings indicate different pathologies. Two frequency sweeps are carried out – one with a continuous tone and another with a pulsed tone. The person's threshold is traced by a stylus linked to the audiometer. *See* Katz (1985).

Bell's palsy an acute facial paralysis of the peripheral type produced by a disorder of the facial nerve (*see* CRANIAL NERVES). Its cause is usually unknown but it can be a result of a viral infection which involves the geniculate ganglion. Bell's palsy occurs often in the middle-aged and elderly. There is a facial paralysis which progresses steadily to a severe weakness and even to total loss of power on one side of the face. The affected side may present with a sagging cheek and it may be impossible to close the eye; in fact, the eye can hardly close and, at times, it is impossible to close because of weakness in the orbicularis oculi (*see* MUSCLES OF FACIAL EXPRESSION). Involvement of the geniculate ganglion can produce loss of tears resulting in a dry eye. The eyes are kept moist with eye drops. *See* Gilroy and Holliday (1982).

Biber test an assessment for comprehension in APHASIA. In the single form of the test, a picture has to be selected showing single word comprehension.

The stimuli can be presented auditorily or visually and the person has to indicate by whatever means whether the heard/seen word corresponds to the picture. A picture is presented with the stimulus word which may be the target word, a related word or an unrelated word and a 'yes/no' response is given if the word corresponds to the picture. In the 'threesomes' version, selection is made from three pictures, two semantically related and an unrelated distractor. The target word is presented auditorily or visually and the person points to the appropriate picture. *See* test manual.

bifid uvula a condition in which two halves of the posterior part of the velum fail to unite. Also known as a uvular cleft, it may be submucus. Hypernasal resonance is often associated with structural malformation. *See also* CLEFT PALATE.

bifurcation a division into two parts or branches such as the point at the bottom of the TRACHEA where the two bronchi (*see* BRONCHUS) divide and lead into the LUNGS.

Big Red Switch a large single plate switch, 5 inches in diameter. It can be used also as a remote switch, i.e. without a cable attaching it to a particular device. When used with a battery-powered receiver or a small appliance receiver, it gives four modes of control: Direct Mode: activates the appliance only when the Big Red is activated; Timed Seconds Mode: by activating the Big Red, the appliance switches on for a predetermined length of time measured in seconds; Timed Minutes Mode: the same as the previous mode but the time is measured in minutes; Latch Mode: one activation of the Big Red turns the appliance on whilst a second activation turns it off.

BIGmack a small portable message system which takes one message of up to 20 seconds and is accessed either by pressing the large plate on the top of the device or by a single switch. It can also activate any battery-operated device or toy and give an auditory reinforcement. It is 5 inches in diameter and 2.25 inches at its highest point and uses an ordinary battery. It is mountable on wheelchair or desktop mounts or can be carried by a shoulder strap. External speakers can also be attached to it. *See* Appendix IV.

bilateral an occurrence which takes place on two sides of a structure. For example, VOCAL NODULES are said to be bilateral as there are nodules on each of the VOCAL FOLDS.

binaural a description of the functioning of the two ears as in normal hearing.

Binet Alfred Binet (1857-1911) believed a child who was slow in learning was similar to a 'normal' child except for some retardation in his mental development. In 1881 the French Government passed a law that all children, including those with learning difficulties, should go to school. Binet was approached to provide a test to ascertain which children required special education. Thus, the first edition of the STANFORD-BINET INTELLIGENCE SCALES was produced. *See* Atkinson et al (1993).

bit acronym for binary digit. This refers to one of the two numbers used in binary notation (i.e. 0, 1). A bit could just be a small part of the computer's memory. Each cell in a computer's memory can store 1 bit. *See* Bishop (1985); Brookshear (1991).

blade in articulatory terms, the part of the TONGUE behind the apex or tip which is used to produce alveolar sounds (*see* ARTICULATION) such as /t,d,s,z/. *See* Ladefoged (1993).

blind experiment an experiment in which the tester and the subject are kept in ignorance of a particular variable.

Blissymbolics developed by Charles Bliss in Canada in 1971, it was based on the concept of semantography. Bliss, born in 1897, was brought up in Austria where 20 languages were spo-

ken. He was concerned about the linguistic confusion produced by so many languages. In the 1960s, he started to devise 'logical writing for an illogical world' (Bliss, 1965). Blissymbolics is a language conveying meaning through pictographic, ideographic and abstract symbols. It has become a popular means for those with communication problems to communicate their needs and wishes. The symbol system has nine shapes to form the basis of all symbols. When combined and drawn in various ways they make up a complete language. It fulfils Bliss's intention of forming a logical system. About 30 years later, it was re-discovered by Shirley McNaughton in Canada when working with non-communicating physically handicapped children. Her team took the most common words required by children and set them out with the symbols on a chart, so that the children could indicate their needs by pointing. Blissymbolics have been used with a multiplicity of children's and adults' disorders. As a system it can be used as an alternative means of communication or to augment the child's unintelligible speech. It was introduced into the UK in 1973. The Blissymbolics Communication Resource Centre (UK) was founded in 1977. The system is very versatile as it can be used by people with various abilities in various different environments. Since the words are always presented with the symbols, even those unfamiliar with the system can understand it. *See* Bailey and Jenkins (1982); Kiernan et al (1982).

block modification a person who stammers is often described as exhibiting blocking behaviour. This is the actual act of stammering, i.e. the repetition of sounds. Van Riper proposed block modification as a therapeutic technique to reduce the amount of blocking behaviour. It is part of the STAMMER MORE FLUENTLY approach, so the criterion for success is not necessarily total fluent speech but an ACCEPTABLE STAMMER where the speaker is happy to speak despite DYSFLUENCY and where the listener is aware of some dysfluency but is not annoyed by it. The first stage of this technique is to identify the stammer, i.e. what it sounds like, then desensitise the person's fear and panic when he anticipates a stammer. Block modification has three stages:

1. Cancellation: after the blocking behaviour has occurred, the speaker corrects what was said.
2. Pull-outs: during blocking behaviour, the speaker stops and repeats the word or phrase in which the blocking took place.
3. Preparatory blocks: blocking behaviour is anticipated and the speaker prepares to speak as fluently as possible.

See Dalton (1983).

Blom-Singer oesophageal prosthesis a device placed in the FISTULA following a LARYNGECTOMY. If successful, the voice can be regained and communication is almost normal. The voice is usually fluent and sounds more normal than OESOPHAGEAL VOICE. It is powered by pneumatic air pressure; the duration in speech is better; the voice is louder and greater change in pitch is possible than with a normal oesophageal voice, in allowing greater scope and variability. If, however, the resulting voice is not liked, the prosthesis can be removed and the tracheo-oesophageal fistula will close completely. *See* Edels (1983).

blood-brain barrier an anatomical and physiological barrier to give protection to the brain cells from dangerous substances and pathogens. If there is any form of trauma to the BRAIN, this can lead to a breakdown of the barrier allowing such harmful substances to attack the brain cells. It could also affect the way in which therapeutic drugs enter the brain to help with tumours in the brain. *See* Tortora and Grabowski (1993).

Bobath method a method of treatment developed by Karl and Berta Bobath to help those with CEREBRAL PALSY. It is based on the inhibition of persisting infantile tonic reflexes and the replacement of these with learned patterns of normal neuromuscular activity.

body language non-verbal form of communication such as gesture, facial expression, bodily movement, etc. which often accompanies speech.

Bodyspek 2000 provides an objective assessment of an infant's hearing. It will identify a significant hearing loss before the child begins to develop language. Electrodes are placed in front of the ear, behind the same ear and at the back of the child's neck. The test starts by setting the sound level to 60dB sound level, all other adjustments then being automatic. The Bodyspek 2000 produces 2000 clicks until the postauricular myogenic response (PAM) is elicited and the test stops automatically. If the child fails at this sound level the child is retested at 80dB. The test usually lasts about ten minutes.

Boehm Test of Basic Concepts (1971, revised 1986) devised by Boehm, it is a standardised assessment which is concerned with the comprehension of concepts. Fifty concepts are divided into four categories: space, time, quantity and miscellaneous concepts. The revised edition includes further subsections of antonyms, synonyms and one in which concepts are combined. The test can be given individually or on a group basis. Children are provided with a picture booklet and are given verbal instructions regarding each task to be carried out. There is also a preschool version which assesses for 26 basic language concepts. It is most appropriate for children between 3 and 5 years of age. By using the test in conjunction with the Boehm Resource Guide for Basic Concept Training, a complete therapeutic programme can be put together for individual children. *See* Boehm (1976, 1986a, b) in Appendix I.

bone CONNECTIVE TISSUE in which collagen fibres are held together by ground substance impregnated with complex calcium salts for great strength. Bone has a matrix, i.e. its ground substance, formed in a concentric tubular pattern. The outer surface has a layer of fibrous tissue known as periosteum. The bones which appear denser are compact bones while those which are more open on the inside are cancellous bone. Classification of the bone is according to shape of which there are five types: long, short, flat, irregular and sesamoid bones. *See* Tortora and Grabowski (1993).

bone conduction *see* PURE-TONE AUDIOMETRY.

bone-conduction hearing aid the sound comes through the air waves and is transmitted to a bone-conductor vibrator placed on the mastoid process behind the EAR. These vibrations produce a signal transmitted to the inner ear through the bones in the skull. It is used when an AIR-CONDUCTION HEARING AID cannot be worn or is ineffective. *See* Miller (1972).

Boston Diagnostic Aphasia Examination (BDAE) devised by Goodglass and Kaplan in 1972 (revised 1983), it is an assessment for APHASIA. It is a formal, standardised assessment which incorporates what the authors describe as the 'three general aims of any aphasia test':

1. Diagnosis of presence and type of aphasic syndrome, leading to inferences concerning cerebral localisation.

2. Measurement of the level of performance over a wide range of both initial determination and detection of change over time.

3. Comprehensive assessment of the assets and liabilities of the patient in all language areas as a guide to therapy.

From a practical point of view, the test does not give hard and fast guidelines for therapy. It highlights all the possible areas where the person may find varying difficulties such as articulation, loss of verbal fluency, word-finding difficulty (*see* LEXICAL-SEMANTIC DEFICIT), repetition, serial speech, loss of SYNTAX, PARAPHASIA, AUDITORY COMPREHENSION, reading and writing. The authors do not accept that there is a disorder called dyspraxia and so they do not use this term. *See* Goodglass and Kaplan (1983); Eisenson (1984); Rosenbek et al (1989); Beech et al (1993).

Boston Naming Test devised by Kaplan, Goodglass and Weintraub in 1983, it is a 'wide-ranging naming vocabulary test'. Its aim is to asses the type of errors made by those with word-finding difficulties in spontaneous speech, and, uses confrontation picture naming to this end. It can be used with children aged between 5.5 and 10.5 years of age, adults with APHASIA, and those with DEMENTIA and ANOMIA. There are sixty black-and-white line drawings, graded in difficulty. Stimulus CUES can be given. *See* Kaplan et al (1983) in Appendix I; Beech et al (1993).

Boston School a group of workers concerned with research into the diagnosis, nature and treatment of aphasic disorders. This research is based on a localisation model in which they believe aphasic patients can be categorised according to which part of the left cerebral hemisphere (*see* CEREBRAL HEMISPHERES) is damaged. The Boston School proposes seven major types of aphasia: (1) Broca's aphasia; (2) Wernicke's aphasia; (3) conduction aphasia; (4) anomia; (5) transcortical sensory aphasia; (6) transcortical motor aphasia; (7) alexia with agraphia (*see* APHASIA 1-7) and four PURE APHASIAS: (1) APHEMIA; (2) PURE WORD DEAFNESS; (3) PURE ALEXIA; (4) PURE AGRAPHIA. *See* Goodglass and Kaplan (1983).

bottom-up (top-down) a cognitive way of processing information. It assumes the person starts with basic information and works on it in such a way that it becomes more complex. Starting with complex information which is broken down into basic information is known as top-down processing. *See* Atkinson et al (1993).

bound morpheme a morpheme (*see* MORPHOLOGY) which cannot exist on its own. For example, the affix 'de-' in a word like 'devise' is a bound morpheme as 'de-' cannot be used as a separate meaningful unit. It is opposed to FREE MORPHEME. *See* Matthews (1974).

bracketing a mode of representation analysis for CONSTITUENT ANALYSIS. Each sentence which is either spoken or written can be analysed into several component parts with the hierarchical relations represented linearly by brackets (see boxed example below). Another way of showing the constituent analysis of the sentence is by branching in a TREE DIAGRAM. *See* Lyons (1981).

bradykinesia *see* PARKINSON'S DISEASE.

bradylalia abnormally slow rate of speech.

brain comprises two CEREBRAL HEMISPHERES – the left and right–connected by the CORPUS CALLOSUM. The motor and sensory areas run in parallel regions on either side of the central fissure down to the lateral fissure. Below the cerebral cortex is the THALAMUS (acts as sensory relay station to cerebral cortex), HYPOTHALAMUS (controls temperature, metabolism and endocrine balance), RETICULAR SYSTEM (arousal system which activates regions of cerebral cortex), CEREBELLUM (controls muscles, balance and coordination of voluntary movement) and the MEDULLA OBLONGATA (controls breathing, swallowing, digestion and heart beat). *See* Barr (1979); Tortora and Grabowski (1993).

brain abscess a collection of pus in the brain substance. It may be caused by bacteria from the ear, usually suppurative otitis media (*see* OTITIS MEDIA), resulting in an abscess occurring in the temporal lobe (*see* CEREBRAL HEMISPHERES). The bacteria can also come from the blood. It acts as a TUMOUR OF THE CENTRAL NERVOUS SYSTEM. It distorts the brain structures by compressing its various parts. The symptoms produced are those of raised INTRACRANIAL PRESSURE, fever, aphasia, epileptic seizures (*see* EPILEPSY), coma and headaches. Diagnosis is by CT (COMPUTED TOMOGRAPHY) scan and a culture of bacteria from the areas given above. Treatment is by surgical drainage and appropriate antibiotic or other chemotherapy. *See* Gilroy and Holliday (1982); Kaye (1991).

brain death there has to be no chance for the person to recover from BRAINSTEM damage and no evidence of brainstem function following tests which will show lack of pupil response to light, lack of corneal reflex to stimulation, lack of oculocephalic reflex, failure of vestibulo-ocular reflex, failure of gag or cough reflex on bronchial stimulation, no motor response in the face or muscles supplied by the CRANIAL NERVES in response to painful stimulus, and failure of response of respiratory movements when the patient is disconnected from a ventilator and the $PaCO_2$ is allowed to rise to 50mmHg. The tests should be carried out by two senior doctors. *See* Kaye (1991).

(	(	(THE)	(DOG)	)	((CHASED)	(	(THE)	(CAT)	)	)	)
		.	.	.	.		.	.	.		
		.	.	.	.		.	.	.	.	
		det	N	NP	V		det	N	NP	VP	S

brain-stem this structure within the brain comprises the MEDULLA OBLONGATA, the PONS and the MIDBRAIN. Each of these three parts has structures particular to each, as well as tracts and fibres which are common to all three. *See* Barr (1979); Kaye (1991).

brain-stem evoked response audiometry *see* AUDITORY BRAIN-STEM RESPONSE (ABR).

brain tumours *see* TUMOURS OF THE CENTRAL NERVOUS SYSTEM.

branch

1. A section of a computer program which is not part of the main routine. It is often called a SUBROUTINE. The branching part of the program appears between branch instructions which direct the program to carry out a particular branch and which then direct the program back to the main routine.
2. In linguistic discussion, a branch links constituents together into a TREE DIAGRAM. *See* Lyons (1981).

breath groups the length of utterance which a person can produce in one breath. Poor breathing may affect the syntactic, phonological and semantic content of what is said. In speech and language therapy, breath groups can be introduced into treatment programmes for those who have DYSARTHRIA or DYSPHONIA. The person is shown how to reduce the number of words used in one breath to a level at which communication is more intelligible. *See* Brosnahan and Malmberg (1976); Robertson and Thomson (1986).

Bringing Unity into Language and Learning Development (BUILLD) devised by Valot, BUILLD is a curriculum guide to the teaching of the MINSPEAK APPLICATION PROGRAM (MAP) – UNITY. It uses a variety of therapeutic techniques for teaching the program, with motivating, functional activities including cooking, art, reading books, writing, playing games and singing songs. Its main aim is to tackle the teaching of multiple associations which specifically address icon associations. The person using Unity will begin with single words and increase the number of words they can use into frequently used phrases and sentences across the different settings. The success of this program is the use of the team approach, i.e. those who work most frequently with the user, including parents, speech and language therapists, occupational and physiotherapists, teachers etc. There are 11 units in the curriculum. *See* Valot (1995).

Bristol Language Development Scales devised by Gutfreund and her colleagues in 1989 for children between 15 months and 5 years with an expressive language difficulty, including those with a language and/or hearing impairment, as well as non-English speaking children. It gives a detailed analysis of the child's expressive language. The therapist has to elicit a language sample which is then transferred onto the transcription sheet. The sample is then analysed using three methods:

1. PRAGMATICS: how the child uses language.
2. SEMANTICS: the meaning of the child's language.
3. SYNTAX: the form of the child's language.

Items within each section are divided into 10 stages of development. The main scale enables the therapist to assess the developmental level of a particular child at a specific age, identify gaps in the overall expressive language profile and diagnose areas of deficiency in the child's expressive language development. There is a syntax-free scale for non-English speakers, hearing-impaired children and children with learning disabilities who use a mixture of words and signs to communicate.The therapy planning form is used to formulate individual treatment plans for each child. It is based on the Bristol Language Development Research Programme led by Gordon Wells. The research 'Language at Home and at School' followed the language development of a group of children from infancy through primary school. Papers from the research project can be found in *'Language, Learning and Education'*. *See* Wells (1985); Gutfreund (1989) in Appendix I; Beech et al (1993).

British Ability Scales an extensive battery of tests for assessing general cognitive abilities. It produces IQ scores and a detailed profile of the child's cognitive abilities in 23 areas of cognitive development. These 23 areas are organised into six major process areas:

1. Speed of information processing.
2. Reasoning.
3. Spatial imagery.
4. Perceptual matching.
5. Short-term memory.
6. Retrieval and application of knowledge.

The test can be administered in separate parts to children in the age range of 2;6–17 years of age. *See* Elliott et al (1990) in Appendix I.

British Picture Vocabulary Scales devised by Dunn and colleagues, it is a formal, standardised assessment to test a person's auditory vocabulary. It is suitable for children with a LEARNING DISABILITY, children who cannot produce an oral or written response, or as a screening test for new school entrants. It should not be used with those with a hearing loss. The child is given a page of four pictures, only one of which corresponds correctly to the auditory stimulus – the child need only finger or eye point. A ceiling score and a basal score must be found. It is quick to administer and can be given either as a detailed test using the 'long form' or as a quick screening test using the 'short form'. *See* Dunn et al (1982) in Appendix I; Beech et al (1993).

British Sign Language (BSL) used by the hard of hearing in the UK. It is a natural language, which has been developed by deaf people, having a grammar of its own, unlike a sign sys-

tem such as MAKATON, which is not grammatical in its structure. However, the grammar of BSL does not match that of spoken English. *See* Kiernan et al (1982).

broad transcription *see* TRANSCRIPTION SYSTEMS.

Broca's aphasia discovered by a French neurologist, Paul Broca, in the nineteenth century. A major APHASIA proposed by the BOSTON SCHOOL for a communication disorder caused by trauma to the brain. The area which Broca discovered, known as Broca's area, is in the left cerebral hemisphere in the third frontal convolution in the precentral gyrus. For a description of the communication difficulties found in Broca's aphasia – *see* APHASIA (1). *See* Goodglass and Kaplan (1983); Rosenbek et al (1989).

bromocriptine a dopamine receptor agonist for idiopathic parkinsonism. It is often given if sinemet is not having any effect or the on/off phenomenon continues while on sinemet. The side effects are the same as those of L-dopa (*see* LEVODOPA). It should not be given to those with severe dementia as it may increase confusion and agitation. It can be used with other anti-parkinsonian drugs. *See* Gilroy and Holliday (1982).

bronchi two divisions of the TRACHEA which lead to the left and right LUNGS respectively. There are three differences between the two bronchi:

1. The right bronchus is shorter than the left.
2. The right bronchus is vertical while the left is almost horizontal.
3. The right bronchus is wide while the left bronchus is narrower.

When the bronchi reach the lungs, they branch again into smaller bronchi or secondary lobar bronchi – one for each lobe of the lungs. These branch, in turn, into tertiary or segmental bronchi, which branch into bronchioles. These bronchioles divide, finally, into terminal bronchioles. The whole system from the initial division at the end of the trachea is known as the bronchial tree. *See* Joseph (1979); Tortora and Grabowski (1993).

BSER brain-stem evoked response audiometry see AUDITORY BRAIN-STEM RESPONSE.

buccal nerve *see* MOUTH.

buccinator *see* MUSCLES OF FACIAL EXPRESSION.

Buddy Button small single plate switches suitable for any device which requires to be activated by a switch from a communication aid to a computer.

buffer part of a peripheral unit where data are stored temporarily when transferred from the computer's memory. The buffer will hold information sent to it and act on it depending on the speed at which the information reaches the unit. *See* Bishop (1985).

bug any error or part of a computer program which does not work as it should. The process in which the bugs are removed from programs is known as debugging. *See* Bishop (1985).

BUILLD *see* BRINGING UNITY INTO LANGUAGE AND LEARNING DEVELOPMENT.

bulbar palsy a palsy caused by a disorder in the pathways of the nuclei which originate in the MEDULLA OBLONGATA. This disease produces weakness in the affected muscles which can deteriorate over a period of time. The disease affects four muscle groups: (1) MUSCLES OF MASTICATION; (2) MUSCLES FOR SWALLOWING; (3) muscles of the tongue; (4) muscles of the face. It is a progressive disease which begins with difficulty of tongue movement, progressing to immobility of the tongue. The orbicularis oris muscles (*see* MUSCLES OF FACIAL EXPRESSION) are affected in the early stages, making it difficult to close the lips and thus producing excessive drooling. The soft palate (*see* MOUTH) fails to close which allows food to be regurgitated down the nose. The final stage of the disease is a failure to swallow and close the jaw. The prognosis is poor and death occurs in 1–2 years due to aspiration pneumonia. If the muscles are affected by an upper motor neuron disease (*see* NEURON) there is spastic rather than flaccid weakness. This is also known as pseudobulbar palsy. There is no cure. The major nursing problem is ensuring adequate nutrition due to the swallowing difficulty. *See* Draper (1980).

bunching a description of the production of sounds in which the tongue is placed towards the back of the mouth under the soft palate to produce back vowels (*see* CARDINAL VOWEL SYSTEM), velar and uvular fricatives [ɣ, x, X, ʁ] (*see* ARTICULATION). *See* Catford (1989).

burst a phenomenon found in acoustic phonetics when there is a sudden peak showing a burst of energy when an abrupt release occurs in plosive sounds (see ARTICULATION). *See* Ladefoged (1993).

Bus Story devised by Catherine Renfrew in 1969 (2nd edition, 1991). The child is told a short story accompanied by 12 illustrations of a sequence of events in the form of a comic strip. The child retells the story, supported by a review of the pictures. This retelling is analysed in respect of the amount of correct information given, sentence length and complexity. The test is standardised in the UK and can be applied to children from 3;0 to 8;0 years. *See* Renfrew (1991).

byte a group of eight BITS. *See* Bishop (1985); Brookshear (1991).

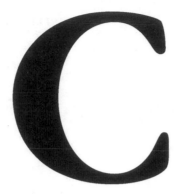

CA *see* CHRONOLOGICAL AGE.

CADL *see* COMMUNICATIVE ABILITIES IN DAILY LIVING.

café-au-lait spots *see* TUMOURS OF THE CENTRAL NERVOUS SYSTEM.

CAMELEON a high-tech communication aid using synthesised speech output (DECTALK). It uses a dynamic display which changes when the client hits a 'category' symbol, and a page of those symbols appears. It has a colour LCD display and can be accessed by a touch screen, switch, direct manual selection or keyboard access. It can also be fitted with an environmental control, a colour monitor or a printer. *See* Appendix IV.

canal any passage or tube-like structure within the body. For example, the ear canal situated in the outer ear (*see* EAR) is an air-filled tube closed at one end by the eardrum. *See* Joseph (1979).

cancellous bone *see* BONE.

cancer a layman's term used to describe the existence of a malignant tumour. There are various types of cancerous growths. They can occur in the brain, the larynx, and, commonly, in the female breast. *See* Kaye (1991); Tortora and Grabowski (1993).

Canon communicator a high-tech communication aid, it is a mini-electronic typewriter which can be used with those who have difficulty being understood because they have inadequate expressive language or none at all. The original keyboard had the 26 letters of the alphabet placed in frequency order, i.e. the most used letters placed around the outside of the keypad with other less used letters placed towards the centre of the keyboard. The keys for the vowels and consonants are of different colours, i.e. consonant keys were on the light-grey keys while the vowels and 'y' were on dark-grey keys. In more modern models, there is an alphabetic keyboard with the same colour differentiation between the keys. Some models also have a memory capacity where messages are placed under the top row of keys on the keypad. Messages are printed out on thermal tape. In the latest device, messages can also be recalled using digitised speech output. Up to a total of 240 seconds recording time can be recorded under the 26 alphabet keys (CC-7S model). The memory of the device can store up to 7000 characters under the 26 alphabet keys (CC-7S/CC-7P models). Phrases can be printed out and, with the CC-7S models, the memory message can be played back as well as printed out. There is also a calculator function. All the communicator's functions can be operated by a single key operation by designating a key at the intersection of a row and column. An optional large display can be connected to either of these new models. It has two 26-character lines with a word wrap-around function. Alternative keyboard covers are available for those with a tremor who may press the wrong key. The communicator itself works off a battery pack which can be recharged. Straps for attaching it to the client's arm or wheelchair are also available. *See* Appendix IV.

Canon typestar an electronic typewriter which has a normal QWERTY keyboard with the usual functions of TAB, SHIFT/SHIFT LOCK, REPEAT (to repeat the last printed character once or several times). As with other kinds of typewriter, it is possible to set margins and tab positions as well as cancelling them. However, the word, phrase or sentence can be edited before it is printed out. It will appear in a small screen in the centre above the keyboard. Characters can be inserted or deleted. A mode key allows different kinds of typeface to be used when printing out text whilst the code key allows the machine to carry out various functions such as centring text between the margins, centring between tabs, indenting a line of text and feeding paper automatically into the typewriter.

capacity the amount of data which can be held on a disk or in any other unit which stores data. *See* Bishop (1985).

Capgras' syndrome a neurotic syndrome. The person has a delusion that a close relative has been replaced by his or her double. It is usually found in SCHIZOPHRENIA.

carbamazepine *see* EPILEPSY.

carcinoma a malignant growth which can appear in any part of the body. Treatment may require surgery, RADIOTHERAPY or chemotherapy. *See* Pracy et al (1974); Kaye (1991).

cardinal vowel system devised by Daniel Jones in about 1914, it provides a set of reference points on the periphery of the vowel area in the mouth to describe vowels in relation to each other. The system has eight primary vowels which act as reference points of tongue and lip position. The diagram for primary cardinal vowels is:

```
front              back

  i                  u
    e              o
      ɛ          ɔ
        a      ɒ
```

In the primary vowel system, the front vowels are unrounded, i.e. the lips are spread, while the back vowels are rounded, i.e. the lips are pouted. As the tongue moves from [i], it moves down and back for the production of the other vowels and is bunched at the back of the mouth for the back vowels. There are four classifications of vertical tongue positions used in this system:

1. Close – the highest position in the mouth [i,u], which allows the vowel to be produced without audible friction.
2. Half-close - the next level [e,o].
3. Half-open - the next level [ɛ,ɔ].
4. Open – the next level [a,ɒ] where the tongue is furthest from the roof of the mouth.

The secondary cardinal vowels are produced by reversing the lip positions which results in the front vowels becoming rounded and the back vowels becoming unrounded. The diagram for secondary vowels is:

```
front              back

  y                  ɯ
    ø              ɣ
      æ          ʌ
        a      ɑ
```

All vowels can be described within the framework of either primary or secondary cardinal vowels. *See* Ladefoged (1993).

Carhart's notch a special feature found on a pure-tone audiogram. It is represented on the audiogram by a dip in bone conduction (*see* PURE-TONE AUDIOMETRY) at 2000 Hz and is associated with OTOSCLEROSIS.

carotid artery one of the main arteries in the neck. As it rises it branches into the external and internal carotid arteries. The external carotid artery serves superficial structures within the neck and head such as the LARYNX, TONGUE, external ear (*see* EAR) and MUSCLES OF MASTICATION. The internal carotid artery supplies the anterior two-thirds of the BRAIN and orbits. *See* Joseph (1979).

Carrow Elicited Language Inventory (CELI) devised by Carrow-Woolfolk in 1974, it is an imitation test which assesses the level of expressive language of children between 3 years and 7 years 11 months. It uses 52 phrase and sentence stimuli containing a range of syntactic constructions and grammatical morphemes presented to the child to imitate directly. It is standardised on a North American population. *See* Carrow-Woolfolk (1974) in Appendix I; Beech et al (1993).

carry-over the generalisation of techniques given to those in therapy to everyday communication.

cartilage a type of connective tissue. There are three types – hyaline, fibrous and elastic. Hyaline is found in the costal cartilages, fibrous is found in discs among the vertebrae while elastic is found in the pinna (*see* EAR) and the EPIGLOTTIS. See Tortora and Grabowski (1993).

case in case-marked languages such as Latin, inflections on nouns signalled grammatical relations such as subject, direct object and indirect object. Case survives in English pronouns, in the distinctions I/me, she/her, he/him, we/us, they/them. *See* Lyons (1968).

case grammar a generative model of grammar devised by Charles Fillmore in the 1960s. It involved a deep structure which was distinct from that in Chomsky's (*see* CHOMSKYAN LINGUISTICS) STANDARD THEORY in having as categories semantically-labelled entities such as agent, benefactive and instrumental for the arguments of the verb. (These categories are the 'cases' of the title of the theory.) Deep-structure verb + case configurations then map onto conventional surface structures in well-defined ways. *See* Steinberg (1982).

case history a summary of the person's illness, disease or disorder from onset to the stage at which the person presents for treatment. In the case of communication disorders, the therapist records the progress of the disorder from its onset to the initial interview. This will include details of the relevant parts of the person's medical history, leisure activities and feelings about their present condition. The amount of information required for a case history is determined by the severity of the disorder which the person has. *See* Byers Brown (1981).

CASP *see* COMMUNICATION ASSESSMENT PROFILE FOR ADULTS WITH A MENTAL HANDICAP.

catarrh a mucinous discharge from a mucous membrane. A symptom of nasal irritation. The most common products in the atmosphere to cause nasal catarrh are dust, and smoke from tobacco. *See* Pracy et al (1974).

category

1. most commonly used in relation to grammatical categories such as noun, verb, adjective, which are classificatory units crucial for the description of language. See Lyons (1968); Huddleston (1976).

2. in the field of ALTERNATIVE AUGMENTATIVE COMMUNICATION (AAC), category refers to the groupings of vocabulary. For example, in a low-tech system such as a picture book, specific pages can be set up in different categories such as 'clothes' where the category picture is placed in the centre of the page and

pictures of the specific clothing placed around the category picture. In a high-tech system, a symbol can represent the type of vocabulary and the second hit or symbol represents the particular item of vocabulary *See also* LANGUAGE, LEARNING AND LIVING (LLL). *See* Beukelman and Mirenda (1992).

catenative a lexical verb which in English pre-modifies another lexical verb is referred to as catenative in some grammatical descriptions, e.g. 'begin' in the following example: he began to despair.

CELF-R Scoring Assistant a software program which allows for scoring the CELF-R assessment on an IBM PC or compatible. It will provide a summary report. *See* Wiig (1988a) in Appendix I.

CELF-R Screening Test a short version of the CELF-R assessment to decide if a more in-depth assessment using the full CELF-R is necessary. As well as the parts which are similar to the CELF-R, there is an optional oral expression subtest for 5;0 to 7;0 years of age and an optional written expression subtest for ages to 8;0 – 16;0. *See* Wiig (1988b) in Appendix I.

CELF-RUK *see* CLINICAL EVALUATION OF LANGUAGE FUNDAMENTALS (REVISED UK VERSION).

central hearing loss a hearing loss produced by a pathological condition occurring along the path of the auditory nerve from the BRAIN-STEM to the cerebral CORTEX. It produces a problem in speech perception rather than just hearing.

central nervous system (CNS) the system within the body which produces reflexes when one part of the body is particularly stimulated. These responses come from the BRAIN via the SPINAL CORD. *See* Taverner (1983); Tortora and Grabowski (1993).

central processor a unit which is used to operate other units. For example, a computer can be described as a central processor for the information which appears on a monitor screen, or for information which goes to a printer. It can also be used to describe a unit which is used to operate ENVIRONMENTAL CONTROLS. *See* Bishop (1985).

central tendency a method of finding out the distribution of scores received from experiments. There are three such measures:

1. Mean – the sum of scores of each person tested, divided by the number of people who took part in the experiment;
2. Mode – the most frequently occurring score;
3. Median – the middle score after all the scores have been put in order.

If all the measures are the same, i.e. mean = mode = median, it is called a symmetrical or normal distribution of scores and can be shown as such on a graph. If the scores diverge, they are said to be skewed. *See* Miller (1975); Clarke and Cooke (1992).

centre in articulatory terms, the part of the tongue between the blade and its back. It is used to produce palatal sounds and is part of the ARTICULATION of the palatoalveolar sounds as the centre of the tongue approaches the hard palate. A description of any vowel which appears in the middle of the CARDINAL VOWEL SYSTEM. The vowel which is right in the centre of the cardinal vowel space is the schwa vowel [ə]. To produce this vowel, the tongue takes up a central position in the mouth. *See* Ladefoged (1993).

centrencephalic epilepsy *see* CONGENITAL NEURONAL DYSFUNCTION.

cephalic usually a suffix to describe disorders in or of the head, for example, microcephalic (an abnormally small head – *see* MICROCEPHALY).

CERA *see* CORTICAL EVOKED RESPONSE AUDIOMETRY.

cerebellar a description of structures found within the CEREBELLUM and of its disorders. These may produce dysarthric (*see* DYSARTHRIA) speech.

cerebellar dysarthria *see* ATAXIC DYSARTHRIA.

cerebellum comprises a cortex of grey matter, a central area of white matter and four pairs of central nuclei. The cerebellum is connected to the MEDULLA OBLONGATA, PONS and the MIDBRAIN by the inferior, middle and cerebellar peduncles respectively. The cerebellum organises the person's motor movements. The synchronous movements of muscles will be affected adversely if there is a lesion to this part of the brain affecting the person's speech producing cerebellar DYSARTHRIA. *See* Barr (1979); Tortora and Grabowski (1993).

cerebral a description of structures or disorders that occur within the BRAIN.

cerebral abscess *see* BRAIN ABSCESS.

cerebral artery an artery which supplies the BRAIN. One of the most important is the middle cerebral artery which is situated in the lateral fissure between the frontal and temporal lobes (*see* CEREBRAL HEMISPHERES). Rupture of this artery or a branch produces a CEREBROVASCULAR ACCIDENT (CVA) as blood spreads over the brain and affects areas such as Broca's area (*see* CEREBRAL HEMISPHERES). This can cause APHASIA. *See* Barr (1979).

cerebral hemispheres the BRAIN has two hemispheres, right and left, connected by the CORPUS CALLOSUM. The folds and convolutions are known as gyri and the intervening grooves are known as sulci. Two of the sulci which appear in the fetus develop into the lateral and parieto-occipital fissures. These fissures with the central and calcarine sulci divide the hemisphere into four lobes – frontal, parietal, temporal and occipital. The frontal lobe extends forward from the central sulcus and upwards from the lateral fissure. The medial surface covers the anterior part of the corpus callosum. The parietal lobe, on the lateral surface, is bounded by the central sulcus and the lateral fissure. On the medial surface, the parietal lobe is bounded by the frontal lobe, corpus callosum, calcarine sulcus and parieto-occipital fissure. The temporal lobe, on the lateral surface, is bounded by the lateral fissure. The inferior surface of the lobe extends to the temporal pole. The occipital lobe starts where the temporal lobe ends and is separated from the parietal lobe by the parieto-occipital fissure. The left hemisphere in the majority of people is the dominant hemisphere (*see* DOMINANCE) and it controls the right side of the body. It contains the language centres of the brain. In particular, Broca's area can be found in the frontal lobe while Wernicke's area can be found in the parietal lobe. Both hemispheres have a motor and sensory region from which signals are sent to the nerves innervating the muscles of movement, touch and smell, etc. The occipital lobe is concerned with vision. The right hemisphere has centres controlling rhythm, artistry, arithmetic and control of muscles used for speaking and eating. *See* Barr (1979).

cerebral infarction *see* CEREBROVASCULAR ACCIDENT.

cerebral palsy a group of disorders of movement and posture due to slow development and non-progressive disorders of the BRAIN. There are several possible causes of cerebral palsy which can occur at various times around the child's birth.

1. During the PRENATAL period, the possible causes are congenital infections, e.g. congenital malformations within the brain, radiation or nutritional deficiency or lack of oxygen.
2. During the PERINATAL period, the possible causes are periventricular haemorrhage, birth asphyxia, birth trauma, hyperbilirubinaemia or venous stasis/thrombosis.

3. During the POSTNATAL period, the possible causes are MENINGITIS, ENCEPHALITIS, trauma or metabolic disorders.

There are four types of cerebral palsy:

1. Spastic cerebral palsy: the most common type of cerebral palsy which accounts for about 70 per cent of children so affected. The damage to the brain, which produces both hemiplegia and bilateral hemiplegia, is centred on the corticospinal tracts (*see* PYRAMIDAL SYSTEM). Bilateral hemiplegia produces a pseudobulbar palsy (*see* BULBAR PALSY) which produces dysarthric characteristics of speech (*see* DYSARTHRIA), impaired swallowing (*see* DYSPHAGIA) and a poor gag reflex.

2. Ataxic cerebral palsy: damage to the brain in the CEREBELLUM which produces HYPOTONIA, a broad base gait, TREMOR and DYSMETRIA. Speech becomes dysarthric (*see* DYSARTHRIA) while intelligence is usually within normal limits.

3. Dyskinetic cerebral palsy: damage to the BRAIN, causing involuntary movements and reduced voluntary movements, is found in the BASAL GANGLIA. There are three subtypes:
   (a) athetosis: slow, writhing movements and severely dysarthric speech caused by damage to the extrapyramidal system in the brain or asphyxia at birth or anoxia to the basal ganglia. There can also be a HEARING LOSS;
   (b) chorea: fast, jerky movements in the upper extremities caused by a disease to the basal ganglia;
   (c) dystonia: increase in muscle tone, no contractures and persistence of primitive reflexes. Distorted postures are maintained for long periods of time and produce rotation, adduction of limbs and extension of the spine. It affects the AGONIST and ANTAGONIST muscles.

4. Mixed cerebral palsy: a form of cerebral palsy which has features of (1)–(3). Those who may be involved with treatment will include the physiotherapist, speech and language therapist, occupational therapist, educational psychologist and, possibly, an ENT surgeon.

See Gilroy and Holliday (1982); Hosking (1982); Illingworth (1987); Kolb and Whishaw (1990); Kaye (1991).

cerebrospinal fluid (CSF) fluid that circulates round the BRAIN coming from the ventricles (*see* THIRD VENTRICLE and FOURTH VENTRICLE) in the brain and the central canal of the SPINAL CORD. Most of the CSF consists of water, protein and a few cells. It also contains sugar and sodium chloride. The CSF is used to diagnose diseases of the MENINGES and CENTRAL NERVOUS SYSTEM. *See* Barr (1979); Kaye (1991).

cerebrovascular accident (CVA) the medical term which encompasses all the different ways in which a stroke occurs. The functioning of the BRAIN is dependent on its blood supply and the oxygen carried in the blood. A quarter of the oxygen we breathe goes to the brain. If the brain is deprived of oxygen for greater than three minutes, cells are damaged. When a CVA occurs, there is interruption of the normal blood supply and irreversible cell damage takes place. There are two disorders which affect the blood supply to the brain – haemorrhage and thrombosis:

1. Brain haemorrhage: a vessel ruptures either in the brain itself or in the subarachnoid space. About 10 per cent of all cerebrovascular accidents are due to haemorrhage. The resultant haematoma (blood clot) produces compression damage of the surrounding brain tissue and by raising the INTRACRANIAL PRESSURE may interfere with brain function at distant sites. In addition, subarachnoid bleeding can occur from a berry aneurysm. These

form usually at junctions in the cerebral arteries (*see* CEREBRAL ARTERY). The vessel wall is weakened and the dilating artery ruptures at the defective site. Ninety per cent of berry aneurysms are found on the CIRCLE OF WILLIS. The rupture of an aneurysm often affects CRANIAL NERVES. The majority of people may have the following symptoms:

   (a) severe generalised headache with pain radiating to the neck;

   (b) nausea and vomiting;

   (c) transient vertigo;

   (d) feeling of faintness and confusion and coma.

2. Arteriovenous malformation: a haphazard network of blood vessels which may be found anywhere in the brain. The part of the brain which is affected is stained brown by numerous small haemorrhages which have occurred in the past. The symptoms include:

   (a) generalised or partial seizures;

   (b) headaches on the side of the malformation;

   (c) a 'bruit' which may be heard over the orbits in the skull;

   (d) 50 per cent of malformations bleed into the SUBARACHNOID SPACE.

Treatment is given for the seizures by anticonvulsant drugs whilst surgery can be used to remove the malformation.

The main cause of infarction is cerebral thrombosis. This is due to formation of a thrombus which blocks the internal carotid and vertebral arteries as well as the cerebral arteries and their branches. Mostly, cerebral infarction follows thrombosis in atherosclerotic vessels.

A less common cause of infarction is embolism. It begins as a thrombus (a) on the wall of the left atrium of a fibrillating heart; (b) on the left ventricular wall after a heart attack; or (c) on the wall of the internal carotid artery (*see* CAROTID ARTERY) due to the forma-

tion of an atheromatous plaque. When it becomes detached it comes to rest in a cerebral artery (*see* CEREBRAL ARTERY). HEMIPLEGIA, unconsciousness or APHASIA occurs within a few seconds of onset. Ninety per cent of all strokes are caused by a blood vessel blockage by thrombus or embolism. *See* Gilroy and Holliday (1982); Kaye (1991).

character letters, numerals and other symbols including spaces used in word processing or in writing a program for a computer. Every character has its own code made up of bits. The codes are those of the ASCII. *See* Chandor et al (1985).

Chatterbox an early high-tech communication aid, it is a speech synthesiser which produces the words typed into it. It uses a QWERTY keyboard and a built-in amplifier unit with rechargeable batteries. There is a 12-character display screen which allows typing errors to be corrected before pressing the 'speech key'. The memory holds 74 sentences and phrases which the person may need to access quickly. These expressions are for emergencies, feeding, shopping and everyday conversation.

chi-square test a statistical test which allows an experimenter to show how well the data fit a theoretical distribution. *See* Porkess (1988).

childhood-onset pervasive developmental disorder a name given in the USA to try to avoid confusion with childhood schizophrenia (*see* CHILDHOOD PSYCHOSES). It was proposed in DSM-III and is supported by many mental health professionals in the USA. The condition differs from SCHIZOPHRENIA in that it does not include DELUSIONS, HALLUCINATIONS or THOUGHT DISORDERS as symptoms. However, children who are diagnosed as having it show difficulties in forming social relationships and produce odd facets to their behaviour. *See* Davison and Neale (1994).

childhood psychoses a group of different disorders with a prevalence of 0.4 per cent. The most common form of childhood psychosis is AUTISM. Less common childhood psychoses are childhood schizophrenia (compare CHILDHOOD-ONSET PERVASIVE DEVELOPMENTAL DISORDER) which produces auditory hallucinations (*see* HALLUCINATIONS) and confusion with accompanying mood disturbances, FLATTENING OF AFFECT, mannerisms and grimacing, while the child's IQ is usually within normal limits; disintegrative psychoses in which the child develops normally until 3–4 years of age after which there is sudden loss of skills as well as of expressive language, and their behaviour regresses; manic-depressive (*see* MANIC-DEPRESSION) psychoses which are very rare before puberty. *See* Davison and Neale (1994).

childhood schizophrenia *see* CHILDHOOD PSYCHOSES.

chlorpromazine drug for treating MANIC-DEPRESSION (*see also* PHENOTHIAZINES).

Chomskyan linguistics the publication of *Syntactic Structures* by Noam Chomsky in 1957 heralded a radical change in linguistic science, both in terms of theoretical innovation and, somewhat later, the claim by Chomsky that linguistics is a branch of cognitive psychology. Chomsky's theory, initially known as transformational generative grammar (*see* TRANSFORMATIONAL GRAMMAR), has itself altered radically since 1957. Its latest manifestation is known as government and binding theory (GB). Chomsky has consistently maintained, however, whatever form his grammatical theory has taken, that the linguist's grammar is at once a characterisation of the language and an account of what the native speaker knows (and has internalised) about his language. *See* Lepschy (1982); Lyons (1991).

chorda tympani nerve *see* TONGUE.

chorea *see* CEREBRAL PALSY (3b).

chromosomes a child receives 22 pairs of chromosomes plus a sex chromosome from each parent. In a male, these chromosomes are an X and a Y, while in the female they are both X chromosomes. As this is an equal division of the chromosomes, the child has half the characteristics of each parent. If there is an abnormality in the chromosomes, certain syndromes can result, e.g. DOWN'S SYNDROME. Some syndromes and diseases are described in terms of the autosomal or sex chromosome abnormality as follows:

1. Dominant autosomal disorder is inherited by several members of the family. There is a 50 per cent chance of children being affected as only one gene is abnormal.

2. Recessive autosomal disorder is inherited by fewer members of the family. There is a lesser chance of children being affected than in (1) as an abnormal gene from each parent is required. Both disorders can be produced by an abnormality of the X chromosome.

3. X-linked recessive disorder appears in males as they have only one X chromosome and so will have the abnormal gene while females who have an abnormal gene in one X chromosome have a second X chromosome which cancels out the first. For an X-linked disorder to be present in females both X chromosomes have to be affected. Disorders produced by this type of chromosomal abnormality include Duchenne Muscular Dystrophy (*see* DYSTROPHY).

See Hosking (1982).

chronic a description of a disease or illness which has a slow progression or its symptoms are slow to evolve. It is opposed to acute (*see* ACUTE (1)).

chronic non-specific laryngitis a condition caused by nasal discharge into the nasopharynx (*see* PHARYNX) and thence to the LARYNX, which becomes irritated. In many cases, the only symptom is persistent HOARSE VOICE. The primary problem, i.e. nasal disorder, should be treated before the secondary problem of the laryngitis. *See* Pracy et al (1974).

chronological age (CA) the natural age of a child or adult. It is used in assessments carried out by various rehabilitation professionals such as speech and language therapists, psychologists, etc. The child's CA can be compared to the AGE EQUIVALENT SCORE obtained in certain assessments. Chronological age is also used by psychologists in the formula to work out an INTELLIGENCE QUOTIENT.

circle of Willis an anastomotic arrangement which joins together the blood supply brought to the brain by the internal carotid arteries (*see* CAROTID ARTERY) and the vertebral-basilar arteries. From this arterial circle come all the cerebral arteries (*see* CEREBRAL ARTERY) which supply the BRAIN. If obstruction occurs in one of the major input arteries, it is possible for blood to flow round the circle of Willis and supply the territory of the blocked artery. *See* Barr (1979); Tortora and Grabowski (1993).

circumvallate papillae *see* TASTE BUDS.

classical conditioning a learning procedure used in BEHAVIOUR THERAPY. It is based on the theory first proposed by Pavlov in his experiments with dogs. He found that dogs could learn a conditioned response (CR). He based his theory on the fact that people can learn certain reactions by giving an unconditioned response (UR) to an unconditioned stimulus (US). His experiments were aimed at finding out if a conditioned response could be learnt from a conditioned stimulus (CS). For example, Pavlov found dogs salivated (UR) when they smelled or tasted meat (US). Pavlov switched on a light when the dogs were given the meat (CS – dogs learn light is only on when given meat) and the dogs salivated (UR). However, he found if the light were switched on, the dogs still salivated (CR – as they had been conditioned to salivate at the meat when the

lights were on). There are three stages in learning a conditioned response to a conditioned stimulus starting from an unconditioned stimulus:

1. Simultaneous conditioning: both the light (CS) and the meat (US) are presented together, thus making the dogs salivate (UR).
2. Delayed conditioning: the light (CS) is switched on for a few seconds before the meat (US) is given to the dogs and is left switched on until the dogs salivate.
3. Trace conditioning: the light (US) is switched on, then switched off before the meat (US) is presented so that only a memory trace of the light remains for the conditioning process to take place. By repetition of placing the CS next to the the US, the association of the two is reinforced. If reinforcement does not take place, extinction of the CR may take place.

See Atkinson et al (1993).

Claudius converse a high-tech device which can be fitted to the telephone and produces speech artificially. 'Claudivs' (Roman spelling of the Roman Emperor who had a speech defect) is an acronym for Calling Line Announcement Using Digitally Integrated Voice Synthesis. It consists of a keypad with 16 buttons which, when pressed, can produce 64 phrases including emergency messages for ambulance, fire or police. Both female and male voices can be produced. It can be used in a face-to-face conversation.

clause in some models of grammar, a clause is a grammatical unit which is smaller than, or co-terminous with, a sentence, but larger than a phrase. Its defining characteristic is that it contains a verb (though some grammatical descriptions would recognise reduced or verbless clauses). Clauses are normally identified as 'main' or 'subordinate' and the functions of subordinate clauses, e.g. adverbial, object, may also be identified. *See* Allerton (1979).

clavicular a description of the use of the chest. For example, some people who have dysarthria may not produce normal ABDOMINAL-DIAPHRAGMATIC RESPIRATION, but, instead, breathe from their chest. This is known as clavicular breathing.

clavicular respiration *see* CLAVICULAR.

cleft palate a congenital condition in which there is failure of the palatal shelves to unite together with the nasal septum. In the normal development of the MOUTH the palatal shelves come together to form the hard palate or roof of the mouth as the TONGUE falls down into the cavity. A cleft palate is the embryological failure of the hard palate to fuse together while the child is *in utero*. A cleft lip is caused by failure of the tissue surrounding the lip to fuse together during the same period. A cleft lip and palate occur when both the hard palate and lip have failed to form. Clefts can occur unilaterally or bilaterally. Most children who have this condition at birth can be helped by surgery. A cleft lip will be repaired around 3 months of age while a cleft in the palate will be closed at 6 months of age. Carrying out an operation at such an early age allows the surgeons to make use of the continual growth in the tissues of the affected areas. Thus, healing is more natural and few scars are left. A submucous cleft palate has a divided uvula or bifid uvula, a whitish line down the midline of the soft palate and a bony notch on the ridge between the soft and hard palates. The muscles of the soft palate do not function correctly and velopharyngeal incompetence (*see* VELOPHARYNGEAL) may result. Occult submucous cleft palate exists when the situation just outlined occurs but the white line is obscured by muscle, the bony notch is not evident and there is no bifid uvula. As

surgical procedures have improved in closing a cleft lip and/or palate, the need for speech therapy to improve the child's articulation is not as great as in the past. However, the therapist's main purpose is to counsel the parents about the child's future speech, efficacy of surgery and to give advice on the best types of feeding techniques available at the time. There may be problems of nasality as well as other articulation problems which will require speech therapy. *See* Edwards and Watson (1980); Grunwell (1993) (analysing cleft palate speech); Sell et al (1994) (screening assessment of cleft palate speech); Sell and Grunwell (1994) (speech and the unoperated cleft palate subject).

client-centered therapy a type of PSYCHOTHERAPY proposed by Carl Rogers which assumes that each person has the motivation and ability to change and the person is the best qualified to decide how the change will occur. The therapist takes little part in the session and listens while individuals explore and analyse their own problems. *See* Atkinson et al (1993).

clinical audiology audiology used to evaluate the effects of a HEARING LOSS on the person's daily life and give him the means to cope with communication.

Clinical Evaluation of Language Fundamentals (revised UK version) devised originally by Wiig, CELF-R aims to assess school-age children to find out the nature and severity of the language difficulties. It comprises eleven subtests including: formulated sentences, word structure, listening to paragraphs, sentence structure, semantic relationships, sentence assembly, oral directions, word associations, word classes, recalling sentences and linguistic concepts. The UK version was put together by a team from the National Hospital's College of Speech Sciences and the Psychological

Corporation and includes UK record forms, a manual supplement (written by the NHCSS panel) and amended stimulus manuals. *See* Wiig (1994) in Appendix I.

clinical psychology a clinical psychologist assesses and treats EMOTIONAL DISORDERS and CONDUCT DISORDERS which occur among those with a LEARNING DISABILITY and/or physically handicap, juvenile delinquents, drug addicts and in families where relationships have broken down. Such psychologists work in hospitals with inpatients and outpatients and in prisons. *See* MacKay (1975).

clonic *see* EPILEPSY.

close vowel *see* CARDINAL VOWEL SYSTEM.

cloze procedure a way of analysing reading processes. It takes the form of a passage of text with different types of words missing which have to be filled in by the client.

clumsy child syndrome a form of general DYSPRAXIA which manifests itself as impaired motor coordination. Difficulties arise in gross motor activities such as jumping, hopping and throwing, as well as in fine motor coordination. Written language may also be affected. It sometimes co-occurs with DEVELOPMENTAL VERBAL DYSPRAXIA. Dressing dyspraxia is also associated with this syndrome. The child has difficulty in orienting clothes when dressing so that shirts or jerseys may be put on upside down or back to front.

cluster reduction *see* PHONOLOGICAL PROCESSES.

cluttering a particular type of DYSFLUENCY in which the main feature is excessive speed of delivery. Resulting speech may at times be incoherent due to transposition and omission of sounds. PROSODY is also affected and these abnormalities may carry over to reading and writing.The individual is often unaware of the problem and unable to monitor his speech. Therapy for this disorder is aimed at relaxing the person and slowing down the speech RATE to a more acceptable level. *See* Dalton and Hardcastle (1989).

CNS *see* CENTRAL NERVOUS SYSTEM.

co-articulation an articulation which occurs almost simultaneously with another articulation. For example, in words such as 'eighth' and 'width', the [t] and [d] become dentalised as the speaker approaches [θ]. Thus, these two words would be pronounced [etθ] and [w+dθ]. Anticipatory co-articulation occurs where the articulators for both sounds move to the place of articulation (*see* ARTICULATION) of the second sound. For example, the word 'shoe' is pronounced with lip-rounding and even the [ʃ] is rounded, thus producing co-articulation. *See* Ladefoged (1993).

cochlea *see* EAR.

cochlear implants devices which are used as substitutes for the hair cells of the organ of Corti (*see* EAR) and which convert sounds into electronic signals which are interpreted by the BRAIN. The sound waves are picked up by a small microphone connected to a small microprocessor where they are converted into electrical signals. These signals go to electrodes placed in the cochlea and trigger nerve impulses in the cochlear branch of the vestibulo-cochlear nerve. The nerve impulses can then follow their normal route to the brain. *See* Atkinson et al (1993); Tortora and Grabowski (1993); Allum-Mecklenberg (1996.

cochlear nerve *see* EAR.

cochlear reflex *see* ELECTROCOCHLEOGRAPHY.

cochlear window *see* EAR.

cocktail party phenomenon the process of picking out what is said in a crowded room, setting aside all other linguistic information. This is known as selective listening. *See* Clark and Clark (1977); Atkinson et al (1993).

45

cocktail party syndrome described first by J.C.P. Williams in 1961, it was found in four unrelated children who had a learning disability, an unusual facial appearance and supravalvular aortic stenosis. It is also known as Williams' syndrome. Some of the most common abnormalities found by Williams and his colleagues were:

1. Mild prenatal growth deficiency and mild microcephaly.
2. Average IQ; friendly, loquacious personality, HOARSE VOICE and mild neurological dysfunction. Perceptual and motor function is more reduced than verbal and memory performance.
3. Facial appearance is marked by prominent lips and open mouth.
4. Cardiovascular anomaly – supravalvular aortic stenosis.

During early infancy, these children tend to be fretful and have feeding problems. During childhood, they tend to be outgoing and loquacious, a personality referred to as 'cocktail party manner'.
See Smith (1985).

coffee jar test a screening procedure developed by Gordon and McKinlay (1980) to identify clumsy children. A number of common objects are included which the child is required to manipulate, e.g. threading beads is one of the tasks.

cognitive behaviour therapy a means of remedying behavioural and emotional disorders by trying to modify the person's thoughts. If cognitive methods are used to modify these thought processes, this is a cognitive therapy. Cognitive behaviour therapy or cognitive behaviour modification has been developed in the field of behaviour therapy. The basic premise is that emotional disorders are caused by maladaptive thought patterns and the main task of therapy is to remediate these processes. There are three main types of cognitive behaviour therapy:

1. Cognitive restructuring methods.
2. Coping skills procedures.
3. Problem-solving therapies.

It is the cognitive restructuring methods which make this type of behaviour therapy stand out from other psychological therapeutic techniques. There are three different cognitive restructuring methods commonly used:

1. Ellis's RATIONAL-EMOTIVE THERAPY.
2. Meichenbaum's SELF-INSTRUCTIONAL TRAINING.
3. BECK'S COGNITIVE THERAPY.

See Rachman and Wilson (1980); Atkinson et al (1993).

CommPac a high-tech system which combines voice synthesiser, SoftKey, touch panel and digitised sound all in a single unit placed below and connected to a notebook computer. There is also the Mini-Commpac which mounts directly under a Gateway 486 subnotebook computer. *See* Appendix IV.

communication the ability to transfer information from one person either to another person or to a group of people. There has been much discussion as to the form the communication process takes. Thus, the speech chain came into being. When a link breaks in this chain, the result is a communication disorder and the therapist has to find ways to mend the links so the chain will function normally. *See* Denes and Pinson (1973).

Communication Assessment Profile for Adults with a Mental Handicap (CASP) devised as a functional communication assessment for adults with a severe to mild LEARNING DISABILITY. However, it is unsuitable for those who have a profound learning disability or a severe visual impairment. The assessment is carried out by carer/key worker and speech and language therapist. There are three parts:

1. Carer's assessment: questionnaire concerning the client's communication abilities and requiring basic infor-

mation about the client's daily life and environment.

2. Therapist's assessment: this concerns the client's communication abilities about event knowledge, hearing and auditory discrimination skills, vocabulary, and comprehension of functional use of everyday objects, comprehension at sentence level and comprehension and expression at sentence level.

3. Joint assessment: both the carer and therapist work together completing the summary of assessments, involving the client wherever possible.

The Communication Environment Rating Scale is completed, giving a broad outline of whether the client's different environments are enabling/encouraging him or her to use his or her communication skills. Priorities for change are also agreed. *See* Beech et al (1993).

communication board a low-tech form of alternative augmentative communication. Thus, it can be used with those who have no or very limited verbal output which may be unintelligible or it may just be used as a temporary means of communication during therapy until the person's communication improves. The board can have pictures, symbols, words or phrases on it depending on what the person can understand best. *See* Enderby (1987); Beukelman and Mirenda (1992).

communication disorder *see* COMMUNICATION.

communication profiles different types of assessment for testing the severity of APHASIA. The profiles examine in particular everyday situations in which those with aphasia may find themselves. Thus, people are tested in various situations such as 'greeting', 'understanding', 'social conventions' and so on. *See* Eisenson (1984).

Communicative Abilities in Daily Living (CADL) devised by Holland, CADL is a test of functional communication

which takes the form of a communication profile. There are ten functional categories: (1) reading, writing and use of numbers; (2) SPEECH ACTS; (3) verbal and non-verbal contexts; (4) role playing; (5) divergencies; (6) relationship-dependent communicative behaviour; (7) non-verbal symbolic communication; (8) DEIXIS; (9) humour, absurdity; (10) use of metaphor. There is an attempt to relate CADL to type, cause and severity of APHASIA. The rating is on a three-point scale. Administration takes the form of a structured interview utilising props and situational contexts. It is designed for all age groups. CADL has two objectives: (1) to gain a valid reflection of communication skills; (2) to obtain a reliable assessment of these skills. It is a test of talking behaviour and communication, assessing more than just propositional and linguistic content. It does not discriminate against those who may use an alternative augmentative communication system. *See* Holland (1980) in Appendix I; Eisenson (1984); Rosenbek et al (1989).

compact a distinctive feature proposed by Jakobson and Halle for marking open vowels. They are denoted by [+COMPACT] while other vowels are [–COMPACT]. The opposite is DIFFUSE. Chomsky and Halle described these vowels as LOW. *See* Hyman (1975).

compact bones *see* BONE.

compatibility a phenomenon which, if it exists, would mean computer programs could be used on two different computers without having to be altered. Normally, it is impossible, for example, to write a program on a BBC computer using BBC BASIC and run it on an Apple microcomputer. However, wordprocessing documents can be copied from IBM PC computers to Apple Mac computers. Apple Macs with the Power PC chip can run any IBM PC computer software.

competence the knowledge individuals have of their own language. In

Chomsky's view, competence, the normally implicit knowledge of the language, is opposed to PERFORMANCE, the implementation of this knowledge in speaking and understanding. *See* Lyons (1968); Fromkin and Rodman (1993).

complement the traditional sense is of an element of SENTENCE or CLAUSE structure which 'completes' the action of the verb. In this sense, it can refer to any obligatory post-verb element. In a more restricted sense, it refers to the 'completing' role of elements of structure following the verb 'to be' (or similar verbs), e.g. he is HAPPY, she was IN THE GARDEN, he is A TAXI DRIVER (the complement is shown in upper case). *See* Lyons (1968).

complementary distribution a type of phonological analysis. When two sounds belong to the same phonological unit or phoneme (*see* PHONOLOGY), they are in complementary distribution. In other words, there is no overlap between the distribution of the sounds, i.e. no overlap in the set of contexts in which the sound is found. *See* Hyman (1975); Fromkin and Rodman (1993).

compliance in terms of the hearing mechanism, compliance refers to the ease with which sounds travel from the tympanic membrane to the middle ear.

compound racemose gland *see* SALIVARY GLANDS.

comprehension the process used by humans to understand forms of communication including speech, written language and gesture. Communication disorders such as APHASIA may have some elements of a comprehension disorder. In aphasia, there is often a distinction made between expressive and receptive disorders. The latter refers to comprehension problems as the way in which the person receives information either visually or auditorily. When children have an expressive language delay or disorder, their comprehension can still be better than

their ability to produce utterances. Many people think that if the child can understand what is said to him, he will be able to produce a similar utterance which may not be the case. *See* Crystal (1993); Fromkin and Rodman (1993).

compulsion neurosis *see* OBSESSIVE-COMPULSIVE DISORDER.

compulsive rituals *see* AUTISM.

computed axial tomography *see* COMPUTED TOMOGRAPHY.

computed tomography (CT) a non-invasive X-ray technique used to locate space occupied by lesions. It differs from ordinary X-ray techniques in that it uses a narrow, moving beam which makes multiple scans of the brain. The results are processed by computer which distinguishes the different densities of brain tissue. Thus, lesions can be highlighted, some having a greater or lesser density than the surrounding brain tissue. A CT scan can pick out haemorrhages, tumours and cysts as well as atrophy, oedema, necrosis and multiple sclerosis. *See* Barr (1979); Draper (1980); Gilroy and Holliday (1982); Kaye (1991).

computer a machine which takes in information, processes it and sends it out in a specific way to units linked to the computer, e.g. printer, monitor or disk drive. There are three types of computer: (1) digital computer; (2) analog computer; (3) hybrid computer. Digital computers include main frame computers, minicomputers and personal/microcomputers. *See* Bishop (1985).

computer-aided learning a system which uses computer programs designed especially for remediation and/or teaching purposes.

computer games some games are designed to be recreational while others are designed to be educational or therapeutic. The former type usually test the person's dexterity and skill to hit or avoid objects moving about a screen or the person's logic, imagination and knowledge. There are three types of game:

1. Strategy, e.g. chess.
2. Adventure, e.g. those where directions have to be followed to find specific items.
3. Arcade e.g. those just for amusement which usually scroll across the screen.

Home computers and personal computers have many such games designed for them and can have joysticks or paddles for playing the game. *See* Chandor et al (1985).

computer graphics the production of pictures from a computer program which appear on a monitor screen and which can be printed out. *See* Chandor et al (1985).

computer memory *see* MEMORY (2).

computer program a set of instructions given in a logical order to help solve almost any problem. The computer accepts instructions written in a specific language. Possible languages which can be used are:

1. BASIC – the most common, simplest and most versatile language.
2. Pascal – a language emphasising structured programming and good programming techniques.
3. COBOL – Common Business Orientated Language. It is internationally accepted as a computer language for commercial use. The American Defence Department were the original sponsors. It is a high-level language for solving problems. The source program is written using statements in English of a standard but readable form.
4. FORTRAN – FORmula TRANslation. It is a problem-solving high-level language for writing programs to cope with mathematical and scientific problems. The source program combines algebraic formulae and English statements of a standard but readable form.

Many of the program listings may have loops, subroutines and certain other commands. Programmers usually begin by drawing a flowchart which they translate into the logical formation of a program. This is mapped onto the instructions of the language they wish to use. As the program is written, the writer may unintentionally incorporate various bugs which he has to try and remove before producing the program commercially. *See* White (1985); Bishop (1985); Brookshear (1991).

concept keyboard an input device for operating software without having to use the computer's QWERTY keyboard. If using a BBC computer, it is plugged into the user port. It is a touch-sensitive pad which comes in A3 and A4 sizes. The overlay is placed on the pad and the required squares are pressed at the appropriate time during the running of the program.

concord the grammatical phenomenon in which a form of one word in a sentence 'agrees' with a corresponding form in another word. For example, in English the subject of a sentence agrees with the verb in the present tense:

1. The dog runs away.
2. The dogs run away.

In (1), the singular form of the verb has the affix '-s' while in (2), the plural form has a zero morph (i.e. no affix) and is just 'run'. *See* Lyons (1968); Fromkin and Rodman (1993).

concrete operations the third stage of PIAGET's theory of the child's cognitive development during the 7–11-year-old period, having overcome the difficulties found during the pre-operational stage. The child's thought processes are now becoming more logical but he can still only understand relationships directly perceived by him (i.e., the child cannot yet think abstractly). During this stage the child can work out hierarchies of classes and subclasses and can also place shapes in order by size without measuring them. *See* Beard (1969).

conditioned response *see* CLASSICAL CONDITIONING.

conditioned stimulus *see* CLASSICAL CONDITIONING.

conditioning tests tests used to assess the hearing of some young children (from about 2;6 years) who are too young to be tested by PURE-TONE AUDIOMETRY. It is based on OPERANT CONDITIONING. The children are told to do a specific action, e.g. put brick in box, put peg in peg board, when they hear a specific sound. The sounds are either pure tones (*see* PURE-TONE AUDIOMETRY) or warbles (*see* WARBLE TONE). When the child responds accurately and consistently then the intensity is reduced until the child's hearing threshold is reduced. The child should receive a reinforcement after a correct response.

conduct disorder persistent socially disapproved behaviour associated with social impairment. The prevalence is 3–9 per cent of school-age children. Conduct disorders are most common in boys (4:1), most children affected come from social classes IV and V. The causes arise from the child's experience of life:

1. Family factors – persistent conflict, divorce, etc.
2. Social factors – poor housing, etc.
3. Educational factors – one-third of these children have learning difficulties, especially with reading, etc.
4. Temperamental factors – unpredictable reactions, irritability, etc.

The most common symptoms include: fighting and bullying, aggression and temper tantrums, defiance and disobedience, destructiveness, lying, stealing, truancy, fire setting and arson. The major types of conduct disorder include:

1. Socialised conduct disorder: children who have failed to acquire socially approved standards of behaviour. However, within the family they can often make warm relationships and are often described as 'likeable rogues'.
2. Unsocialised conduct disorder: a more severe disorder in which children form poor peer relationships. They are frequently self-destructive, aggressive and seem keen to be punished. Family life is always discordant, discipline harsh and little affection is shown to the children, who thus experience rejection.
3. Mixed conduct and emotional disorder: children are indifferent to stress, resulting in abnormal behaviour.

Many children with a conduct disorder are restless and overactive for a short period of time but a small number are extremely and persistently overactive. Such children have problems from an early age. All psychotherapies (*see* PSYCHOTHERAPY) can be used to treat this condition. *See* Rutter (1975); Davison and Neale (1994).

conduction the transmission of sounds from one point to another.

conduction aphasia a major type of APHASIA described by the BOSTON SCHOOL. It is caused by damage to the ARCUATE FASCICULUS in the left hemisphere (*see* CEREBRAL HEMISPHERES). For a discussion of the communication problems in conduction aphasia – *see* APHASIA (3). *See* Goodglass and Kaplan (1983) in Appendix I; Rosenbek et al (1989).

conductive hearing loss a HEARING LOSS caused by a pathology affecting the conduction of sound through the outer ear and/or middle ear into the inner ear (*see* EAR).

confabulation a symptom of amnesia. The person who tries not to accept he has memory problems fills in the gaps in his memory with made-up information. *See* Davison and Neale (1994).

configuration the way in which the computer is set up to accept information and run programs or operate printers, disk drives and other peripheral units. For example, when the BBC Master 128 is configured for use in ADFS, it has to be reconfigured to accept disks designed for use with the BBC B which uses the DFS filing system, or it may be that the computer has to be configured for the use of a parallel printer. *See* Bishop (1985).

congenital disorder a disorder which appears at birth, perhaps as a result of a problem during the PRENATAL, PERINATAL or POSTNATAL periods or an inherited trait. It is opposed to a DEVELOPMENTAL DISORDER which occurs during childhood.

congenital hearing loss a hearing loss which occurs before the period of language development (*see* ACQUISITION). It can be caused by various diseases during the PRENATAL and PERINATAL periods.

congenital muscular dystrophy a congenital myopathy. A range of disorders of muscles which present as progressive weakness of muscles. The severe physical breakdown of the muscle is similar to other forms of DYSTROPHY. Treatment is given through PHYSIOTHERAPY. *See* Gilroy and Holliday (1982); Hosking (1982).

congenital neuronal dysfunction a condition which produces sudden, abnormal discharges of neurons in the brain, producing epileptic convulsions. This occurs in the RETICULAR SYSTEM in the centrencephalon. Thus, the type of EPILEPSY produced is known as centrencephalic epilepsy. *See* Draper (1980).

connected speech a particular type of speech. It describes the way in which conversation and different kinds of utterances are put together. It is opposed to speaking with single words and phrases which can function differently in general conversation. Prosodic features (*see* PROSODY) used in flowing speech are especially important. *See* Cruttendern (1994).

connective tissue (CT) tissue made up in a ground substance comprising fibres. There are two types determined by the type and quantity of fibres in the ground substance – packing connective tissue and supporting tissue. In the former there are two subgroups – reticular tissue and loose/dense CT, while the latter comprises BONE and CARTILAGE. *See* Tortora and Grabowski (1993).

consonant a sound which is not a vowel (*see* CARDINAL VOWEL SYSTEM). Such sounds have specific descriptions for the way they are articulated. They are described in terms of their voicing, place of articulation and manner of articulation (*see* ARTICULATION). *See* Ladefoged (1993).

consonant cluster a grouping of two or more abutting consonants in different parts of a word:

1. Word-initially – 'step', 'grape', 'blame', etc.
2. Word-medially – 'birthday', 'temper', 'ember', etc.
3. Word-finally – 'lamps', 'damp', 'jingle', etc.

Grunwell (1987) suggests rules for producing consonant clusters based on Cruttenden (1994). For example, for two-place initial clusters: C1, C2: '(1) where C1 is /s/, C2 must be one of /ptkmnwlj(f)/ (eg sphinx); (2) where C2 is one of /wrlj/, C1 may be one of a large number of consonants predominantly obstruents, including /ptkbdgfθ/ etc.' Other rules can be found for three-place clusters. *See* Grunwell (1987).

consonantal any sound or movement in the VOCAL TRACT which involves obstruction or some degree of constriction to the airflow. A DISTINCTIVE FEATURE used to differentiate sounds into two groups. [+CONSONANTAL] sounds are produced with an obstruction in the airstream when it reaches the mouth and are produced with low acoustic energy; [−CONSONANTAL] sounds are produced with little or no obstruction and high acoustic energy. *See* Hyman (1975).

constituent analysis the analysis of the hierarchical structure of sentences. The rules that follow exemplify a (highly simplified) account of the constituent structure of English sentences using phrase structure rules:

S $\longrightarrow$ NP + VP
NP $\longrightarrow$ (det) + (adj) + N
VP $\longrightarrow$ V + (NP)
PrepP $\longrightarrow$ Prep + NP

The rules define the hierarchical structure of English sentences. The symbols and abbreviations represent the constituents:

S = sentence
NP = noun phrase
VP = verb phrase
PrepP = prepositional phrase
det = determiner
adj = adjective
N = noun
V = verb
Aux = auxiliary
$\longrightarrow$ = 'consists of'

The first rule means a 'sentence consists of a noun phrase plus a verb phrase'. The brackets in the following rules mean the constituents in the brackets are optional. These rules are often called rewrite rules as the left-hand side of the formula can be rewritten in the form on the right-hand side. There may be only one symbol on the left while any number of symbols can appear on the right. The '+' symbol is the ordering symbol, so in the first rule a verb phrase must follow a noun phrase. This type of analysis can be shown graphically by use of branches in a TREE DIAGRAM or by BRACKETING. *See* Brown and Miller (1991).

constriction narrowing in the VOCAL TRACT. It is used when making a CONSONANT sound. *See* Catford (1977).

constructional apraxia impairment in producing two- or three-dimensional designs by copying, drawing or in construction either to command or spontaneously. There is difficulty with spatial orientation and body orientation. Difficulty with dressing, exemplified by putting clothes on back to front or inside out is related to an orientation problem rather than a motor disorder. Those who have right-sided lesions will neglect dressing the left side of the body or put both legs in the same pant leg. *See* Kolb and Whishaw (1990).

constructs *see* PERSONAL CONSTRUCT THEORY.

contact ulcers growths that appear on the vocal folds producing hoarse voice. The symptoms of contact ulcers are:

1. Extreme localised and generalised tension of the folds.
2. Explosive speech patterns.
3. Sudden glottal stops.
4. Restricted pitch.
5. Habitual throat clearing.

They are produced by the hard cartilaginous surfaces of the vocal processes hitting the opposite fold. Therapy takes the form of reducing the effort in phonation, reducing the pitch level of the voice, slowing down speech RATE with a relaxed mouth and jaw and at a lower volume, as well as stopping the use of hard glottal attack. *See* Greene and Mathieson (1989); Fawcus (1991).

continuant a distinctive feature proposed by Chomsky and Halle to distinguish sounds produced from friction [+CONT] from those produced without [–CONT]. This phonological description is equivalent to the articulatory description of a fricative (*see* ARTICULATION). *See* Hyman (1975).

continuous stationery paper designed for use with a printer. It is made up of several hundred sheets of paper folded along perforations. Down each side of the paper are strips with holes so that it will fit into the tractor feed on the printer. These can be torn off when printing is completed. *See* Chandor et al (1985).

contour *see* SUPRASEGMENTAL PHON-OLOGY.

contrastive analysis a phonological analysis of a person's sound system (*see* PHONOLOGY) which involves the comparison of one sound system with another. The sound system of a young child can be compared with that of an adult so as to find out what sound(s) the child is lacking. In the same way, it can be used with children whose sound system is disordered. By comparing the children's disordered sound system to a normal sound system, it is possible to find out what sounds they have and which are lacking in their system. However, Cruttenden (1972) believes this analysis is inappropriate, if not impossible, to use because the child's acquisition of sounds is so erratic. He states: 'Child language is so unfixed, so constantly changing that it is doubtful whether the term is appropriate'. If this type of analysis is used by the clinician, the variation in the child's acquisition of sounds should be taken into account. By using this form of analysis, it is possible to find out if there is a regular error pattern since the therapist can work out in which part of the word(s) the sound substitution, omission, distortion or addition takes place. *See* Grunwell (1987).

contrecoup effect *see* HEAD INJURY.

control group one of two groups which take part in an experiment, the other group being the experimental group. The control group is regarded as the group of 'normal' subjects against which the performance of the experimental group will be compared. Control groups and experimental groups are used in INDEPENDENT GROUP DESIGN. It is also called the control condition. *See* Miller (1975); Porkess (1988).

Convaid an early high-tech device used as an alternative augmentative communication system. It has a built-in synthesiser which produces an adult male or female voice and a child's voice. There is a touch-keyboard of 64 squares. When one of these squares is pressed, the synthesiser produces the word. There is also an alarm square to call for attention.

conversion reaction the sudden impairment of muscular and sensory functions associated with psychological factors. The arms and legs can become weak, blindness can occur and those affected no longer feel pain although they are physiologically normal. People may also become dysphonic (*see* DYSPHONIA). The effects of a stress-provoking situation produce these symptoms or a nervous reaction following a long period of excitement which suddenly ends. *See* Fawcus (1991) (for conversion reaction and dysphonia); Davison and Neale (1994).

convulsion the sudden onset of seizure-like, involuntary movements, e.g. grand-mal epilepsy (*see* EPILEPSY), FEBRILE CONVULSIONS. *See* Gilroy and Holliday (1982).

coprolalia the significant increase of abusive and obscene language without any real reason.

copula a grammatical description of a verb linking two parts of a sentence, usually the subject and the complement. In a majority of cases the copulative verb in English is 'to be':

1. The men are tall.
but there can be other verbs used in the same way:
2. He felt very well
3. You look great!

See Lyons (1968); Fromkin and Rodman (1993).

cordectomy the surgical removal of a VOCAL FOLD for tumours on the fold. When one fold is removed, the one which remains will usually compensate completely. If this does not happen, a TEFLON INJECTION might be required to enable this compensation to occur.

coronal a DISTINCTIVE FEATURE proposed by Chomsky and Halle to distinguish sounds produced with the tip of the tongue [+COR] from those which are not [–COR]. This phonological description is similar to the articulatory description of alveolar, dental and palatoalveolar consonants (*see* ARTICULATION). *See* Hyman (1975).

coronoid process *see* MANDIBLE.

corpus callosum the part of the BRAIN which links the two CEREBRAL HEMISPHERES and covers the lateral ventricle (*see* THIRD VENTRICLE). Its main body is about 8 cm long and it carries information from one hemisphere to the other. *See* Barr (1979).

correlation the statistical relationship of two variables. It has the symbol 'r' to show the correlation. The range of correlation is from 0 to 1. The closer to the value of '1', the nearer is the correlation between the two variables. *See* Miller (1975); Tortora and Grabowski (1993).

cortex a layer of grey matter which covers the two CEREBRAL HEMISPHERES. It is shaped into folds. Its total weight accounts for about 40 per cent of the weight of the brain. It is full of neurons and fibres, and is 1–4 mm thick. *See* Barr (1979); Tortora and Grabowski (1993).

cortical a term for describing structures or disorders found in or near the cortex.

cortical evoked response audiometry (CERA) an audiometric test to check the late responses of the CORTEX. The results are displayed as stage III on the graph of auditory evoked responses. The electrodes have a similar placement to that for the AUDITORY BRAIN-STEM RESPONSE TEST. The person is given a series of tone bursts with slow rise and fall on each frequency. It is non-invasive, frequency specific and gives an objective measure of the person's response. Although it is a very slow test to administer, it comes very close to the hearing threshold. *See* Jacobson and Hyde (1985).

corticosteroids used for treating inflammatory diseases by reducing the inflammatory reaction and preventing the adverse effects of prolonged pressure. *See* Tortora and Grabowski (1993).

counselling a method of helping people to overcome their problems and help them to help themselves. The aim is to allow the person to come to terms with their own problems and work out what they can do rather than for the therapist to work out the solution to their problems. Often, the relationship between the person and the counsellor is particularly important rather than the type of counselling adhered to by the therapist. Carl Rogers proposed three important attributes for the counsellor:

1. Congruence, i.e. the counsellor has to demonstrate 'genuineness or authenticity'.
2. Unconditional positive regard, i.e. 'prizing, warmth, non-possessive warmth, or, most commonly, respect'.
3. Empathic understanding, i.e. 'a very special way of being with another person'. (Nelson-Jones 1982)

Communication is the all-important factor in helping people to come to terms with their problems. Other approaches have been considered but the therapist's personality is the most important factor. *See* Nelson-Jones (1982); Dalton (1994).

count nouns nouns which the language treats as separable entities, as evidenced by their use with numerals, e.g. one boy, two boys; one book, two books, etc. It is opposed to MASS NOUNS. *See* Palmer (1976).

counterbalancing a process used in the REPEATED MEASURES DESIGN in which the two groups are tested under the same conditions. If the two groups were to carry out both conditions in the same order, the results could be affected by their feelings of tiredness, etc. Thus, the subjects are split equally and each group carries out both conditions separately and then they change over. *See* Miller (1975).

CR conditioned response (*see* CLASSICAL CONDITIONING).

cranial nerves nerves that leave the BRAIN to innervate different muscles throughout the body. There are 12 nerves with the following functions:

I   Olfactory – sense of smell

II Optic – vision

III Oculomotor – supplies extraocular muscles

IV Trochlear – supplies superior oblique muscles

V   Trigeminal – comprises three parts:
   i ophthalmic
   ii maxillary (upper jaw)
   iii mandibular (lower jaw)

VI Abducens – supplies lateral rectus

VII Facial – supplies muscles of facial expression (motor component)

VIII Vestibulocochlear – supplies balance and hearing

IX Glossopharyngeal – supplies general sensation and taste; supplies sensory component and pharyngeal plexus

X   Vagus – supplies parasympathetic component of cardiac oesophageal and pulmonary plexi; sensory component supplies the superior laryngeal nerves and recurrent laryngeal nerves

XI Accessory – supplies the spinal and cervical areas of the spine

XII Hypoglossal – supplies all intrinsic and extrinsic muscles of the tongue except the palatoglossus (*see* MOUTH).

Motor nerve fibres originating in the BRAIN cross over in the brain to supply muscles on the opposite side of the body. Thus, if a CEREBROVASCULAR ACCIDENT occurs in the left CEREBRAL HEMISPHERE, there will be a HEMIPLEGIA down the right side, as the nerves from the left hemisphere will be affected. *See* Gilroy and Holliday (1982); Tortora and Grabowski (1993).

creaky voice a description of a person's voice which contains very low pitch. This occurs usually in males. The arytenoid cartilages (*see* ARYTENOIDS) hold one end of the folds tightly closed, which produces irregular vibrations at a low pitch. The sound produced may be called laryngealised. *See* Ladefoged (1993).

cretinism a congenital condition caused by an abnormality in the thyroid gland (*see* TRACHEA) and the amount of hormone it secretes. The clinical features may include: LEARNING DISABILITY, general sluggishness, anaemia, small stature, coarse skin, large tongue, low temperature, slow pulse and chronic constipation. Treatment consists of the provision of thyroid extract at an early stage which produces a good prognosis for physical development, but is probably of little value for improving the learning disability. *See* Clarke and Clarke (1974); Tortora and Grabowski (1993).

Creutzfeldt-Jakob disease see JACOB-CREUTZFELDT DISEASE.

cri-du-chat syndrome a syndrome described first by Lejeune and his colleagues in 1963. The following disorders are found:

1. Low birth weight, slow growth and high-pitched cat-like cry (produced by abnormal laryngeal development which disappears gradually as the child becomes older).
2. LEARNING DISABILITY and hypotonia.
3. MICROCEPHALY, round face, epicanthal folds, strabismus (often divergent), low set and/or poorly formed, facial asymmetry.
4. Congenital heart disease.
5. Abnormal hands with simian crease, distal axial triradius and slightly short metacarpals.

See Hosking (1982); Smith (1985).

cricoarytenoid *see* LARYNX.

cricoid cartilage *see* LARYNX.

cross-hearing a phenomenon in which sounds heard in one ear could have come from the outer ear via bone conduction or the air around the head.

This can cause confusion when testing a person's hearing.

CS (conditioned stimulus) *see* CLASSICAL CONDITIONING.

CSF *see* CEREBROSPINAL FLUID.

CT *see* CONNECTIVE TISSUE.

CT scan (computed tomography scan) *see* COMPUTED TOMOGRAPHY.

cued speech devised by Cornett in 1966 as an alternative augmentative communication system. It is not a sign language as such, but rather an oral approach supported by hand signs. The instructor can show the person the sound orally while the shape made by the hand clearly 'shows' which sound has been made. *See* Kiernan et al (1982).

cues techniques used by the therapist to help the person succeed in therapy. These cues may be:

1. Signing, i.e. giving a clue to the correct response by gesture.
2. Semantic, i.e. giving the meaning of the word.
3. Phonemic, i.e. giving the first sound of the correct response.
4. Repetition, i.e. the therapist gives the response which is repeated.
5. Visual, i.e. the therapist produces a picture of the correct response, perhaps with some distractors so that there is certainty about the correct response.

See Rosenbek et al (1989).

cuneiform cartilages found in the LARYNX. There are two cartilages. They look like small mounds and appear in the aryepiglottic fold. *See* Tortora and Grabowski (1993).

cursor the symbol (often a small flashing rectangle or horizontal or vertical line) which indicates the position on the screen where characters or graphics symbols will next appear when the program displays them. The cursor can move to any point on the screen. *See* Bishop (1985); Brookshear (1991).

Cushing's disease *See* DEPRESSION.

CV, CVC *See* PHONOTACTICS.

CVA *See* CEREBROVASCULAR ACCIDENT.

cyanosis a condition due to the presence of more than 5 g of reduced haemoglobin in the circulation. It imparts a blue colour to lips, tongue, nose and finger nails. It may be due to conditions such as chronic bronchitis, emphysema, pneumonia or heart disease. *See* Tortora and Grabowski (1993).

cytomegalovirus a highly infectious viral condition which infects nervous tissue. It is one of the diseases which can produce disorders in children, if the mother has it during the PRENATAL stage of the child's development. It can result in LEARNING DISABILITY, CEREBRAL PALSY and other handicaps. It is part of the TORCH classification of conditions which can affect the fetus during the prenatal period. *See* Hosking (1982).

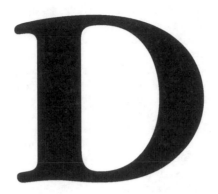

dactylology *see* FINGER SPELLING.

DAF *see* DELAYED AUDITORY FEEDBACK.

daisywheel printer a type of printer which produces printouts or hard copy by means of a wheel or thimble placed on the print unit with spokes emanating from the centre with characters at their ends which are hit by a hammer against a ribbon. The print wheel looks like a daisy, hence the name daisywheel printer. *See* Bishop (1985).

damping a reduction of the amplitude of vibrations in a vibrating object. For example, a tuning fork begins to vibrate when it is struck against an object and resonates at a particular frequency. If the tuning fork is touched when it is vibrating, the amplitude of the vibrations is reduced and dies away.

Dandy-Walker malformation also known as Dandy-Walker cyst, this is due to obstruction from birth of the foramina of Majendie and Lushka with resultant enlargement of the ventricles. This results in an abnormally large head and is associated with HYDROCEPHALUS while the brain tissue around it fails to grow adequately. *See* Hosking (1982); Kaye (1991).

data a grouping of characters, symbols and words into a text or values operated on by a computer program but not the program itself. They can be contrasted with information which is often said to come from the analysis of the data. Any collection of numeric or other information. *See* Bishop (1985); Brookshear (1991).

data transmission the process of sending data from computer to computer by electronic means. This usually involves the use of MODEMS. *See* Chandor et al (1985).

DAVE *see* DIGITALLY AIDED VOICE EMULATOR.

DDK rates *see* DIADOCHOKINESIS.

deaf a description of people who cannot use their hearing as a primary channel of communication even with amplification. *See* Nowell (1985).

death instinct *see* PSYCHOANALYSIS.

debugging the process of finding and correcting errors in a computer program which may prevent it from being run. Errors can be of two types – those which are produced because of lack of logic in the writing of the program and those which are produced by a mistake in the codes used during the program. The latter are known as syntax errors. These can be caused by failing to use the correct command word (*see* BASIC) or the failure to use the correct punctuation in a line of the program. *See* Bishop (1985).

declarative sentence a sentence which makes a statement. It contrasts with interrogative and imperative in the classification of sentence types, e.g. the man went into town. *See* Lyons (1968).

DECtalk speech synthesis used with some high-tech communication aids including TOUCH TALKERS, DELTA TALKERS, the LIBERATOR COMMUNICATION AID, CAMELEON, ORAC and DYNAVOX. It produces ten voices – four male, four female, a child's voice and one which can be either male or female. Each voice can be modified within specific parameters to allow inflection and other speech characteristics. *See* Keller (1994).

deep dyslexia *see* ACQUIRED DYSLEXIA.

deep structure *see* CASE GRAMMAR; TRANSFORMATIONAL GRAMMAR.

defence mechanisms processes, proposed by Freud among others, to allow people to protect themselves against anxiety-provoking situations. These mechanisms will thus involve some degree of self-deception. Defence mechanisms are regarded as the 'normal' way of coping with stress (*see* HYSTERIA), as long as the person does face the stressful situation. They become an abnormal response when they become the dominant way of coping with problems. The defence mechanisms often cited are:

1. Repression: painful memories and various impulses are repressed by the person.
2. Rationalisation: where logical motives are worked out by the person so that they seem to have acted rationally.
3. Reaction formation: where a person tries to hide a motive by going to the opposite extreme.
4. Projection: where people, in trying to ignore their own undesirable qualities, project them to an extreme degree onto someone else.
5. Intellectualisation: where a person deals with undesirable topics, e.g. death, in an abstract and intellectual way to become detached from the situation.

6. Denial: where the person denies that the anxiety-provoking situation exists.
7. Displacement: where if a motive cannot be gratified in one form, the person tries to overcome using another channel.

See Atkinson et al (1993).

degeneration the progressive wasting of part of the body or structures within the body caused by disease. Nerves in the peripheral nervous and CENTRAL NERVOUS SYSTEM can degenerate by Wallerian degeneration. Its opposite is regeneration. *See* Barr (1979); Kolb and Whishaw (1990).

deglutition *see* SWALLOWING.

degrees of freedom *see t*-TEST.

deixis a linguistic term for those features of sentence/clause structure which relate that sentence to specific temporal or locational features of the situation of the utterance. Deictic words include: here/there, now/then, I/you, etc. *See* Lyons (1968); Fromkin and Rodman (1993).

Déjérine's syndrome *see* ACQUIRED DYSLEXIA (3).

delayed auditory feedback (DAF) an electronic device which is often used to improve a stammerer's fluency. While it can have this effect on the dysfluent person, it has an opposite effect on the fluent person. Under normal conditions, when people speak they can hear it through their auditory feedback system as the sound travels to the ear through the bones in the skull. This chain of events is broken when using a DAF machine as there is a delay inserted between the person speaking and hearing what is said. This delay will slow down the RATE of speech so that the speaker can check what has been said before continuing. As DYSFLUENCY can be produced by a very fast rate of speech, if the person slows down, he can often speak more fluently. It can also be used with other communication disorders where the rate of speech may be very fast, such as some forms of DYSARTHRIA or DYSPHONIA.

delayed conditioning *see* CLASSICAL CONDITIONING (2).

delayed echolalia *see* ECHOLALIA.

delayed release a distinctive feature proposed by Chomsky and Halle. It distinguishes sounds produced by gradual release as in the case of the fricative part of affricates (*see* ARTICULATION) which are all described as [+delayed release]. It is also used in ARTICULATORY PHONETICS. *See* Hyman (1975).

Delta Talker a high-tech communication aid with digitised speech output and synthetic voice. It uses MINSPEAK to organise vocabulary to store into the device. It has a memory of two and a half minutes for digitised speech and 256K of memory for synthetic voice. It has similar features to the ALPHA TALKER and the LIBERATOR COMMUNICATION AID in that it uses Icon Prediction to show where messages are stored and Predictive Selection where locations without messages are dead. This allows the device to have a predictive scan facility.There are also auditory prompts for those who have visual impairment. It has a visual display unit of two lines where accessed vocabulary will appear whether stored using digitised or synthetic outputs. The overlays can be reduced to 8 and 32 locations. The device allows for direct selection either manually or by optical headpointing, single, dual or two-switch scanning as well as using multi-switch such as a joystick. *See* Appendix IV.

delusion false, unreasonable beliefs which the person holds and will not waver from under any amount of reasoned argument. Such delusions have a strong element of meaning to them. These are often called primary delusions. If people have secondary delusions, they follow a similar pattern but they try to find a reasonable explana-tion for other abnormal experiences such as HALLUCINATIONS, illusions, etc. *See* Stafford-Clark and Smith (1983); Atkinson et al (1993); Davison and Neale (1994).

dementia the progressive loss of function of brain cells producing changes in a person's character especially in old age. The damage may be caused by trauma, infections to the CENTRAL NERVOUS SYSTEM, tumours (*see* TUMOURS OF THE CENTRAL NERVOUS SYSTEM), metabolic disorders, infarctions or haemorrhages (*see* CEREBROVASCULAR ACCIDENT). The principal dementias are ALZHEIMER'S DISEASE or senile dementia, MULTI-INFARCT DEMENTIA, PICK'S DISEASE, NORMAL PRESSURE HYDROCEP-HALUS, JAKOB-CREUTZFELDT DISEASE and HUNTINGTON'S DISEASE. There is global loss of functioning affecting intelligence, learning, memory, motor skills and social skills. Its progress is slow but inexorable. The prevalence of dementia is 5 per cent of people by 65 years of age and 15–20 per cent of people by the age of 80 years. It can occur in children though rarely. *See* Gilroy and Holliday (1982); Stafford-Clark and Smith (1983); Kolb and Whishaw (1990); Davison and Neale (1994).

demonstrative pronouns deictic words which refer the person reading or hearing them to a specific object or person near to or removed from the speaker. Such pronouns include 'this/that'. *See* Lyons (1968).

dendrite a type of neuron which is short, chubby and has branches emanating at one end while at the other there is a long axon. *See* Kolb and Whishaw (1990); Tortora and Grabowski (1993).

dental *see* ARTICULATION.

dependent clause *see* CLAUSE.

depression an affective disorder. Its precise cause is unknown but it is thought it could be a combination of factors including genetic, sex, life stress, biochemical as well as cognitive problems, with one or two being more prominent than the others. It affects three areas: mood, response to stimulation and functioning of the AUTONOMIC NERVOUS SYSTEM. These problems have all been summed up succinctly by Stafford-Clark: 'Unable to sleep, to eat, to work efficiently, to hope or to enjoy any of the simple pleasures of life, he may all too often despair of his plight, to die may then seem to him to be all that is left' (Stafford-Clark and Smith, 1983, p. 107). There are three types of depression:

1. Simple/minor depression: a general slowing down in activity with people feeling sad, miserable, and worried, resulting in a loss of interest in everyday activities. It does not appear as a medical problem.
2. Endogenous/major depression: the person has a permanently depressed mood, feelings of hopelessness, helplessness, worthlessness, poor sleep and appetite regimes, due to anxiety.
3. Psychotic depression: a major characteristic is delusions plus a severely depressed mood, severe weight loss and a high risk of suicide. Psychotic depression has as a contributory factor Cushing's disease which is a disorder of the adrenal glands producing an abnormal amount of cortisol.

Depression in itself is a unipolar disorder while manic-depression is a bipolar disorder. It can be treated by tricyclic ANTI-DEPRESSANT DRUGS, MONOAMINE OXIDASE INHIBITORS, ELECTROCONVULSIVE THERAPY, PSYCHOSURGERY, LITHIUM and various forms of PSYCHOTHERAPY. *See* Stafford-Clark and Smith (1983); Kolb and Whishaw (1990); Atkinson et al (1993); Davison and Neale (1994).

depressor anguli labii inferioris *see* MUSCLES OF FACIAL EXPRESSION.

Derbyshire Language Scheme (DLS) devised by Masidlover and Knowles in 1977 (revised 1987) for use with children who have a language delay/disorder. It has non-standardised assessment procedures to test the severity of the delay and teaching procedures based on the preceding assessment. It is based on the natural communication of the child by playing with toys and looking at pictures. Language is taught and assessed through play. The criterion for success is the child using what he has learnt during the therapy sessions at home and in the community. The assessment is divided into two parts: the Rapid Screening test and the Detailed Test of Comprehension. The results of these assessments can be placed onto an assessment summary. There is a progress record to show graphically the child's performance, and to reveal areas of language development which still require therapy. *See* Masidlover and Knowles (1987) in Appendix I; Beech et al (1993).

descriptive grammar the basic linguistic knowledge of a language. It does not prescribe how one should speak but how it is possible to speak and understand as well as about the sounds, words, phrases, sentences of a particular language. *See* Fromkin and Rodman (1993).

descriptive statistics a part of statistics which analyses the scores obtained from experiments using bar charts, HISTOGRAMS, measures of CENTRAL TENDENCY, STANDARD DEVIATION, PERCENTILES SCORES and Z SCORES. *See* Miller (1975); Porkess (1988).

Detailed Test of Comprehension (DTC) an assessment procedure used in the DERBYSHIRE LANGUAGE SCHEME. It is used after the RAPID SCREENING TEST has been administered so that the therapist can assess more accurately the problems which the child has in comprehension and expressive language. These two aspects of communication are tested in natural contexts using everyday toys and pictures. The authors introduce the concept of information-carrying words, i.e. how many words the child requires to understand a command. In the example below, the sentences are from different levels of the DTC. In other words, the child has to show his comprehension at different levels by ignoring similar distractors. When testing the child's expressive language, the therapist writes down everything the child says during the test even if it is unconnected with the toys or pictures used in the test – see boxed example below. *See* Masidlover and Knowles (1987) in Appendix I.

determiner a constituent which precedes a noun to show differences in meaning between nouns, e.g. quantity and number. Usually a determiner is one of the articles, either definite or indefinite, but it can also be a personal, possessive or demonstrative pronoun or a word signifying quantity. The determiner marks a NOUN PHRASE and usually appears at the beginning of a noun phrase. *See* Strang (1968).

developmental aphasia *see* APHASIA.

developmental disorder any disorder which occurs after birth and progresses during childhood. *See* Davison and Neale (1994).

developmental dyslexia a reading and writing disorder which occurs in children who have average or above average intelligence. In general, the child has difficulty in learning to spell. The term dyslexia is used to describe only a child whose reading and spelling are unexpectedly poor. The BANGOR DYSLEXIA TEST is a screening test to find out the severity of the disorder. *See* Hornsby (1984); Ellis (1993).

developmental psychology the study of human development and behaviour from birth through childhood, adolescence and into adulthood and old age, perhaps concentrating on a particular part of the developmental process e.g. language development. *See* Atkinson et al (1993).

developmental verbal apraxia a disorder found in children with symptoms similar to those found in ACQUIRED APRAXIA. Thus, there is an inability to make articulatory speech sounds voluntarily; there is struggling to get the target sound; producing single words may not be a problem but there is a failure to produce them in a pattern. *See* Miller (1986); Byers Brown and Edwards (1989); Beukelman and Mirenda (1992) (AAC and developmental apraxia of speech); Stackhouse (1992); Stackhouse and Snowling (1992).

developmental verbal dyspraxia a term used to describe articulatory dyspraxia in childhood more precisely. It looks at this problem in a holistic way and the child as a complete person. It is seen as a syndrome which has some of the following symptoms:

1. Soft neurological signs (e.g. clumsiness).
2. Delayed lateralisation of cerebral function.
3. Predominance in males.
4. Some feeding problems.
5. Oral apraxia – poor lip posture, tongue control, slow DDK rates, and problems with oral sensorimotor feedback.
6. Speech – delayed speech development, resistant to therapy and unintelligible.

INSTRUCTION	No. of item	Comp. Level
Wash the teddy	TEDDY	0
WASH the TEDDY	CLOTH, BRUSH, TEDDY, DOLL	2
WASH the TEDDY'S FOOT	SAME AS ABOVE	3
WASH the LITTLE TEDDY'S FOOT	LITTLE TEDDY, BIG TEDDY	4
	LITTLE DOLL, CLOTH, BRUSH	

7. Articulation – inconsistent vs rigid pattern, phonetic experimentation, non-English articulation, errors in polysyllabic words, breakdown in continuous speech, perseveration, intrusive schwa, sound omissions, voice, place and manner errors (*see* ARTICULATION), vowel distortion and some dysarthric features.
8. PROSODY – inappropriate stress and intonation, variable speech, use of monotone.
9. Resonance – fluctuating nasality.
10. Incoordination of the VOCAL TRACT – DYS-PHONIA, dysprosody, disorder of resonance.
11. Language – history of delayed language development, verbal comprehension often ahead of expressive language skills, phonological disability, restricted use of syntax and disordered language development.
12. Learning difficulty – often significant discrepancy between verbal and performance tasks, problems with reading, spelling, writing and drawing, poor auditory memory, sequencing difficulties, cross-modality difficulties and selective attention problems.

See Gordon and McKinley (1980).

deviant language language which does not fit into a normal developmental sequence. Abnormalities may relate to phonation, SUPRASEGMENTAL PHONOLOGY and/or segmental features (*see* PHONOLOGY), SYNTAX or SEMANTICS or a combination of all these.

deviation *see* CONDUCT DISORDER; STANDARD DEVIATION.

devoiced sounds which are devoiced are those which are usually voiced but because of their environment lose some of their voicing. This often occurs with the voiced plosives /b,d,g/ (*see* ARTICULATION) when used WORD-FINALLY, e.g. big, bad, etc. In narrow transcription (*see* TRANSCRIPTION SYSTEMS (2)), this process is represented by the DIACRITIC placed under the affected sound. *See* Cruttenden (1994).

diachronic linguistics one of the types of descriptive linguistics proposed by de SAUSSURE in 1913. It studies the historical changes in language over time. Thus, a linguist studying language using this procedure would look at the progression of English from Old English to Middle English to Modern English. This is also known as historical linguistics. It is opposed to synchronic linguistics (*see* SAUSSURE). *See* Lyons (1968); Culler (1986).

diacritic in narrow transcription (*see* TRANSCRIPTION SYSTEMS (2)), markings have to be placed above or below the sound to show any particular features which are used in its production. For example, [ʰ] is the diacritic placed above and in the gap between the sounds to show aspiration, e.g. [pʰɨn]. These diacritics also show intonation contours and mark stress in a word or sentence in SUPRASEGMENTAL PHONOLOGY. In transcribing the speech of either children with phonological delay/disorder or those with DYSARTHRIA, the speech therapist will have to know the diacritics used to mark the characteristics of such speech. *See* Abercrombie (1967); Fromkin and Rodman (1993); Ladefoged (1993).

diadochokinesis (DDK) the average rates used by people to move their articulators in producing certain sequences of sounds and facial movements. The sequences are produced in all positions in the mouth, e.g. /p,p,p,/, /t,t,t/, /k,k,k/, /p,t,k,p,t,k/, /oo..ee..oo..ee/, etc. This test can be used with both adults and children. Its opposite is ADIADOCHOKINESIS. *See* Canning and Rose (1974) (children); Robertson and Thomson (1986) (adults).

diagnosis the identification of the person's presenting condition by the therapist after thorough examination, investigation and assessment. It is important to make sure that the decision is correct and no other diagnosis is likely. If it is uncertain which communication disorder the person has, a differential diagnosis takes place. It may be that an adult would be referred for assessment but there is no comment made about the existence of a communication disorder. Assuming the the person has had a stroke (*see* CEREBROVASCULAR ACCIDENT), for example, he could have, among others, either APHASIA, DYSARTHRIA or dyspraxia (*see* ACQUIRED DYSPRAXIA). To make sure the correct treatment is given each of these conditions would have to be assessed and the results analysed. Similarly when a young child is referred, he may well have an articulation or phonological delay or language delay. The therapist would have to test for each possible condition and, after analysing the results, decide what the person's problem is. In situations where someone may have the characteristics of two disorders, the therapist has to decide which is the more major problem for treating. As one is treated, the other may begin to show improvement. *See* Byers Brown (1981).

diagnosogenic theory of stuttering a theory proposed by Wendell Johnson that stuttering behaviour is the result of the attitude of the listener to the normal dysfluencies of the child.

diagnostic audiometry the testing of a person's hearing to find out the severity and type of HEARING LOSS, e.g. CONDUCTIVE HEARING LOSS, SENSORINEURAL HEARING LOSS, etc. *See* Katz (1985).

Diagnostic Statistical Manual (DSM) the classification of mental disorders used in the USA. The latest edition is DSM-IV. In its expanded form this stands for '*Diagnostic and Statistical Manual of Mental Disorders*, 4th edition. It is published by the American Psychiatric Association and is the official diagnostic system used extensively by mental health professionals. The first diagnostic system was published in 1952 (DSM-I) with successive versions in 1968 (DSM-II), 1980 (DSM-III), 1987 (DSM-IIIR); 1991 the DSM-IV

options book and a draft version of the complete DSM-IV in 1993. The main change in DSM-IV is the introduction of a multi-axial classification system with five axes concerning clinical syndromes, personality disorders, general medical conditions, psychosocial and environmental problems and axis 5 which is a global assessment of functioning scale (GAF Scale) where consideration has to be given to psychological, social and occupational functioning on a hypothetical continuum of mental health/illness. There are places on the scale of 0/1 (inadequate information), 10 (persistent danger of severely hurting self or others (e.g. recurrent violence) OR (persistent inability to maintain minimal personal hygiene OR serious suicidal act with clear expectation of death) up to 100 (superior functioning in a wide range of activities, life's problems never seem to get out of hand, is sought out by others because of the many positive qualities. No symptoms.). *See* Davison and Neale (1994).

dialect language variations in grammar and vocabulary used in particular areas of a country or by particular social groups within an area. It may include regular usage but it will also contain elements which are peculiar to that region of the country. For example, in Aberdeenshire (Scotland), all whwords begin with /f/. Thus, 'what' becomes /fɪt/. Common everyday phrases change, e.g. 'how are you' becomes 'fit like'. Other dialectal variations include 'loon' for 'boy' and 'quine' for 'girl'. *See* Trudgill (1974); Fromkin and Rodman (1993).

diaphragm *see* ABDOMINAL-DIAPHRAGMATIC RESPIRATION.

diastematomyelia a rare condition in which a bony projection produces a cleft of the spinal cord. There is a weakness in the muscles of the legs and deformity of the feet. Sensory impairment may also exist. Surgery can provide relief from some of the symptoms in some cases. *See* Gilroy and Holliday (1982); Kaye (1991).

diazepam a drug with sedative and hypnotic properties.

dichotic listening stimulation of both ears with different stimuli. Dichotic listening was studied extensively by Doreen Kimura in the early 1960s while working at the Montreal Neurological Institute. She presented spoken digits simultaneously, one of which was heard in each ear through headphones connected to a stereo tape recorder. Each person was given three pairs of digits and asked to recall as many of the six digits as possible in any order. Kimura was interested in the auditory processing of those with temporal lobe lesions. She found that all subjects, regardless of the site of lesion, recalled more of the digits which had been presented to the right ear than those presented to the left ear. The same was found in normal control subjects. Thus, Kimura concluded that, when different stimuli are presented simultaneously to each ear, the pathway from the right ear to the speaking hemisphere has preferred access, and the ipsilateral pathway from the left ear is relatively suppressed. *See* Kolb and Whishaw (1990); Fromkin and Rodman (1993).

diencephalon a structure in the brain also known as the forebrain, which appears immediately above the MIDBRAIN. It has two segments which become the CEREBRAL HEMISPHERES. As they grow forwards, they form the frontal lobes (*see* CEREBRAL HEMISPHERES), growing backwards to form the occipital lobes (*see* CEREBRAL HEMISPHERES) and to the sides to form the temporal lobes (*see* CEREBRAL HEMISPHERES). The structures of the THALAMUS, HYPOTHALAMUS and THIRD VENTRICLE are also found in this area. *See* Barr (1979); Kolb and Whishaw (1990); Tortora and Grabowski (1993).

difference limen for intensity (DLI) the smallest change in the intensity of a pure tone which can just be heard.

Those who have normal hearing usually have difficulty in deciding on small changes in intensity when the intensity level is near threshold. As intensity increases, the DLI decreases. *See* Katz (1985).

differential diagnosis *see* DIAGNOSIS.

diffuse a distinctive feature proposed by Jakobson and Halle for marking close vowels [+DIFFUSE] (*see* CARDINAL VOWEL SYSTEM). It is opposed to COMPACT. Chomsky and Halle changed it to HIGH. *See* Hyman (1975).

digastric muscles *see* MUSCLES FOR SWALLOWING.

digital subtraction angiography a modern technique in which a radio-opaque contrast medium can be injected into an arm vein. By computer enhancement the background can be subtracted leaving good quality pictures of the arteries alone. This avoids having to inject into arteries directly – a technique which can be dangerous to the person. *See* Kaye (1991); Tortora and Grabowski (1993).

Digitally Aided Voice Emulator (DAVE) a high-tech, portable communication aid. Users can have 16 two-second messages stored so that they can recall them by use of a single switch. There is a tabletop version with a scanning display unit built into the main case while another model can be mounted onto a wheelchair. DAVE has a microphone which is used to program in the sixteen messages. A switch is used to allow the unit to record the message. The same switch, when put in the correct position, allows the messages to be played back. *See* Appendix IV.

digitised speech an electronic form of speech used by high-tech AAC systems. It differs from SYNTHETIC SPEECH in that it is a human voice which is stored onto a computer chip inside the device. However, it does take a lot of memory in the device although it does replicate closely the human voice which is used for the storing. Devices which use solely digitised speech include the ALPHA TALKER, INTRO TALKER, WALKER TALKER and MACAW. Other devices such as the DELTA TALKER and the ORAC have a combination of digitised speech and SYNTHETIC SPEECH. *See* Beukelman and Mirenda (1992).

diglossia a label proposed for the linguistic situation in some countries, e.g. Greece. It refers to a situation in which two varieties of a language co-occur. However, both varieties have different uses. Usually one is used for formal occasions while the other is used colloquially. *See* Trudgill (1974).

digraph the actual visual shape of a vowel sound [œ]. *See* Cruttenden (1994).

diphthong a type of vowel in which the tongue and/or lips move during the duration of the vowel segments within the same syllable. In received pronunciation (RP) there are many diphthongs, e.g. /meɪk/, /tʃeə/, whereas in Scottish-English such diphthongs are produced as pure vowels. However, they do have diphthongs in common with RP such as /naɪn/, /haʊs/, /naɪf/ etc. The production of diphthongs can be explained using the CARDINAL VOWEL SYSTEM. The phonetician can start at one sound, e.g. [a] and show the glide to another, e.g. [ɪ] to produce [aɪ]. *See* Catford (1989).

direct object in CONSTITUENT ANALYSIS, a term applied to the syntactic relation that obtains between the main verb and, usually, the noun phrase that follows it within the VP and that is dominated by a VP node. In (1), the 'cup' is the direct object of 'broke':

1. The child broke the cup.

See Lyons (1968); Fromkin and Rodman (1993).

Director an environmental control system which can be operated by communication aids. It can be operated by the ALPHA TALKER, DELTA TALKER, TOUCH TALKER, LIGHT TALKER and LIBERATOR COMMUNICATION AID. The Director learns any infra-red signal from an infra-red hand control. In this way, the communication aid user can have total control of their environment from accessing a few symbol sequences. For example, it can learn all the functions to operate a television, i.e. switch on/off, turn volume up/down, change channel, use teletext etc. In conjunction with the X-10 system, it is possible to turn on and off lamps, radiators or any devices which work off mains electricity. The Director can also operate curtains opening and closing, door opening and closing etc. *See* Appendix IV.

discontinuous a distinctive feature proposed by Jakobson and Halle to distinguish sounds which are made with a complete closure in the vocal tract [+DIS-CONTINUOUS] i.e. plosives (*see* ARTICULATION) from those which are not [−DISCONTINUOUS], i.e. fricatives (*see* ARTICULATION) or vowels (*see* CARDINAL VOWEL SYSTEM). *See* Hyman (1975).

discourse analysis the analysis of linguistic units larger than a sentence. A discourse is a continuous utterance in which more than one sentence is represented, e.g. a story told by a child or adult. The data are analysed in an attempt to identify linguistic regularities about the sentence. *See* Fromkin and Rodman (1993).

disintegrative psychoses *see* CHILDHOOD PSYCHOSES.

disk disks are used for saving computer programs (*see also* BASIC) for future use, as well as text, databases and spreadsheets. When disks are bought, they are usually unformatted. While unformatted, the disks can be used in most machines as long as the disk is the correct size to fit the disk drive. There are three sizes of floppy disk: 5.25 inches, 3 inches and 3.5 inches. While the disks remain unformatted the operator will be unable to save any information on them. Therefore, the disks will have to be formatted. The procedure for formatting will be explained in the computer's manual. Computer disks are similar to music disks which have to have tracks put on them to accept the music. The formatting process does this for computer disks. This process divides the disk into sectors and produces tracks on them. *See* Bishop (1985); Brookshear (1991).

disk drive the unit which is attached to a computer so that information can be saved onto a computer DISK and loaded back into the computer's memory when required. Disks are placed in a disk drive which rotates the disk at a particular speed and can read from or write the information to the disk. Some disk drives have switches at the back which will have to be changed to the correct number of tracks or an error message will appear on the monitor screen and the switch position changed to the correct number of tracks. The commands used to operate the disk drive are SAVE, LOAD, RUN and DELETE (*see* BASIC). There is usually a single disk drive used but it is possible to have a double disk drive which makes copying from one disk to another much easier. Computers such as the BBC Master Compact, the Archimedes and Amstrad PCs and PCWs have integral disk drives (i.e. they are already fitted at the side of the monitor or the control box on which the monitor stands). As well as these external disk drives, more and more computers are being supplied with internal disk drives known as hard disk drives. These are small disks placed one above the other onto which a large amount of computer information can be stored. *See* Bishop (1985); Brookshear (1991).

dissimilation a process in which a neighbouring sound influences another sound but, unlike assimilation, the influence changes the sound. This occurs in DIACHRONIC LINGUISTICS to show phonetic changes in language. *See* Brosnahan and Malmberg (1976); Fromkin and Rodman (1993).

dissociative disorders those who have these types of disorders find it difficult to recall important personal events or may temporarily forget their identity or even assume a new identity. They are also liable to wander far away from their customary environment. There are four main dissociative disorders: dissociative amnesia where the the person is suddenly unable to recall important personal information especially after a traumatic event – this forgetfulness is quite different from normal forgetfulness; dissociative fugue where the person not only forgets totally what is happening but suddenly moves from home and work and takes on a different identity; multiple personality disorder where a person can have at least two separate ego states, which can act in different ways or have different feelings either independently of each other, or together at different times; depersonalisation disorder where the way the person perceives the self is disconcertingly and disruptively altered. *See* Davison and Neale (1994).

distinctive feature phonological descriptions of the way in which sounds are produced. The terms placed in square brackets are in binary notation which shows two polar ends, e.g. [+CONTINUANT], [−CONTINUANT]. Jakobson and Halle (1956) and Chomsky and Halle (1968) proposed many such features. Jakobson and Halle's distinctive features were acoustic in formation:

acute	grave.
compact	plain.
diffuse	sharp.
flat	checked.
lax	unchecked.
mellow	tense.
discontinuous	strident.

Chomsky and Halle's distinctive features follow articulatory positions for producing sounds:

coronal	high.
continuant	low.
anterior	back.
strident	nasal.
voice	lateral.

sonorant   round.
delayed release   distributed.

See Hyman (1975); Fromkin and Rodman (1993).

distocclusion a type of malocclusion found in a person's teeth.

distraction tests tests used with very young children (6–18 months of age) who are unable to cope with PURE-TONE AUDIOMETRY. Children sit on their mother's knee. A person sits in front of the child and produces toys to distract him while the audiologist stands behind him and produces tones by a warble device, rattle, etc. The tester has to observe the child's reaction to the tones. This reaction usually involves the child turning his head to the side on which the tone is presented. The only problem is that the child could respond to other stimuli in his immediate environment. *See* Hodgson (1985).

distributed a distinctive feature proposed by Chomsky and Halle to distinguish sounds produced with a stricture such as bilabial and palatoalveolar fricatives (*see* ARTICULATION) [+DISTRIBUTED] from those which are not made at this place of articulation [−DISTRIBUTED]. *See* Hyman (1975).

disyllable two syllables which make up a phonetic unit. It is contrasted to monosyllable. *See* Catford (1977).

divergent thinking a thinking process which allows the person to move off in different directions encompassing several aspects of a particular subject. This can often lead to novel or original ways of thinking. *See* Taylor et al (1982); Kolb and Whishaw (1990).

dizygotic twins who are not identical since they come from different egg cells and are not genetically similar, whereas identical twins come from a single egg cell and have the same heredity. The latter are also known as monozygotic twins. *See* Atkinson et al (1993); Tortora and Grabowski (1993); Davison and Neale (1994).

DLS *see* DERBYSHIRE LANGUAGE SCHEME.

dominance the two CEREBRAL HEMISPHERES are important because they contain particular centres to allow humans to communicate, become artistic or read and write and so on. However, one of these hemispheres is more dominant than the other – this is the hemisphere which contains the language centres. In 98 per cent of right-handed people, language skills are in the left hemisphere, and in 60 per cent of left-handed people language skills are controlled by the left hemisphere. So, four out of five people with damage to the left hemisphere are likely to have their language affected. Sperry (Nobel Prize Winner, 1981) carried out experiments where the two hemispheres were split so that he could find out accurately the specialisation of each hemisphere. In one of his experiments, he flashed the word 'nut' onto the left side of a screen for one-tenth of a second. The subject's gaze was fixed on the centre of the screen. The visual image goes to the right side of the brain which controls the left side of the body. He was able to pick up the nut with his left hand but he could not say what the word was because the left hemisphere did not receive any information. The subject could not report what his left hand had picked up because of the same lack of information to the left hemisphere and his hands were hidden from him by the screen. By carrying out similar experiments, Sperry was able to highlight the specialisation of the two hemispheres of the brain. *See* Atkinson et al (1993).

dorsum the back of the tongue which produces sounds such as velars and palatals (*see* ARTICULATION) by coming close to the hard and soft palates (*see* MOUTH). *See* Catford (1977).

dot matrix printers printers which forms letters or graphics with a system of dots on the paper made up by a matrix of wires or styluses. Thermal paper as well as ordinary paper can be used with these printers with an ink ribbon. *See* Bishop (1985).

double blind procedure a procedure used when carrying out experiments. Neither the subject of the experiment nor the person administering the test procedures knows what the experiment is about or when the experimental condition is taking place. This procedure is often used in research into the effectiveness of drugs when a placebo or a drug is given. In such cases, neither the subject nor the person conducting the test procedures knows if the subject is being given the placebo or the drug. *See* Atkinson et al (1993); Davison and Neale (1994).

Down's syndrome in the mid-1860s, Dr. Langdon Down identified the characteristics of this syndrome to which he gave his name. It is produced by trisomy 21, i.e. an extra part of a chromosome is present on the long arm of chromosome 21. Thus, a person who has Down's syndrome has 47 chromosomes instead of 46. People who have this condition comprise 22 per cent of the whole population of those with learning disabilities in Great Britain. There is an equal distribution throughout the world. One in 666 live births results in Down's syndrome. The physical features that characterise Down's syndrome are:

1. Epicanthic folds, i.e. slanting eyes.
2. HYPOTONIA, i.e. floppy limbs.
3. Square-shaped face.
4. Small nose and ears.
5. Tongue that protrudes more than in those who do not have Down's syndrome.
6. Teeth appear late.
7. Little fingers curve inwards.
8. A wide gap between big and second toes.

Neurological problems such as epilepsy are very rare, milestones are almost always delayed, intelligence is low, there are heart malformations and the individuals are prone to upper respiratory tract infection. The same developmental sequences in babbling are similar between those who do not have Down's syndrome and those who do. As far as phonological development is concerned, the rate of acquisition is slower in Down's syndrome although the sound system follows a similar sequence of development. It has been found that development of one-word utterances is delayed by about one year in Down's syndrome. Such children usually produce first words around 2 years of age at which age the proportion of meaningful utterances in the Down's syndrome child is less than 5 per cent; this increases slightly at around 4 years of age. When Down's syndrome children reach the two- to three-word utterances, they express similar semantic relationships to those of other children. This stage is reached at about 4–5 years of age. When producing more complex utterances, the Down's syndrome child's syntax is deficient although it does seem to increase using MEAN LENGTH OF UTTERANCE as the child grows older. When considering PRAGMATICS, the main type of illocutionary sentences used are declaratives, imperatives and questions. *See* Cunningham (1982); Bishop and Mogford (1993); Davison and Neale (1994).

drive often described as an internal motivational force. *See* Atkinson et al (1993).

DTC *see* DETAILED TEST OF COMPREHENSION.

duration the length of time, in milliseconds, used to produce sounds. *See* Catford (1977).

dynamic display a general term for communication aids that use displays which change following each hit. The symbols are electronically generated on the touch screen. For example, if the user hits the symbol for 'clothes', the screen will change to a page of symbols for 'clothes'. There are various devices which use this system, such as the CAMELEON and the DYNAVOX.

A second type of dynamic display is where the symbols remain static but the indicators for choosing the symbols change. For example, if the user chooses the 'drinks' symbol, the only symbols which will light up are those associated with the 'drinks' category. This system operates on the ALPHA TALKER, DELTA TALKER and the LIBERATOR COMMUNICATION AID. See Beukelman and Mirenda (1992).

dynamic memory see RANDOM ACCESS MEMORY.

DynaVox a high-tech communication aid with synthetic speech (DECtalk) using a dynamic display. Graphic symbols designed exclusively for the device, DynaSyms, are used. These symbols change each time the client touches one. The symbol appears on the top area of the touch screen. When the complete phrase or sentence is accessed, the top line is pressed and the device speaks out the whole message. DynaWrite is a software package which allows the user to spell in longer messages using word prediction. It follows grammatical rules, personal preference and a built-in 40 000 word dictionary. A combined software package using DynaSyms and DynaWrite is also available. DynaCard is a credit card-sized memory card providing up to 4 million characters of memory. DynaVox 2 has a coloured display as well as a monochrome version, 8 MB and 20 MB memory cards, built-in infra-red environmental control unit with word prediction and word processing, and is lighter in weight. See Appendix IV.

dysarthrias a group of disorders which stem from defined neurological conditions and which manifest abnormalities of RESPIRATION, PHONATION, RESONANCE and ARTICULATION. There are four main types although clear differentiation is not always possible:

1. Dyskinetic dysarthria:
   (a) Hyperkinetic type: this occurs in myoclonic and choreiform disorders. PROSOSDY is severely affected particularly in relation to rate and rhythm. There is deletion of sounds and word segments due to incoordination of the articulators. Reduced velar movement gives rise to hypernasal resonance.
   (b) Hypokinetic type: this occurs most frequently in PARKINSON'S DISEASE. Articulation is poor but this is due more to the difficulty in controlling rate and range of movement in ongoing speech than to specific articulatory weakness. On a word-to-word basis, speech may be clear but there is rapid deterioration in connected speech.

2. Spastic dysarthria: originates in the upper motor neurons. All parameters of speech are affected; respiration is poor, spasticity of the vocal folds results in hoarseness, intonation patterns are restricted and stress is equal and excessive. The congenital form is associated with CEREBRAL PALSY when it is also known as congenital suprabulbar paresis.

3. Peripheral dysarthria: also known as flaccid dysarthria and lower motor neuron dysarthria. The principal speech characteristics are: hypernasality; nasal emission of air; continuous breathiness during phonation and audible inspiration. The consonants are also distorted and the person speaks in short phrases because of breathing problems.

4. Mixed dysarthria: occurs in those who have an impairment in more than one motor system. Possible causes of this condition are tumours, trauma and degenerative conditions such as MOTOR NEURON DISEASE and MULTIPLE SCLEROSIS etc.

The speech disorders of those who have these forms of dysarthria will be characteristic of the motor speech disturbances characterised in the individual motor system disturbances outlined in (1)–(3) above. *See* Darley et al (1975); Murdoch and Hudson-Tennent (1994) (acquired dysarthria in childhood).

dysequilibrium syndrome a neurological condition resulting from renal dialysis. It is thought to occur when dialysis rapidly alters the blood comportment and there is production of a gradient of electrolytes from brain to blood. This results in fluid shift into the brain. It happens towards the end of the dialysis process and is characterised by signs and symptoms of increased intracranial pressure followed by spontaneous recovery. *See* Gilroy and Holliday (1982).

dysfluency the general term used to describe stammering/stuttering behaviour as well as cluttering. It can describe either the speech of someone who stammers or has other types of disorder, e.g. Parkinsonian speech. It can also describe other forms of speech which include a lot of repetitions, hesitations and so on. It is also called non-fluency. When a speaker hesitates during a conversation for effect or while thinking of something else to say, this is described as normal dysfluency or normal non-fluency. *See* Dalton (1983, 1994).

dysgraphia as an ACQUIRED DISORDER caused by a trauma to the brain such as stroke or head injury, it affects writing and is associated with APHASIA. Such disorders in writing may mirror other disorders caused by aphasia, e.g. anomia, agrammatism. However, the condition may involve only minor spelling mistakes or difficulty in copying and writing to dictation. Writing disorders are not always associated with aphasia. As a developmental disorder, it is usually associated with DYSLEXIA. *See* Eisenson (1984); Hornsby (1984); Ellis (1993).

dyskinetic cerebral palsy *see* CEREBRAL PALSY.

dyslalia a historical term for articulation disorder which is no longer in use.

dyslexia a widely used description for someone who has difficulty with reading, writing and spelling. For a child, it is the unexpected failure to learn to read and write as he reaches the appropriate age (*see* DEVELOPMENTAL DYSLEXIA) while for an adult, it refers, usually, to the difficulty found in reading after a stroke or head injury or other trauma to the brain (*see* ACQUIRED DYSLEXIA). *See* Eisenson (1984); Hornsby (1984); Kolb and Whishaw (1990); Ellis (1993).

dysmetria the loss of the ability to work out the distance between the person and the object. It is caused by damage to the CEREBELLUM. *See* Gilroy and Holliday (1982).

dysphagia a disorder in swallowing caused by a trauma to the brain such as a stroke or head injury or brain tumour, etc. It can also be caused by degenerative diseases or lesions to the upper motor or lower motor neurons. These causes produce difficulty in swallowing liquid. Dysphagia can also be caused by organic and anatomical disorders such as structural abnormalities, e.g. cleft palate, disease, radiography, surgery (e.g. partial/total glossectomy), neck or facial trauma and burns. When these occur the client can have difficulty swallowing solids. Therapy depends on what the client cannot swallow and which part of the swallowing system does not function. *See* Silverman and Elfant (1979).

dysphasia *see* APHASIA.

dysphonia disorders of respiration, pitch intensity and/or resonance which impair communication. Aetiology may be organic, behavioural or psychogenic. Organic-based disorders include structural anomalies, neurological and endocrinological disease. Behaviourally based disorders include excessive muscular tension misuse and abuse. Psychogenic disorders include conversion dysphonia, delayed pubertal voice and trans-sexual conflict. *See* Greene and Mathieson (1989); Fawcus (1991); Dalton (1994).

dyspraxia *see* APRAXIA; ACQUIRED APRAXIA; DEVELOPMENTAL VERBAL APRAXIA; DEVELOPMENTAL VERBAL DYSPRAXIA.

dysprosody inappropriate production of suprasegmental features of speech, i.e. intonation, pause, stress and rate.

dystonia the abnormal movement or posture caused by a disorder affecting the agonist and antagonist muscles. Dystonia musculorum deformans is a movement disorder in the axial and limb muscles. It can be inherited as an autosomal dominant or recessive trait (*see* CHROMOSOMES). The condition progresses from a mild movement disorder to involvement of the lower limbs and in its final form to inability to walk. There is no specific drug therapy. However, there is often spontaneous remission. Acute dystonic reaction is caused by the sudden onset of dystonic movements in the facial muscles and a movement disorder in the eyes. Meige's disease affects movements of face, mouth and jaw. This is also known as Breugel's disease. *See* Gilroy and Holliday (1982); Kaye (1991).

dystrophy usually describes the weakness and degeneration of muscle fibres caused by genetically controlled myopathies. There are several dystrophies all of which have different characteristics:

1. Duchenne muscular dystrophy: a sex-linked recessive disease (*see* CHROMOSOMES) which is progressive. It occurs predominately in males in the ratio 20:100 000. Children are normal at birth and reach their early milestones at a normal rate although there may be some delay in standing and walking. The child develops a clumsy, waddling gait and has difficulty in climbing stairs. GOWER'S SIGN appears at this stage. By about 10 years of age, the child may be confined to a wheelchair. Prognosis is not good, death can occur in the person's teens or early twenties.

2. Facioscapulohumeral dystrophy: an autosomal dominant disease (*see* CHROMOSOMES). It begins between 10 and 20 years of age. The person has minimal disability.

3. Scapuloperoneal dystrophy: an autosomal dominant or sex-linked recessive disease (*see* CHROMOSOMES). It occurs in early childhood. No treatment is required as there is a full life expectancy.

4. Limb girdle dystrophy: an autosomal recessive disease (*see* CHROMOSOMES). It occurs between 10 and 20 years of age. The person may be confined to a wheelchair after 40 years of age.

5. Distal dystrophy: an autosomal dominant disease (*see* CHROMOSOMES). It occurs in adults. There is full life expectancy.

6. Oculopharyngeal dystrophy: an autosomal dominant disease (*see* CHROMOSOMES). It occurs in the middle years and it is slowly progressive.

See Gilroy and Holliday (1982); Kaye (1991).

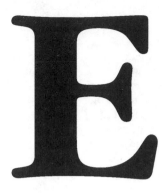

E-tran frame *see* EYE TRANSFER COMMUNICATION SYSTEMS.

ear the ear comprises three parts:

1. Outer ear: it comprises three parts:
   (a) Auricle or pinna: whilst the most visible part of the ear, it is the least important for hearing in humans. It is formed by elastic CONNECTIVE TISSUE which is covered by skin. It gathers sound waves from the environment and is most efficient at gathering high-frequency sounds.
   (b) The external auditory canal extends inwards from the auricle to the tympanic membrane. In adults, it goes inwards and at a slightly upward angle while in children it goes downwards at an acute angle. This canal is lined with skin while the outer third has glands that secrete wax which protects its lining and prevents foreign bodies from entering the ear. The inner two-thirds is encased in bone and is also lined with skin. Its function is to act as a resonator for frequencies between 2000 and 5500 Hz and helps to transport sound to the tympanic membrane.
   (c) Tympanic membrane: the external auditory canal ends in a concave disc made up of three layers.

The first layer comprises skin continuous with the auditory canal; the second layer is rough fibrous connective tissue and contributes most to the vibrating of the tympanic membrane when sounds hit it; the third layer consists of mucous membrane continuous with the inner ear. The normal tympanic membrane is a pearly grey, semi-transparent ring of tissue held together by the annulus. Its function is primarily a mobile link in the auditory chain. The surface of the tympanic membrane is greater than the round window.

2. Middle ear: this part of the ear transmits sound waves from the medium of the air from the outer ear to the fluid of the inner ear. It comprises six walls. The inner wall contains the basal turn. It opens into the eustachian tube (anterior side). It is connected to the nasopharynx (*see* PHARYNX). It is covered by a mucous membrane whilst the eustachian tube is lined with hair follicles. The tube is usually closed in adults and opens only when the person sneezes or swallows etc. In children, it is shorter and more horizontal and open. As it is open, infection can get into it quite easily. There are two windows: the oval window is above the promontory while

the round window is below the promontory. The stapes rests in the oval window while there is a tough elastic membrane in the round window. The canals in the inner ear all extend from the oval window. The three ossicles in the middle ear are the malleus (hammer), the incus (anvil) and the stapes (stirrup). These are the smallest bones in the body and are formed at birth. The action of the ossicles provides amplification for the middle ear. They bring the vibrations from a large area (the tympanic membrane) and focus them on a small area (the oval window). The size of the tympanic membrane is 17 times that of the oval window. There are two main muscles in the middle ear:

(a) The stapedius muscle attaches to the neck of the stapes. When it contracts it pulls it out of the oval window and to the side, tenses the oval window and causes less vibration. The nerve supply comes from the facial nerve (cranial nerve VII).

(b) Tensor tympani: It is attached to the malleus. When it contracts it tenses the tympanic membrane causing less sound to be transmitted. It is supplied by the trigeminal nerve (see CRANIAL NERVE V). Both muscles work reflexively and bilaterally even if the sound only goes in one ear.

3. Inner ear: a bony structure which forms a snail-like shell and three semicircular canals. It sends messages to the brain for hearing and balance. The vestibular mechanism allows a person to balance. The auditory mechanism is contained in the cochlea. It is filled with fluid in various sacks. When the cochlea is unwound it forms three tubes – the scala vestibuli contains perilymph as does the scala tympani while the scala media contains endolymph. The scala tympani ends in the round window while the scala vestibuli ends in the oval window.

Between the scala media and the scala vestibuli is Reissner's membrane while the basilar membrane is between the scala media and the scala tympani. The organ of Corti is found in the basilar membrane.

See Denes and Pinson (1973); Tortora and Grabowski (1993).

eardrum *see* EAR (tympanic membrane).

EAT *see* EDINBURGH ARTICULATION TEST.

echolalia a phenomenon found in many communication disorders where people repeat almost word for word what the therapist says to them. Delayed echolalia occurs when the repetition of the word, phrase or sentence is made after an interval of time has passed or after another person's utterances. *See* Eisenson (1984).

ECochG *see* ELECTROCOCHLEOGRAPHY.

ECT *see* ELECTROCONVULSIVE THERAPY.

Edinburgh Articulation Test (EAT) devised by Antony in 1971, it is a standardised test of articulation which an be used with children of 3 to 6 years of age. It includes:

1. A quantitative score which provides a standard score and an articulatory age;

2. A qualitative profile based on a degree of immaturity of the articulatory realisations, together with the provision for noting atypical articulation.

The test is presented in the form of a picture-naming task and phonetic transcription is made of the child's responses. *See* Antony et al (1971) in Appendix I; Beech et al (1993).

Edinburgh Functional Communication Profile (EFCP) a test for assessing someone's functional communication. There are twelve interaction situations, grouped into six communicative contexts: (1) greeting; (2) acknowledging; (3) responding; (4) requesting; (5) propositions; and (6) verbal problem-solving. It is designed to be used with elderly clients as well as aphasic clients who have difficulty in coping with aspects of daily communication. Rating is on a seven-point scale of carefully defined responses. Administration takes the form of observations either by therapist, spouse or medical staff. The profile looks at people's total communication including the use of signing, computers, etc., to help them communicate, for which they still receive credit. It can also discriminate between the non-language modes used by the person. *See* Skinner et al (1984) in Appendix I; Beech et al (1993).

Edinburgh Maskering a device to help principally those with dysfluent speech. Earphones are linked into a control box which has a volume control on it. When switched on there is a white sound noise which blocks out dysfluent people's feedback systems, so that they cannot hear what they are saying. If such people cannot monitor their speech, then they can become more fluent. *See* Adams and Lang (1992) (use with Parkinson's disease).

education of hearing-impaired children there are three main educational approaches to help the child who has a hearing loss:

1. The oral approach: the child is only allowed to use spoken communication which may include finger spelling or lip reading. Two approaches within the oral approach are:
   (a) acoupedic approach: the emphasis is placed totally on hearing for teaching speech and language. Its aim is to integrate those with a degree of hearing loss into the 'hearing' world. It was devised by Pollack;
   (b) multisensory approach: both hearing and visual stimuli are used. The child is encouraged to use lip reading but no sign languages or systems are allowed. When language is being taught it should be in a meaningful context. However, lip reading can be confusing as some sounds are very difficult to see while others are

quite understandable. Its efficacy depends on the speaker making the sounds as clear as possible and the conversation must take place in good light. As it is not a language system, it is not a particularly good way for a child to develop language. The main aim is to prevent the child from becoming a 'deaf ghetto' (Van Uden, 1970).

2. The manual approach: the child can use sign languages such as British Sign Language or sign systems such as the Paget-Gorman sign system. Van Uden's comment already quoted is perhaps the best argument against this approach. However, it can expand the child's communication capabilities as sign languages do have their own language systems. Many deaf parents ask for their children to be taught BSL as it is less ambiguous than lip reading.

3. Total communication: the child is encouraged to use aspects of both the oral and manual approaches to develop speech and language. No one approach is emphasised more than another. This approach may include other types of communication:
   (a) Rochester Method: an oral approach used with finger spelling.
   (b) CUED SPEECH.

See Northern and Downs (1984); Bench (1992).

educational audiology the testing of children so that those diagnosed as having a hearing loss will have suitable education and treatment given to them.

educational psychology an educational psychologist assesses and treats children in school who have learning problems (e.g. reading problems, DEVELOPMENTAL DYSLEXIA or emotional disorders (e.g. ELECTIVE MUTISM, AUTISM), or CONDUCT DISORDERS. Educational psychologists are also involved in special education. They counsel parents and teachers as well as other professionals about the causes of the child's problems at school. *See* Atkinson et al (1993).

EEG *see* ELECTROENCEPHALOGRAPHY.

EFCP *see* EDINBURGH FUNCTIONAL COMMUNICATION PROFILE.

ego *see* PERSONALITY.

egocentric speech *see* PRE-OPERATIONAL STAGE.

egocentricity *see* PRE-OPERATIONAL STAGE.

egressive airstream *see* AIRSTREAMS.

ejective a sound which is produced by a glottalic airstream (*see* AIRSTREAMS (3)). The sequence of movements required for producing an ejective is:

1. Close the glottis (compare lifting a heavy weight).
2. Make an obstruction in the mouth, e.g. at lips [p] or at the soft palate [k].
3. Move the larynx up (feel the air compressed in the mouth).
4. Release the closure.
5. If the obstruction is at the lips a voiceless ejective [p¹] is produced or if the obstruction is at the soft palate a voiceless ejective [k¹] is produced.

See Catford (1989).

elective mutism a condition in which some children choose not to speak in certain situations, most commonly at school. However, although they may not speak at school, they may speak at home as well as to members of their class outside school but refuse to speak to the same friends when in school and elsewhere. The incidence is 8:10 000 children, with the sexes being equally affected. There are several possible causes for this condition including SEPARATION ANXIETY, SIBLING RIVALRY, overprotective mothers, family history of mental disease, and severe NEUROSIS or DEPRESSION. It may also be caused by an articulation or phonological problem which children can have and for which they have been teased or mocked since they first spoke in school Reinforcement can occur if other children or parents speak about the condition in front of the child to the teacher or therapist. It is an emotional disorder, which for some children may just take the form of shyness which can be overcome without many problems. However, in its severe form, it can become a lasting disorder revealing an abnormal temperament which appears as apathetic (*see* APATHY), morose, unprepossessing, withdrawn, timid, anxious or fearful. Since it results in a communication disorder, it can be treated by a speech therapist as long as it is recognised there may be underlying psychological factors. PSYCHOTHERAPY in the form of BEHAVIOUR THERAPY or PSYCHOANALYSIS has been successful with such children. The child should be desensitised to the situation in which he does not speak. This can take some time but, following this, the child should be put in as many speaking situations as possible to gain confidence. Whispering should be allowed although the use of the child's normal voice should be encouraged as soon as possible. *See* Rutter (1975); Davison and Neale (1994).

electrocochleography (ECochG) an objective test to ascertain hearing threshold. Three electrodes are placed on the head – the active electrode is placed on the promontory in the inner ear (*see* EAR), while another electrode is placed on the ear lobe and the earth is placed on the forehead. It picks up the potential generated in the cochlea (*see* EAR) and auditory nerve. It is rapid; each ear can be tested individually and the state of the client is not affected. However, children may need to be anaesthetised. An ENT surgeon is required to place the electrode in the ear. It cannot test individual frequencies.

electroconvulsive therapy (ECT) a treatment procedure used with those who have DEPRESSION. Most clients are given a low electrical current to the non-dominant cerebral hemisphere (*see* DOMINANCE) which is intended to relieve any confused state after the treatment is finished. It is just as effective if given unilaterally or bilaterally. People are anaesthetised intravenously with succinylcholine or suxamethonium. After the session has ended, normal breathing has been restored and consciousness fully regained, the person cannot remember anything of the treatment although the memory of what occurred prior to treatment is intact. Treatments usually take place once or twice per week. PSYCHOTHERAPY is also required. It has been found that using both forms of treatment at the same time provides the most beneficial treatment programme. *See* Stafford-Clark and Smith (1983); Kolb and Whishaw (1990); Atkinson et al (1993); Davison and Neale (1994).

electroencephalography (EEG) a technique for studying the electrical activity within the BRAIN. This emanates from the cerebral cortex. The waves are plotted on an electroencephalogram by an electroencephalograph. There are four types of wave which can appear on the printout:

1. Alpha waves appear at a frequency of 10–12 cycles per second and appear in most people while awake.
2. Beta waves appear between frequencies of 15 and 60 cycles per second and occur while the nervous system is functioning.
3. Theta waves appear at frequencies of 5–8 cycles per second and occur when the person is under emotional stress.
4. Delta waves appear at frequencies of 1–5 cycles per second and occur while the person is asleep. If they occur while the client is awake, this could indicate brain damage.

EEG is used in the diagnosis of EPILEPSY, TUMOURS OF THE CENTRAL NERVOUS SYSTEM, infectious diseases, such as MENINGITIS, and trauma. *See* Tortora and Grabowski (1993).

electronic book an alternative input system to the BBC microcomputer (*see* ACORN COMPUTERS). It is an A4 ring binder which can be connected to the computer. Inside the back cover, there are twelve touch-sensitive cells. An overlay is placed on top, the operator touches the required picture or word and the computer responds appropriately.

elicitation the process of obtaining data, e.g. words, syllables, phrases, sentences, to form a sample of a person's use of language. In speech and language therapy, elicitation often takes the form of formal and informal assessments.

elision a process by which some words in contexts can lose a sound or syllable in certain environments, e.g. ladies an' gentlemen. *See* Cruttenden (1994).

ellipsis the omission in context of elements of sentences. Responses to questions in English, for example, normally omit subjects and/or auxiliary verbs. For example:
A: What have you been doing?
B: Watching television.
In (B), the sentence lacks both a subject and an auxiliary verb. The full form would be:
B: I have been watching the television.
Many children use this form of sentence and so, during the assessment of language delay or language disorder, it is sometimes uncertain if the child is producing ellipsis and really knows the omitted part, or has produced what appears to be an elliptic sentence because he has not reached that stage of language acquisition to be able to produce complex sentences. *See* Lyons (1968).

embedding CLAUSES that are placed within a sentence are embedded sentences. The basic sentence is known as the matrix sentence. If a relative clause is placed within the utterance, it is central embedding.

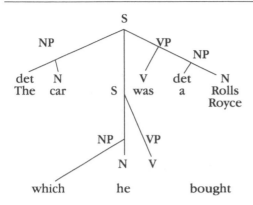

(1) The car which he bought was a Rolls Royce.

See Huddleston (1976).

embryo the developing human from fertilisation to the end of the second month of pregnancy. During this time, known as the embryonic period, the embryonic membranes form around the embryo. A specialised part of the membranes is the placenta, the function of which is to produce an oxygen and nutrient passage into the fetal blood from the mother and the passage of carbon dioxide and other products of metabolism back into the mother. The umbilical cord develops at this time and contains the fetal artery and veins which allow blood to flow between the fetus and placenta. After the second month, the developing human becomes a fetus and from the third month, the time *in utero* is called the fetal period. *See* Haines and Mohiuddin (1972); Tortora and Grabowski (1993).

embryology the study of the developing human fertilised ovum from fertilisation to the end of the second month of pregnancy. *See* Haines and Mohiuddin (1972); Tortora and Grabowski (1993).

EMOS *see* ENHANCED MINSPEAK OPERATING SYSTEM.

emotional disorders found in children who have DEPRESSION or ANXIETY. Both these factors produce obsessional (*see* OBSESSIVE-COMPULSIVE DISORDERS), phobic (*see* PHOBIAS) and psychosomatic symptoms. The prevalence rate is 2.5–5.5 per cent of all children, with an equal incidence between the sexes, although as children grow older there is a gradual increase in the number of female children affected. It is unlikely that there is one sole cause for emotional disorders but rather several intermingled such as SEPARATION ANXIETY, developmental fears and phobias (*see* FEARS AND PHOBIAS IN PRE-SCHOOL CHILDREN), developmental rituals (*see* AUTISM), etc., life events producing stress, e.g. loss, overwhelming traumatic events, family influences involving unconscious conflict and the use of defence mechanisms, e.g. id vs ego, SIBLING RIVALRY, OEDIPUS COMPLEX, etc. PSYCHOTHERAPY has been shown to be useful in treating these disorders. *See* Rutter (1975); Atkinson et al (1993); Davison and Neale (1994).

encephalitis the result of a viral infection which invades the CENTRAL NERVOUS SYSTEM. The virus produces a fever, convulsions and coma. Treatment takes the form of antiviral agents, steroids and anticonvulsants. EEG is used as a means of diagnosis. *See* Gilroy and Holliday (1982); Kolb and Whishaw (1990).

encephalitis lethargica a type of ENCEPHALITIS due to an influenzal virus which was a cause of postencephalitic parkinsonism, found during the worldwide epidemic of 1917–1928. *See* Gilroy and Holliday (1982).

encopresis incontinence of faeces. This may be due to a failure to learn bowel control or a response to psychological stress. *See* Rutter (1975).

encounter groups a form of SENSITIVITY TRAINING used with those who lack social skills. The members of the group pair off and spend about one minute telling each other the most important facts about themselves, followed by two things of which they are proud and two things of which they are ashamed. *See* Trower at al (1978); Davison and Neale (1994).

endocrine system this system comprises glands which do not have ducts and secrete hormones directly into the bloodstream. The endocrine glands include the pituitary and thyroid glands, four parathyroids, two adrenal glands, two gonad glands and the pancreas which can function in both the endocrine and exocrine systems. The secretion by these glands is known as a hormone. *See* Green (1978); Atkinson et al (1993); Tortora and Grabowski (1993).

endocrine voice disorders some communication disorders are caused by a disorder of the endocrine system. Dysphonia is such a disorder:

1. Castrati voice.
2. Eunochoid voice: responds to hormone treatment.
3. Incomplete vocal mutation: a failure of the voice to break at the normal time – it either breaks earlier or later than average. The voice may become hoarse or weak, its range is very low and chest resonance is limited. The person will probably complain of vocal fatigue because of trying to lower the voice. The vocal folds show a varying degree of hyperaemia, congestion and irritation. The folds also show a 'mutational triangle' where they fail to adduct. Treatment takes the form of voice therapy, hormone treatment and PSYCHOTHERAPY;
4. Delayed maturation of pituitary gland of thyrogenic origin.
5. Puberphonia: the persistent falsetto voice in a male who has developed a larynx of normal adult proportions. It may be caused by psychological factors such as neuroses, a denial of adolescence, or a defect in the vocal folds resulting from the habitual misuse or an endocrine imbalance. A person will possibly require both speech therapy to lower the voice and psychological intervention.
6. Precocious vocal mutation: the person shows true sexual precocity before 8 years of age.

7. Perverse mutation: occurs in females when the change from the infantile female voice to an abnormal male voice takes place by the excessive secretion of androgenic hormones.
8. Perello: after 6 months of pregnancy, there are physiological changes in breathing and a slight thickening of vocal folds which become oedematous. This can also happen when menstruation occurs.
9. Menopausal voice changes: the adrenocortical activity after the overian oestrogens have been reduced. This can produce a decrease in the fundamental frequency (Fo) (*see* ACOUSTIC PHONETICS), the glottal membrane becomes thicker, the mass of the vocal folds increases in size and there is a decrease in voice pitch.
10. Hemaphroditic voice: occurs in SCHIZOPHRENIA.
11. Voice disorders caused by thyroid disorder:
    (a) cretinism: the person has a larynx similar to that of an infant. The voice is without intonation and has a very limited range of less than one octave.
    (b) myxoedema: hypothyroidism produces voice loss. It could be referred to as hyperfunctional dysphonia. The person puts on weight, there is a decrease in the activity of the basal mechanism, the face becomes dry and puffy, there is a loss of hair and a bowing of the vocal folds.
    (c) hyperthyroidism: slight weakness and huskiness in the voice but nothing really noteworthy.

All these causes can be treated by voice therapy and relaxation. *See* Greene and Mathieson (1989); Fawcus (1991).

endogenous depression *see* DEPRESSION.

endolymph *see* EAR.

English Picture Vocabulary Test (EPVT) devised by Brimer and Dunn, this is a formal, standardised test to find out the extent of a child's 'listening vocabulary'. The child is asked to choose the correct picture from a selection of four and the resulting score measures what the child can understand semantically. *See* Brimer and Dunn (1962, 1973) in Appendix I.

Enhanced Minspeak Operating System (EMOS) this is an updated operating system for Touch Talkers and Light Talkers. It allows for text editing using left and right cursor keys and scrolling in both communication or storage modes. The conversation workspace expands from 40 characters to 255 characters and text and speech markers are maintained with written text in workspace. While users can still have 8-, 32- and 128-location overlays, they can also use any size and shape of location in a 128-location 'alternative' overlay. If icons (symbols) are moved, all the vocabulary is moved with the icon and does not need to be reprogrammed. When the user reviews vocabulary in the device, the sequence and message appears on the same screen. The improved computer emulation allows the user to store emulator commands under eleven of the function keys. When storing an item of vocabulary, the programmer can stop storing, speak to someone or switch off the device and come back to it later and carry on in the middle of the storage procedure.

ENT (ear, nose and throat) *See* Pracy et al (1974).

environmental deprivation a possible cause of LANGUAGE DELAY. When taking a CASE HISTORY, the therapist should establish to what extent the mother plays with the child or takes time to talk with him about pictures and toys or how frequently she or his father tells the child stories. Unless the child has the experience of talking through play, then he may have difficulty in acquiring language. *See* Garvey (1977); Kolb and Whishaw (1990).

epenthesis a sound which is inserted in the middle of a word as a form of intrusion. It occurs a lot in historical linguistics and CONNECTED SPEECH.

epiglottis a structure at the top of the LARYNX and behind the hyoid bone (*see* MUSCLES OF MASTICATION). It is a leaf-shaped piece of cartilage which is attached to the thyroid cartilage (*see* LARYNX). The larger part opens and closes like a trap door. As the larynx moves up during swallowing, the epiglottis closes off the larynx, thus forcing the food to move down the OESOPHAGUS. *See* Tortora and Grabowski (1993).

epilepsy epilepsy is not a disease in itself but a symptom of a disease. While the symptoms last, there is an abnormal amount of electrical activity reaching the cerebral cortex from a focal site in the BRAIN. It occurs in the following diseases: CONGENITAL NEURONAL DYSFUNCTION, SYSTEMIC METABOLIC DISORDER and STRUCTURAL BRAIN DAMAGE. The symptom shows itself in different ways:

1. Grand-mal epilepsy: a generalised seizure which begins with the feeling of agitation whilst the 'attack' is sudden. The person suddenly collapses and will probably turn a shade of 'blue' because of cyanosis. During the tonic phase, people let out a cry, grit their teeth while their body becomes rigid. They may bite their tongue. This stage lasts about 30 seconds. The clonic phase begins with people waving their limbs wildly without control and they may become incontinent of urine or faeces. Eventually, they fall into a deep sleep and waken normally. They may be unable to remember any of these events.

2. Petit-mal epilepsy: found mainly among children. They have a momentary loss of attention, i.e. one or two seconds, during which they either blink or stare into space. It often looks as if they have poor or limited attention. At worst, it can occur hundreds of times a day but may be controlled by drugs. There is no collapse and

recovery follows immediately with no other side effects. It is always due to congenital neuronal dysfunction. There can be remittance in adolescence. It is much more common than grand-mal epilepsy.

3. Status epilepticus: a series of fits between which the client does not recover consciousness. It can last for hours and requires immediate treatment with drugs. Those with this form of epilepsy may have been removed suddenly from a drug regime or have removed themselves from it or may have STRUCTURAL BRAIN DISEASE. Generalised seizures take place in the form of grand-mal, petit-mal attacks, or tonic/clonic seizures or myoclonus.

4. Myoclonus: shock-like contractions of muscles or muscle groups. It is caused by electrical discharges from different levels of the CENTRAL NERVOUS SYSTEM. It can also occur in the metabolic encephalopathies, including hypoxia, hepatic and uraemic encephalopathy and in many infections and degenerative diseases of the BRAIN, BRAIN-STEM and SPINAL CORD.

In a review of the literature concerning language and epilepsy, Lebrun concludes that various types of language orientated activities, especially reading, can cause paroxysmal brain discharges. Epileptic fits may also interfere with verbal behaviour. The popular drug treatment for adults who have epilepsy is phenytoin, but it can produce facial hair, acne rash, thickness of facial features and may cause hypertrophy of the gums. Carbamazepine is given if phenytoin causes problems from its side effects. However, carbamazepine has a range of side effects particularly on the bone marrow and must be used with caution. Sodium valproate can reduce grand-mal and petit-mal seizures but it may cause and increase in weight and gastro-intestinal problems. Its side effects include drowsiness, headache, photophobia,

dizziness, hiccoughs, bone marrow suppression and vomiting. Diazepam is given intravenously for those who have status epilepticus. The side effects of diazepam include somnolence, lightheadedness and increased muscle weakness. *See* Gilroy and Holliday (1982); Lebrun (1988); Kolb and Whishaw (1990).

epithelium epithelial cells form themselves into membranes which can be of one layer or several layers. The former is simple epithelium while the latter is stratified epithelium. The three types of epithelium which form themselves into these membranes are:

1. Squamous cells: cells that are flat and thickened at the nucleus.
2. Cuboidal cells: cells that are similar in height and width and are many sided.
3. Columnar cells: cells that are polygonal in shape, height is greater than width.

These three types differ in their appearance depending on whether they form simple or stratified epithelial membranes. *See* Leeson et al (1985); Tortora and Grabowski (1993).

EPVT *see* ENGLISH PICTURE VOCABULARY TEST.

ethmoid bone *see* NOSE.

eustachian tube *see* EAR.

EvalPAC a high-tech means of evaluating and training a user to use communication aids. By actuating one key, the display on the SpeechPAC lists options for accessing such as standard keyboard, expanded keyboard, scanning, joystick, light pointer or morse code. When the option desired is chosen the EvalPAC switches automatically to that input. Alphabetical overlays and blank overlays are provided. The blank overlays can be designed using pictures or symbols, etc. When the user decides on the type of overlay to be used, he chooses the picture for a particular message and types in the message to store it in EvalPAC's memory. There are 15 levels which can be programmed to allow the user several programs in the memory at any one time. Time delays allow for users who have difficulty in accessing the memory quickly. The EvalPAC is in a self-contained case with the SpeechPAC in the base and the overlays are in the top facing the user. *See* Appendix IV.

exceptional children children who are particularly talented and gifted. It is also used to describe children who have learning difficulties so that the stigma of being described as 'retarded' would be removed.

Exeter Visual Training Device produced by Tudor and Selley (1974), it is a palatal training device designed to stimulate movement of the soft palate and thus treat hypernasality. The Exeter visual speech aid provides feedback about palatal movement.

exophora a term used to refer to a pronominal form in a construction which relies for its reference on the extra-linguistic context. Exophoric reference is usually contrasted with anaphoric pronominal reference, in which the referent is identified from a previous linguistic mention. *See* Allerton (1979).

expansion the rewrite rules used in constituent analysis are also known as expansion rules since one constituent is expanded into a description of several constituents, e.g. NP→(det)+(adj)+N. *See* Lyons (1968).

experimental hypothesis *See* ALTERNATE HYPOTHESIS.

experimental psychology experimentation is used by many types of psychologist, especially behaviourist and cognitive psychologists. They use experiments to find out how people react to various types of stimuli, how they learn and how they use their memory, their emotional responses and how they are motivated to take action. *See* Atkinson et al (1993).

expressive aphasia *see* APHASIA (1).

expressive language communication by means of the spoken or written word. This is possible where COMPREHENSION is impaired, not the resulting language,

although the resulting language is likely to be pragmatically inappropriate. Conversely, there can be a deficit of expressive language with normal comprehension.

expressive-receptive aphasia *see* APHASIA.

Extended Standard Theory *see* TRANSFORMATIONAL GRAMMAR.

external auditory canal *see* EAR.

external carotid artery *see* CAROTID ARTERY.

extraneous movements movement which is inappropriate to the situation as in the case of some types of stammering where stereotyped movement of limbs accompanies efforts to speak. It also occurs as tics and choreiform movement in some neuropathological conditions. *See* Gilroy and Holliday (1982); Dalton (1983).

extrapyramidal system a system of fibres which operates outside the PYRAMIDAL (corticospinal) SYSTEM. Neurons originate in the BASAL GANGLIA. It modulates background for the motor system. *See* Barr (1979); Kolb and Whishaw (1990); Tortora and Grabowski (1993).

extrinsic muscles of the tongue there are three extrinsic muscles of the tongue:

1. Genioglossus muscle: it runs from the superior genial tubercle of the mandible and inserts itself under the tongue. It is supplied by the lingual artery, lingual vein and CRANIAL NERVE IX. This nerve supplies the surface of the posterior one-third of the tongue, the circumvallate papillae (*see* TASTE BUDS).

2. Styloglossus muscle: it runs from the STYLOID PROCESS to the tongue. It pulls the tongue backwards and upwards. It is supplied by the lingual nerve and CRANIAL NERVE Viii.

3. Hypoglossus muscle: it runs from the hyoid bone (*see* MUSCLES FOR SWALLOWING) to the tongue and pulls it backwards and downwards. It is supplied by the hypoglossal nerve (CRANIAL NERVE XII).

See Tortora and Grabowski (1993).

eye contact some people who have a stammer or a voice disorder are so embarrassed when they speak that they fail to look directly at the therapist or person to whom they are talking. It is an important part of deictic (*see* DEIXIS) communication. *See* Dalton (1983).

eye transfer communication systems these systems can be used to find out if the user can communicate, to train a user who may be given a more sophisticated communication aid in the future, or as a means for a user to communicate his needs. The system comprises a transparent panel to which any type of stimulus, e.g. symbols, pictures, words/phrases, etc., is attached on three fully adjustable standing bases. The base can either be mounted on wheels, a weighted base or a clamp base which can be attached to any surface edge.

Eyetyper model 200 a high-tech communication system operated by direct eye contact between the client and the machine. The keyboard has a lens, a light and eight eye-gaze sensors plus a large display panel. The sensors can be used in two, four or eight combinations. A glance can produce a word, phrase or symbol which will appear on the display panel and can be produced by the built-in speech synthesiser. Different overlays can be used. It can be interfaced to a computer, a modem, a printer or other environmental control devices.

EZ keys a software system for use with specific communication aids. It uses word prediction, abbreviation expansion, a built-in reader for giving presentations and instant phrases organised in groups or topics of vocabulary. EZ keys for Windows allows for mouse emulation even if the person is just using the communication aid. All types of accessing are available including switches to infra-red input and Touch Screen. It allows the person to control the environment through their environmental control, and a modem can also be used. There are versions to run in DOS or WINDOWS. *See* Appendix IV.

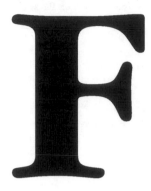

facial nerve   *see* CRANIAL NERVES.

facilitated communication   an approach in ALTERNATIVE AUGMENTATIVE COMMUNICATION first used by Crossley in 1977 with her client Anne MacDonald, a young girl with cerebral palsy whose experiences during her rehabilitation are documented in the book *'Annie's Coming Out'*. Facilitated communication assumes competence in communication rather than impairment. It is also to be assumed by the facilitators that those with autism will produce a meaningful and even quite complex message. To facilitate the person's communication, the person's hand, arm or even finger is held over a keyboard. The keyboard, with letters or symbols, is gradually introduced to the person by direct questions e.g. 'show me the letter "t"', or 'show me the picture of the "house"' etc. Positive feedback is given when the correct letter or symbol is hit. The person is gradually asked to make more complex messages such as entering their name or following a cloze procedure exercise where the person has to fill in the blanks. The person is then encouraged to make longer and more complex statements using facilitation. The prompts are slowly removed although the physical support remains as long as the per-

son wishes it. *See* Crossley (1988); Beukelman and Mirenda (1992); Jones (1995a).

facilitation   the act of enabling a natural process. In speech and language therapy, facilitation is used with various client groups who have some degree of communication impairment to help them relearn or improve their communicative skills. The importance of facilitation in all types of communication disorder cannot be underestimated, not only with conditions such as APHASIA or childhood speech and language disorders but also in the use of augmentative communication where a person has to learn how to use their respective communication system. *See* Eisenson (1984) (facilitation for aphasia); Beukelman and Mirenda (1992).

facioscapulohumeral muscular dystrophy   *see* DYSTROPHY.

factor analysis   *see* TRAIT APPROACH.

failure to thrive   a description of children who have poor physical development, usually caused by a failure to receive social and physical stimulation. *See* Kempe and Kempe (1978); Reber (1985).

false vocal folds   ventricular folds. The superior part of the thyroarytenoid muscle lying above the VOCAL FOLDS. Their normal function is adduction when swallowing, but they function as vocal folds in some types of voice disorder, e.g. ventricular band voice. *See* Greene and Mathieson (1989); Tortora and Grabowski (1993).

falx cerebri a sickle-shaped structure within the BRAIN acting as a vertical partition along the longitudinal fissure of the CEREBRAL HEMISPHERES. Its dura is attached to the crista galli of the ethmoid bone at the front, to the midline of the vault as far back as the internal protuberance, and to the tentorium cerebelli. This midline fold of dura mater separates the two cerebral hemispheres. *See* Barr (1979); Tortora and Grabowski (1993).

family therapy the family goes regularly to see a therapist who observes how the family interact with each other. Atkinson et al suggest 'the basic premise of family therapy is that the problem shown by the identified patient is that something is wrong with the entire family; the *family system* is not operating properly'(Atkinson et al, 1993 p. 692). Each member of the family is directed in ways of how to improve their interaction with each other. The therapist may also go to the family's home for similar reasons. *See* Barker (1981); Atkinson et al (1993); Sauber et al (1993); Davison and Neale (1994).

fascia Two types of fascia exist which form sheets of tough material to divide muscle groups:

1. Superficial fascia: loose CONNECTIVE TISSUE found deep in the skin that often contains a varying quantity of fat. If the tissue consists mainly of fat, it is called adipose or fatty tissue.
2. Deep fascia: dense connective tissue found in a continuous layer below the superficial fascia and formed in sheets. It can form part of a flat muscle which is then called an aponeurosis.

See Tortora and Grabowski (1993).

fasciculus a bundle or a group of nerve or muscle fibres, e.g. ARCUATE FASCICULUS. *See* Tortora and Grabowski (1993).

FAST *see* FRENCHAY APHASIA SCREENING TEST.
fauces *see* MOUTH.
FCP *see* FUNCTIONAL COMMUNICATION PROFILE.
fear thermometer *see* SYSTEMATIC DESENSITISATION.
fears and phobias in pre-school children EMOTIONAL DISORDERS which can affect young children. At the age of 2 years, children can be afraid of ghosts, witches and the supernatural which they hear about in fairy stories; at about 3 years of age, they have a fear of small animals, which may turn into a fear of any size of animal or anything furry, while at the age of 4 years, they often become self-conscious and have feelings which may make them frightened. They may also have the fear of losing someone close to them, e.g. a parent, especially after the death of one parent or close relative, or they may even fear that they themselves may die. Similarly after a divorce in the family, they may become very frightened that the other parent will disappear. If the family has to move house, the child may have a fear of leaving his friends and making new friends. All fears become phobias when they become extreme and begin to interfere with the everyday life of the child. For example, a phobia of the dark may arise because the child has been shut in the cupboard either accidentally or intentionally. As the child is so vulnerable at this early age to such events, his most fearful symptom, i.e. fear of the dark, becomes a phobia. Such phobias may even be reinforced by parents who agree with the phobia because they are frightened by the same stimulus. Thus, children learn to be phobic because the parent is frightened by the same thing, e.g. mice. Children do have their own devices for dealing with fears and phobias. Some follow ritualistic routines, e.g. walking on the lines of the pavement, so that they will not be harmed, or they have favourite toys or objects, e.g. safety

blanket, they believe will keep them safe. BEHAVIOUR THERAPY has been successfully used with such a disorder. *See* Rutter (1975); Atkinson et al (1993).

febrile convulsions fits which occur during a fever associated with an acute systemic infection. They are not caused by infection to the CENTRAL NERVOUS SYSTEM. Many children with this condition have a history of neurological or developmental abnormality. The movements during these convulsions are of the tonic and clonic (*see* EPILEPSY) type. If the child has febrile convulsions as such, there is a good prognosis. When convulsions last for longer than 30 minutes, the brain is deprived of oxygen and scarring can produce a permanent focus for epilepsy in adulthood. Drug treatment is often not needed. Children should always be kept cool following a convulsion. It occurs in 3 per cent of all children, the highest incidence being between 10 months and 2 years of age. About 30 per cent have a family history. *See* Gilroy and Holliday (1982).

feedback the means by which behaviour is monitored. Internal feedback provides information before and during the event; external feedback after the event. In relation to speech, auditory, visual, kinaesthetic and tactile feedback play an important part in communication. Many communication disorders are a result of poor monitoring by the speaker. Such disorders can include stammering (*see* STAMMER, DYSFLUENCY), DYSPHONIA, PHONOLOGICAL DISORDER and learning problems such as those encountered by children learning to read using the phonic approach. DELAYED AUDITORY FEEDBACK is used with those who speak at a very fast rate to try and slow down their speech in such conditions as stammering. *See* Brosnahan and Malmberg (1976).

Feeding Check List devised by Warner (1981), it takes the form of a series of questions relevant to the child's eating behaviour and is designed to improve it. It can be used by a caregiver or therapist. It comprises five sections: general; head and trunk control; food and feeding utensils; control of tongue and lips for feeding and drinking; and general features. Each of these sections has questions which are to be answered with a 'yes/no' response. *See* Warner (1981).

felicity conditions if a speech act, as a communicative activity, is to achieve its derived function then certain circumstances, known as felicity conditions, must pertain. So, for example, if the speech act is intended to assert the truth of the proposition expressed by the utterance, sincerity conditions, such as the speaker is not lying, should prevail. More crucially perhaps, in declarative speech acts such as those involved in christening, preparatory conditions ensure that the speaker has the requisite authority to perform the speech acts. *See* Clark and Clark (1977).

festinant gait *see* PARKINSON'S DISEASE.

fetal alcohol syndrome a condition first recognised by Lemoine and his colleagues in France in 1968 and confirmed by Jones and his colleagues in 1973. The child will have fetal alcohol syndrome if the mother has been drinking excess alcohol during pregnancy. It can produce learning disability and give the child a particular facial appearance – a small nose, slit eyes and a convex top lip. The child is often irritable, hypertonic (*see* HYPERTONIA) and has tremor and tonic seizures. *See* Gilroy and Holliday (1982); Smith (1985); Tortora and Grabowski (1993).

fibreoptic laryngoscope a device made of a large number of glass fibres which are flexible and allow inspection of the recesses of the nose and throat. The person's nose is anaesthetised so that the tube can be passed along the floor of the nose, down the back of the nasopharynx, oropharynx and laryngopharynx (*see* PHARYNX) to the VELOPHA-RYNGEAL area where any muscle weakness or damage to the LARYNX is observed. *See* Edels (1983); Beech et al (1993).

fibrous meningiomas a type of meningioma (*see* TUMOURS OF THE CENTRAL NERVOUS SYSTEM) which results from CONNECTIVE TISSUE elements and consists of strands of intertwining spindle cells with long fibrils. *See* Gilroy and Holliday (1982).

field

1. In computer terms, part of a record which contains information. A database is made up of records all of which contain fields such as the person's 'name', 'address', 'date of birth', etc. *See* Bishop (1985).

2. *see* SEMANTIC FIELD.

figure and ground when a stimulus is presented with two or more distinct areas, e.g. a painting, part of it is perceived as figure while the rest is ground. Figure refers to the objects of interest and appears in front of the ground. This is the most basic form of perceptual organisation. *See* Atkinson et al (1993).

file in computer terms, information is normally stored on a disk in a file with a filename. Each file is given a name so that it can be easily identified by the system software. The file name is given when a program or text from a WORD PROCESSOR is stored on disk. In some forms of BASIC, the command word 'save' is typed followed by the name of the file. In other systems such as an Apple Macintosh or IBM PC or compatible using Windows, the word 'save' is chosen from a pull-down menu using a MOUSE, while to retrieve the file either the word 'load' followed by the file name is typed in or the word 'open' is chosen from pull-down menus. With some word processors, the inverted commas may not be necessary. It is possible to find out what files are on a disk by typing *CAT, CATALOG, DIR or *.,

depending on the type of computer and operating system, or by opening a window when using Microsoft Windows applications or an Apple Macintosh computer. In some word processors, files can be printed out straight from the disk without loading them into the computer's memory. *See* Bishop (1985); Brookshear (1991).

filiform *see* TASTE BUDS.

filing system many microcomputers have different filing systems for storing information on disks allowing easy access to files. The most popular microcomputer used in education and rehabilitation services in the UK is the BBC series of computers. The BBC B uses the disk filing system (DFS) while the Master series uses the Advanced Disk Filing System (ADFS). The latter uses directories which are similar to an all-embracing title. Within a directory, there could be 'subdirectories' which are similar to subtitles, and within these, there can be more 'sub-directories'. The system is similar to a filing cabinet in any office. On the front of the drawer is the name which describes what all the files in the drawer concern, e.g. finance. In the drawer, there may be several files concerning different aspects of a person's finances, e.g. income, expenditure, etc., while within these files, there may be more detailed files of information concerning these areas of finance, e.g. mortgage, rates, bank statement, etc. The ADFS system is designed to make it easy to recall programs written to it. For those using Microsoft Windows 95 or an Apple Macintosh computer, pictures of folders appear in an open window. When each folder is opened the individual documents appear, which in turn can be opened with a MOUSE. *See* Bishop (1985); Brookshear (1991); BBC Master 128 manual.

filled pause a gap between utterances which has been filled by a hesitation, e.g. 'er', 'ur', 'eh', etc. Otherwise these gaps would remain silent. *See* Clark and Clark (1977).

filter an electronic method of producing part of an acoustic analysis. It reduces the amplitude of a sound but at the same time allows others to pass through with little or no reduction in their amplitude. The frequencies which do pass through are called the bandwidth of the filter. *See* Fry (1979).

finger spelling a form of communication used with those who have a hearing loss. Words are spelled out on the fingers, each finger formation forming one letter. It can be used in conjunction with BSL where only one finger spelling is given to represent the initial letter of a word for which there may not be a sign or it may just be used as a shorthand form. It is sometimes called 'visible speech' or dactylology. *See* Beukelman and Mirenda (1992).

FingerFoniks a high-tech communication aid with digitised speech and synthetic voice. The sounds of the letters are produced by pressing the letters on the keyboard. Messages can be stored into the device. *See* Appendix IV.

First Word Language Programme developed by Gillham (1979), it is a language programme used with children who have language delay or disorder, those with learning difficulties and those who cannot produce speech for physical reasons. The child is taught using short structured sessions either once a day or more often. There is also the possibility of using informal settings for therapy where they occur. The therapist should keep records of the progress made by the children. *See* Gillham (1979).

first word stage a stage in a child's development of language. It lasts from about 1 to almost 2 years of age. A child's one-word utterances are sentences of one word which name objects, describe actions, make requests or, with correct intonation, express emotional states or surprise at seeing something unexpected. The sort of items used at this stage are:

1. Familiar things, objects: (a) important people, e.g. dada, mama (b) animals; (c) clothing; (d) household items; (e) body parts.
2. Actions/events: (a) name of movers (agents); (b) movables (objects affected by action); (c) some children pay particular attention to names of objects while others to names of people.
3. Intonation used meaningfully (occurs later during this stage): (a) recurrence; (b) negation; (c) location.

Although the child may not use these completely with meaning, the meaning can be taken from their use of gesture and the context of the utterance. *See* Cruttenden (1979).

'fis' phenomenon a common condition in language development. It occurs when a child does not accept the adult imitation of his own immature version of a word. The name derives from the observations of Berko and Brown (1960) in relation to the imitation of a child's realisation of /fɪʃ/ as /fɪs/. *See* Clark and Clark (1977).

fistula a hole or opening which remains after surgery e.g. after surgery to close a cleft palate. *See* Edwards and Watson (1980).

fit a layman's term for a seizure (*see* EPILEPSY).

flaccid dysarthria *see* DYSARTHRIAS (3).

flaccidity a description of a child or adult whose muscles are hypotonic, making it difficult for the individual to stand or sit upright. It may also produce dysarthric characteristics of speech (*see* DYSARTHRIAS). See Tortora and Grabowski (1993).

flap *see* ARTICULATION.

flat a distinctive feature proposed by Jakobson and Halle to distinguish sounds produced with lip-rounding (*see* CARDINAL VOWEL SYSTEM) [+FLAT] from those which are produced with spread lips [−FLAT]. *See* Hyman (1975).

flattening of affect a phenomenon found in several conditions including SCHIZOPHRENIA in which the person fails to produce an emotional response to almost any stimulus. The person stares into empty space and has weakness in facial muscles (*see* MUSCLES OF FACIAL EXPRESSION). The voice shows no prosodic features (*see* PROSODY). *See* Davison and Neale (1994).

flexion a description of the forward movement of joints, e.g. head moving forward on neck, etc. *See* Tortora and Grabowski (1993).

flooding a therapeutic technique devised by Stomfl and Lewis (1967) used in BEHAVIOUR THERAPY. The person is placed in the most feared situation for a long period of time without the possibility of escape. It is opposed to SYSTEMATIC DESENSITISATION. Some people can recover faster under flooding although it can be highly traumatic. *See* Purser (1982); Atkinson et al (1993).

floppy disk *see* DISK.

fluency a description of normal speech which has little or no non-fluency or DYSFLUENCY. There may be hesitation while the speaker thinks of his next utterance, i.e. normal non-fluency. Fluency is the ultimate aim of all who stammer. *See* Dalton (1983).

fluent aphasia *see* APHASIA (2).

Fo indicator an indicator to improve three different aspects of speech production: pitch of the voice, intonation and phonation. Fo represents fundamental frequency (*see* ACOUSTIC PHONETICS). A contact microphone is held against the throat and the fundamental frequency, indicated by the movement of the vocal folds, is measured by the pointer. The frequency range is 50–550 Hz. The upper and lower limits of the frequency range are indicated by the use of red and green lamps which are set by red and green controls respectively. It can be used with children who have a hearing loss whose sounds are not always used at an acceptable pitch level.

focal sites a specific part of the brain from where symptoms of diseases and disorders can occur. In APHASIA, for example, the focal sites could be Broca's and Wernicke's areas (*see* CEREBRAL HEMISPHERES), etc., or the site in the brain from which the electrical discharges emanate in EPILEPSY. *See* Gilroy and Holliday (1982); Kaye (1991).

font the kind of typeface produced by different kinds of printer or printing processes. If daisywheel printers are used, the font for all characters will be the same, as they are all on the print wheel unless the user has a wheel containing different typefaces, while dot matrix, bubble (ink) jet or laser printers can use different kinds of typeface direct from the computer as their print heads are made up of styluses. The word 'fount' can also be used to describe the same process. *See* Chandor et al (1985).

foramen a description of an opening or passage within the body. Several are called foramina. *See* Tortora and Grabowski (1993).

forced alternative a type of question which makes the person give a response to two or more alternatives, e.g. do you want tea or coffee? *See* Crystal et al (1989).

forebrain *see* DIENCEPHALON.

form in its most general sense, linguistic form is the patterning of elements that make up structure. Linguistic forms are patterns or structures themselves, e.g. SENTENCES, NOUN PHRASES, verbs. In this sense, form is contrasted to FUNCTION. *See* Lyons (1968).

formal assessments *see* ASSESSMENTS.

formal operations the final stage of cognitive development as proposed by PIAGET. It begins at about 11 years of age, when the child can understand abstract relationships and may begin to think in terms of possibilities. He will use hypothetico-deductive reasoning for working out these possibilities. This is probably the least controversial part of Piaget's theory as it is a familiar thought process for most people in everyday life. *See* Beard (1969); Boden (1994).

formant *see* SPECTROGRAPHY.

fortis a description of sounds which are produced with a strong egressive airstream (*see* AIRSTREAMS). They require also more muscle power to produce the sound. It is usually the voiceless consonants which are fortis, e.g. [f], while voiced ones are described as LENIS, e.g. [v]. *See* Cruttenden (1994).

FourTalk a very basic communication aid for someone just starting to use high-tech devices. There are two models: the FourTalk 16 with 1 location with 16 seconds record time or 2 locations with 8 seconds or 4 channels with 4 seconds record time in each location respectively; and the FourTalk 32 which has the same number of possible locations each with double the time of the FourTalk 16 for each location. It can be accessed by direct manual selection and single or double switch. *See* Appendix IV.

fourth ventricle a structure within the BRAIN which acts as a canal in the HIND-BRAIN. It has a diamond-shaped floor while its roof is tent-like and covered by the CEREBELLUM. The floor is covered with symmetrical elevations caused by the grey matter of the CRANIAL NERVES. Dilatation of this ventricle by fluid produces HYDROCEPHALUS. *See* Barr (1979); Kolb and Whishaw (1990); Tortora and Grabowski (1993).

Fox a portable environmental control, it has unique coded radio signals, rechargeable batteries, two external switch sockets for single or two-switch scanning and can be mounted on wheelchairs etc. It can scan from 0.75 to 5 seconds and has status indicators allowing the user to see what devices are on in any room. It can be used to control mains electricity, door opening, telephone and infra-red equipment. *See* Appendix IV.

fragile X syndrome a sex-linked chromosome disorder (*see* CHROMOSOMES). It can produce varying degrees of learning disability with the facial appearance of large forehead, large mouth and ill-formed ears. Carriers can be affected. The child's expressive language is superior to comprehension while perseveration may also be found. *See* Tortora and Grabowski (1993).

free association a part of PSYCHOANALYSIS. The person is encouraged to say everything which is in his mind however irrelevant, shameful or stupid it may seem. If the person stops or hesitates, it is assumed by the therapist that the person is hiding some sensitive information which is worth further investigation. It was first used by Freud (*see* PSYCHOANALYSIS; PERSONALITY). *See* Atkinson et al (1993).

free field audiometry an audiometric test for very young children who cannot use earphones. It usually takes place in two rooms. The person sits in one, equidistant from two loudspeakers. Live or pre-recorded voices are presented. However, the child's ears cannot be tested individually. It is part of speech audiometry.

free variation a phonological description of the distribution of sounds or phonemes (*see* PHONOLOGY). It occurs when two sounds appear in the same position of the word without changing its meaning. For example, the 'r' sounds found in some varieties of English are freely interchangeable in the word 'burns' which can be either [bɑrnz] or [bʌrnz]. In a phonological delay or disorder, the child can produce a sound in the same position of many of the words he uses. Such a sound is said to be in free variation in this child's sound system (*see* PHONOLOGY). *See* Grunwell (1987).

Frenchay Aphasia Screening Test (FAST) devised by Enderby and her collegues in 1987 to establish the existence of APHASIA. It examines COMPREHENSION and EXPRESSIVE LANGUAGE as well as comprehension of reading and writing. Scores are compared with a cut-off score and results obtained which determine if speech therapy is required. *See* Enderby et al (1987) in Appendix I; Beech et al (1993).

Frenchay Dysarthria Assessment devised by Enderby in 1980 (revised 1988), it is a formal standardised test which indicates the severity and type of DYSARTHRIA. The assessment covers eight sections: reflex, respiration, lips, jaw, palate, laryngeal, tongue and intelligibility. All eight sections are scored on a nine-point scale. The test takes about 30 minutes to administer. Enderby believes it has fulfilled six criteria: it is applicable to therapy; it can demonstrate changes in the person's speech; it is easy and short to administer; it has been standardised; no training is necessary for administering it; and the results are easy to understand both by speech therapists and by other professionals. The computerised Frenchay Dysarthria Assessment runs on an Apple computer II, II Plus and IIe. *See* Enderby (1988) in Appendix I; Beech et al (1993).

frenulum *see* TONGUE.

Freud *see* PSYCHOANALYSIS; PERSONALITY.

fricative *see* ARTICULATION.

Friedreich's ataxia a degenerative disorder affecting the tracts of the SPINAL CORD. It occurs during adolescence and early adulthood. The condition is inherited as an autosomal recessive trait (*see* CHROMOSOMES). It produces dysarthric characteristics of speech (*see* DYSARTHRIAS), spastic gait and INTENTION TREMOR. The CEREBROSPINAL FLUID is normal. It is progressive, those with the condition may not be able to walk 5 years after the symptoms have appeared, while death may occur 10–20 years later, usually due to respiration problems. *See* Gilroy and Holliday (1982).

frontal lobe *see* CEREBRAL HEMISPHERES.

fronting in ARTICULATORY PHONETICS, sounds which are produced at the front of the mouth. This includes the front vowels in the CARDINAL VOWEL SYSTEM and the consonants made by the tip and the blade of the tongue. In generative phonology, these sounds are described as [+anterior] or [+coronal]. It describes also a phonological process proposed by David Stampe (*see* PHONOLOGICAL PROCESSES). *See* Grunwell (1987); Ladefoged (1993).

function when contrasted with FORM, function refers to the role which a linguistic element plays in a structure. So a NOUN PHRASE can function as a subject, an object or a complement in a clause structure. *See* Lyons (1968).

function key most microcomputers have function keys which are marked (f0, f1, f2, etc.). They are given specific functions in various application programs such as word processors. There are often between nine and twelve keys and, in combination with other keys, they can cope with many functions. Some pieces of therapeutic software use function keys to reduce the number of key inputs required to operate the computer. Such a piece of software is the PREDICTIVE ADAPTIVE LEXICON (PAL) produced by the Micro Centre of Dundee University. *See* Bishop (1985).

function words members of a closed class of grammatical categories such as determiner, auxiliary, conjunction. The categories of which these words are members contain few members (hence 'closed class') and their role is largely grammatical rather than semantic. *See* Palmer (1976).

functional analysis *see* OPERANT CONDITIONING.

functional communication the social role of language in society. Specifically, it is the appropriateness with which language is used in various contexts. 'As language is used to establish interpersonal relationships, regulate the behaviour of others, satisfy material needs or desires, explore and organise environments and exchange messages and information (Halliday in Cole, 1982), therapy for the language impaired also needs to focus upon such functions' (Green, 1984). Thus, the therapist should devise context-orientated therapy for these people. *See* Green (1984); Clinical Forum in *Aphasiology,* 6;1 (1992); Crockford and Lesser (1994) (functional communication and aphasia).

Functional Communication Profile (FCP) a test of FUNCTIONAL COMMUNICATION, devised by Sarno in 1969 for all age groups. It tests five functions: movement, speaking, understanding, reading and other aspects of communication. The 45 items divided into these five functional categories have been selected according to what are considered functions of everyday urban life. The rating which is based on a nine-point scale is very subjective. Administration takes the form of an unstructured interview. It can be used for prognosis and is designed for all age groups. The profile describes residual skills rather than deficits, and yields a quantifiable measure of functional communication regardless of severity of impairment. It is a test primarily of language in a natural setting rather than all modes of communication. *See* Sarno (1969); Rosenbek et al (1989).

functional dysphonia a disorder of phonation to which no known organic cause can be directly attributed. There are different types of functional dysphonia:

1. Misuse and abuse of the person's voice which produces VOCAL NODULES, CONTACT ULCERS, etc.
2. Learned patterns of maladaptive behaviour.
3. Psychogenic causes: (a) in those with a psychiatric history, having psychoso-matic symptoms and who are vulnerable to physical and mental stress; (b) in those with no history of psychiatric problems but who have prolonged life stress.

See Fawcus (1991).

Functional Performance Record (FPR) devised by Mulhall in 1989, it is an assessment of behaviours of those people who have physical, social or psychological impairments. An assessment is made allowing the therapist to set goals and monitor progress. It has a numerical and descriptive means of giving information. It does not provide a diagnosis or reasons why people behave as they do nor does it provide an aetiology or any other type of classification.

There are three components:

1. The checklist: a 46-page booklet containing 777 items in 27 areas of functioning which can be assessed individually or in any combination. These areas of functioning include activity level, aggression, attention span, feeding, hearing, incontinence, memory, movement of limbs and trunk, reading skills, speech and language production, speech and language reception, toileting, etc.
2. The FPR software: individual client disk – an automated version of the checklist. A database can be made which performs all the functions of the individual client disk.
3. The handbook: contains information for using the FPR.

See Mulhall (1989) in Appendix I.

fundamental frequency *see* ACOUSTIC PHONETICS.

fungiform *see* TASTE BUDS.

G

gag reflex the description of the act of swallowing caused by stimulation of the walls of the oropharynx (*see* PHARYNX). *See* Joseph (1979).

galvanic skin response (GSR) a method for measuring electrical skin responses to presented stimuli using a galvanometer. *See* Taylor et al (1982); Atkinson et al (1993); Davison and Neale (1994).

generalisation *see* CARRY-OVER.

generative grammar a grammar consisting of a set of rules which define or generate all and only the grammatical sentences of a language. The term was introduced into linguistics by Noam Chomsky (*see* CHOMSKYAN LINGUISTICS) in his book *Syntactic Structures* (1957). For a natural language, Chomsky proposed that a generative grammar should not only define the set of grammatical sentences, but should assign structural descriptions to the sentences. While the goals of Chomskyan grammar have remained the same, their form has changed several times since 1957. The most novel and significant feature of early generative grammar was the notion of a transformational rule (*see* TRANSFORMATIONAL GRAMMAR), a device for formally linking related sentence types such as active and passive. In the most recent form of Chomskyan generative grammar, referred to as Government and Binding Theory, transformations play a much more restricted role. *See* Huddleston (1976); Lyons (1991).

generative phonology a phonological theory in which phonological changes are used to describe sound changes in particular contexts or environments of the word. For example, the rule which allows for vowels to be nasalised before nasal consonants would appear thus:

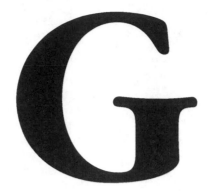

$$\begin{bmatrix} + \text{voc} \\ - \text{cons} \end{bmatrix} \longrightarrow [+ \text{nas}] \ \Big/ - \begin{bmatrix} + \text{cons} \\ + \text{nas} \end{bmatrix}$$

(Grunwell, 1987)

The terms used in square brackets are distinctive features. An explanation of this rule is: a sound that is voiced but is not a consonant (i.e. a vowel) becomes nasalised in the context preceding a nasalised consonant. Such rules can be useful for a speech therapist in that the child's representation of a sound can be compared with the adult target sound by working out the differences of the features used by the child compared with the adult in particular contexts. The input side of the rule has the child's pronunciation described in the form of distinctive features while the output of the rule shows the adult's pronunciation, i.e. the one regarded as being normal. If the rule is context-sensitive, i.e. the error occurs in the same position of the word consistently, the therapist can find out if the child is making a consistent error in a particular part of the word. Grunwell gives an example where /f/ is pronounced as a homorganic affricate in word-initial position:

'feet'   [pfɪt]
'fence'   [pfɛş]
'fish'   [pfɛɱ]

The rule describing this error is:

$$\begin{bmatrix} +cont \\ +ant \\ -cor \\ +strid \\ -voice \end{bmatrix} \rightarrow \begin{bmatrix} -cont \\ +del\ rel \end{bmatrix} / - \begin{bmatrix} +voc \\ -cons \end{bmatrix}$$

An explanation of this rule is: a sound which is a fricative-type [+cont], made towards the front of the mouth [+ant], not made with the tongue tip [−cor], a strong sound [+strid]) and unvoiced [−voice] becomes a non-fricative sound [−cont] and has a longer release time than a single consonant [+del rel] in the context of coming before a vowel. Generative phonology is quite widely used in analysing child speech and its application to omissions, substitutions, distortions and transposition is:

- change feature specifications (i.e. change segments)
- delete segments, compare omission
- insert segments, compare additions
- interchange (reorder or permute) segments (i.e. metathesis), compare transpositions
- coalesce segments

(Grunwell, 1987)

These phonological rules describe patterns of errors. Thus if the therapist decides to use rule-based therapy, then the generative framework for analysing a child's speech may well be useful. See Grunwell (1987).

geniculate ganglion found in CRANIAL NERVE VII, it houses the cells which pick up the sense of taste. It attaches to the lingual branch of the mandibular nerve, the fibres of which go to the taste buds on the front two-thirds of the tongue. See Barr (1979); Tortora and Grabowski (1993).

genioglossus muscle see EXTRINSIC MUSCLES OF THE TONGUE.

genital stage see PSYCHOSEXUAL STAGES OF DEVELOPMENT.

genitive the form of a word which represents possession. There are two forms for possession in English, the use of affixes and the use of the word 'of':

(1) The man's car is brown.
(2) The car of the man is brown.

See Lyons (1968).

genotype the particular set of genes carried by one organism. It contains all the hereditary factors which can be passed down through the generations. See Taylor et al (1982); Atkinson et al (1993).

gerontology the study of the ageing process. See AGEING.

Gerstmann's syndrome a disorder arising from a lesion in the left parietal lobe (see CEREBRAL HEMISPHERES) in the region of the ANGULAR GYRUS. The classic symptoms are: finger agnosia, PURE AGRAPHIA, ACALCULIA and right–left confusion. CONSTRUCTIONAL APRAXIA has also been reported. See Kolb and Whishaw (1990).

Gestalt psychology a particular study in psychology founded by Max Wertheimer in the early part of this century. He and his followers were interested in groupings of visual stimuli and how they were perceived. FIGURE AND GROUND is one part of Gestalt psychology as is the way objects are grouped together where proximity and closure are important to the way we perceive these objects. See Reber (1985); Atkinson et al (1993); Davison and Neale (1994).

Gestural Reorganisation a therapeutic programme to improve an aphasic person's speech by linking meaningful gestures with spoken words and phrases. *See* Rosenbek et al (1989).

gestures fine or gross body movement, facial expression, eye movements and postures used for communication. This can also be termed non-verbal communication. This type of communication can be systematised although many people who rely on non-verbal communication have their own system which is only known to family members or a few close friends. The gestures which are used can also be very similar and their meaning only changes because of the context in which they are used. It has been found that, with practice, aphasic (*see* APHASIA) patients can cope with gesture and use it effectively for communication, although some therapists dispute its efficacy. Those with aphasia who have a HEMIPLEGIA may have difficulty with using gesture. *See* Stuart-Smith and Wilks (1979); Beukelman and Mirenda (1992).

gifted used to describe children who show particular talent or aptitude which exceeds their chronological age. *See* Silver (1992).

GILCU *see* GRADUAL INCREASE IN LENGTH AND COMPLEXITY OF UTTERANCE.

Gilles de la Tourette Syndrome an inheritable, metabolic disorder which produces tics. These tics begin in the face and, in time, increase and begin to affect the shoulders and upper limbs. As breathing becomes poor, the person's speech is affected. There are only minor neurological signs. The disease does not interfere with the person's life expectancy. Prognosis is good for those who are treated with haloperidol. It is also known as tic convulsif. This neurotic syndrome can take the form of obscene language, violent vocalisations and motor tics. These symptoms usually appear all at once. The condition begins before 12 years of age (75 per cent of cases) or before 20 years (96 per cent of cases). The incidence is 2:1 in favour of males.

It can be a life-long illness although antipsychotic drugs, e.g. haloperidol, can suppress the obscene language and odd motor tics. *See* Kolb and Whishaw (1990); Davison and Neale (1994).

Glasgow Coma Scale an objective scale which is used in the assessment of those who have had a head injury. It gives a numerical value to the three most important responses which medical staff try to elicit from a head-injured patient – eye opening, the best verbal response and the best motor response. For eye opening, there is a scale of 1–4, for best verbal response there is a score of 1–5 while for best motor response there is a scale of 1–6. When calculated, a total score of 3–15 is produced. If the score is less than 8 a severe head injury exists, if the score is between 9 and 12, the head injury is moderate while a score of 13–15 indicates a minor head injury. *See* Kolb and Whishaw (1990); Kaye (1991).

glide when in transcription, there are two symbols next to each other, phonologically, they are a part of the same phonological unit, e.g. diphthong. *See* Cruttenden (1994).

glioma the commonest type of intracerebral tumour. It can occur at any age, with increasing frequency up to 65 years of age. *See* Gilroy and Holliday (1982).

global aphasia *see* APHASIA (6); Mark et al (1992).

glossal a description of structures and disorders with tongue involvement.

glossectomy the surgical removal of part or all of the tongue due to disease, trauma or natural wasting. Resulting speech may be quite intelligible, though it may be produced at a slower rate. Exercises similar to those given in some types of DYSARTHRIA are useful. Counselling prior to surgery is very important. *See* Travis (1971); Green et al (1994).

glossolalia the phenomenon of 'speaking in tongues' used by various religious sects. It may also occur under hypnosis.

glossopharyngeal nerve *see* CRANIAL NERVES

glottal constrictions. total adduction of the glottis for producing EJECTIVES and IMPLOSIVES. It is a distinctive feature to mark place of articulation proposed by Chomsky and Halle. *See* Ladefoged (1993).

glottal stop the sound which occurs when the folds come closely together and are opened suddenly during a period of silence. It is represented by [ʔ]. In some varieties of Scottish-English, a glottal stop is very prevalent. In Glasgow, for example, it appears in words such as 'butter', [bʌʔə] and 'bottle', [bɔʔl]. *See* Ladefoged (1993).

glottalic airstream *see* IMPLOSIVE; EJECTIVE.

glottis the space which appears when the VOCAL FOLDS open. The space alters in size and shape depending on the type of sound which is produced. When the sound is voiced the vocal folds are open and vibrating whilst if it is voiceless the folds are closed. Breathy voice is produced by opening the folds slightly allowing the folds to vibrate while at the same time a lot of air rushes through the glottis. Creaky voice is produced by the folds vibrating only at one end while the other end is held together by the arytenoid cartilages (*see* ARYTENOIDS). This produces a low pitched sound. This type of voice can also be described as laryngealised. *See* Ladefoged (1993); Tortora and Grabowski (1993).

glue ear *see* OTITIS MEDIA (3).

Goldman-Fristoe Articulation Test this test is designed to discover which sounds a child has difficulty in producing. However, this test is different from the EDINBURGH ARTICULATION TEST in that the authors have put the emphasis on finding out in which part of the word the child makes an error. The results are scored in three columns headed word-initially, word-medially and word-finally. Not only are 'sound-in-

words' tested but also 'sounds-in-sentences'. In this subtest, the child has to listen and look at two sets of pictures while the therapist tells him the story. The child has to retell the story to the therapist producing as many of the words used by the therapist as he can recall. The scoring is carried out as in the first part of the test. *See* Goldman and Fristoe (1972) in Appendix I.

Goldman-Fristoe-Woodcock Auditory Skills Test Battery devised by Goldman and colleagues to diagnose an individual's ability to hear clearly under difficult conditions. It can be used with individuals between the ages of 3 and 85 years of age. There are twelve areas of measurement of auditory skills including: Auditory Selective Attention Test, Diagnostic Auditory Discrimination Test, various Auditory Memory tests and various sound symbol tests. *See* Goldman et al (1976) in Appendix I; Beech et al (1993).

Goodenough-Harris Drawing test devised by Goodenough and Harris in 1963, this is a test in which the child is asked to draw a man or a woman or a picture of him/herself. Scoring is of 73 characteristics specified in the Manual. The drawings can also be compared to twelve ranked drawings for each of the two scales of Man and Woman. The Manual includes restandardisation data of the Goodenough Draw-a-Man Test, the Draw-a-Woman Scale and an experimental Self-Drawing Scale. It covers an age range of 3;0–15;0 years. The test offers a relatively quick method of assessing general and cognitive development. *See* Goodenough and Harris (1963) in Appendix I.

Gower's sign a symptom found in Duchenne muscular dystrophy (*see* DYSTROPHY). During this disease, the person can have difficulty in standing from either a sitting or a lying position. Gower's sign is the means used by the person to establish a standing position. The person rolls over and pulls himself onto his hands and knees, then pushes up until he has a firm base on his hands and feet. The last stage is to make his feet walk up towards his hands until he can stand upright. *See* Gilroy and Holliday (1982).

Graded Naming Test devised by McKenna and Warrington in 1983, it is an assessment for adults with naming problems as a result of brain damage. The person is required to name 30 black and white drawings which are arranged in a hierarchy of difficulty. Raw scores can be interpreted by comparing them to the pre-morbid vocabulary of the person. The test was standardised on both normal volunteers and clients aged between 20 and 76 years of age who have extracerebral disorders. *See* McKenna and Warrington (1983) in Appendix I; Beech et al (1993).

Gradual Increase in Length and Complexity of Utterance (GILCU) a structured programme to establish fluency in the MONTEREY FLUENCY PROGRAMME (MFP) for those who STAMMER. The therapist asks the person to say one word fluently and then extends this through the highly structured programme until the person can speak fluently in the three modes of the MFP. Fluent speech is reinforced by saying the word 'good'; for those under 12 years, coloured tokens are used for additional reinforcement. *See* Monterey Fluency Programme.

grand-mal epilepsy *see* EPILEPSY.

granulation tissue a granular formation which can occur during healing, for example, in the arytenoid region. *See* Tortora and Grabowski (1993).

grave a DISTINCTIVE FEATURE proposed by Jakobson and Halle to distinguish sounds made at the back of the mouth such as back vowels, velars and labials [+GRAVE] (*see* ARTICULATION) from those made at the front of the mouth [–GRAVE]. It is opposed to ACUTE. *See* Hyman (1975).

greater horn of hyoid *see* PHARYNX.

greater wing of sphenoid *see* MUSCLES OF MASTICATION.

Griffith's Test a test for developmental milestones devised by Griffiths, it involves four elements of the child's development which have to be closely observed:

1. Does the child kick vigorously?
2. Does the child enjoy the bath?
3. Does the child push the feet against the parent's hand?
4. Does the child have strong arm movements?

All children from 1 to 3 months of age may be assessed by this test. *See* Illingworth (1987).

groove a description of the TONGUE when it has a groove along the central longitudinal line of the tongue. It is used for some fricatives (*see* ARTICULATION) such as [s,z,S,Z]. It is opposed to SLIT. *See* Catford (1989).

group design a design used for experiments. It is opposed to single case studies where statistical analysis attempts to show the effects of variables on single people. On the other hand, the group design is aimed at showing the effects of variables on groups of subjects which are either put into independent group designs, repeated measures or matched subjects design. *See* Miller (1975).

group therapy now used quite widely in place of individual therapy. It has many advantages:

1. Patients discover others with similar problems, thus creating support for one another.
2. Conversational situations can be created for context-oriented therapy so that the group can produce some functional communication.
3. More intensive therapy can be given.
4. Carry-over or maintenance is more likely.
5. A more stimulating environment is created, yet the patient is less tired than when given individual therapy

since the burden of responding is spread around the group.

6. The patient finds a social purpose.
7. The patient becomes more involved in therapy.
8. A potentially more effective learning situation is created.

Group therapy is used mainly with those who stammer, or have an aphasia or dysarthria, as well as children who have phonological problems. *See* Fawcus (1989, 1992); Clinical Forum in *Aphasiology* (1991) 5;6; Atkinson et al (1993); Bollinger et al (1993) (group therapy in aphasia); Davison and Neale (1994).

Guillain-Barré syndrome a condition produced by the ascending demyelination of the peripheral nerves. It is thought to be a virus originally and may respond to steroids. It results in motor weakness with associated pains in the shoulders and back. Breathing can be affected and a tracheotomy should be undertaken. In very severe cases, there can be DYSARTHRIA, APHASIA and diplopia. The paralysis ascends through the body. *See* Gilroy and Holliday (1982).

Guthrie test a test to screen newly born babies to check for such conditions as PHENYLKETONURIA. The heel is given a prick to remove some blood for examination. *See* Hosking (1982).

Gyrus, gyri the CEREBRAL HEMISPHERES are covered in grooves due to folding of the CORTEX during development. The gyri are the elevated areas while the sulci (*see* SULCUS) are the fissures. *See* Barr (1979); Kolb and Whishaw (1990).

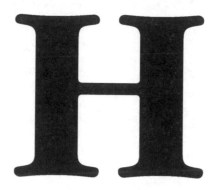

habilitation the process of therapy which aims to help the subject to recover to a level which allows him to function adequately within the community.

hallucination the person believes by using his senses that there is something in close proximity when there is nothing at all. However, it has a quality for the person. Auditory hallucination occurs when the person believes he hears a sound when nothing exists. Hallucinations occur in SCHIZOPHRENIA when those with the condition believe they sense audible thoughts, voices arguing and commenting. *See* Kolb and Whishaw (1990); Atkinson et al (1993); Davison and Neale (1994).

hallux *see* PLANTAR RESPONSE.

hamulus *see* PHARYNX.

haptic perception a combination of tactile perception and proprioception concerned with an individual's sense of his body in relation to space. Some children and adults with certain types of language disorder, mainly of a dyspraxic nature, appear to be deficient in respect of perceptuomotor functioning.

hard copy information which is both printed out on paper as well as appearing on a monitor screen. It is opposed to SOFT COPY. *See* Bishop (1985).

hard of hearing a description of a person whose hearing, though impaired, is used as a primary modality for auditory speech perception and language acquisition.

hardware the actual units which make up a computerised system such as the computer itself, the monitor, the disk drive, printer and any other peripheral unit. Its opposite is SOFTWARE. *See* Bishop (1985); Brookshear (1991).

harmonic *see* ACOUSTIC PHONETICS.

harsh voice a type of DYSPHONIA with the essential feature being tension in the VOCAL FOLDS. The cause can be behavioural such as excessive tension. Therapy is aimed at decreasing tension in the person generally, as well as particularly in the vocal folds. General relaxation or relaxation through suggestion can be used effectively so that the person can learn how to relax spontaneously when in stress-provoking situations. The YAWN/SIGH or chewing approach can be used to decrease tension in the vocal folds. *See* Fawcus (1991).

head injury trauma to the BRAIN which can have widespread effects on the person's daily life. A closed head injury is caused by the brain being knocked against the skull. This is known as the contrecoup effect. In essence, the brain is a mass of tissue surrounded by fluid, so any heavy blow to the head, e.g. punch, hitting it on the ground from a fall, will result in it moving rapidly to the back or side of the skull. Such sudden movement can cause the blood vessels to rupture. The consequences are concussion and bruising which causes haemorrhages and clots. Focal deficits produce HEMIPLEGIA, various degrees of APHASIA or DYSARTHRIA or acquired dyspraxia and problems as a result of damage to the CRANIAL NERVES. Global deficits produce loss of consciousness, disinhibition and memory deficits. Later complications can include post-concussion syndrome, HYDROCEPHALUS, DEMENTIA and fits. Medical treatment takes the form of steroids. The person with minor symptoms has a good prognosis but those severely impaired need a structured therapeutic programme, preferably in a rehabilitation unit. Those who have a head injury will probably require therapeutic intervention from various therapies such as OCCUPATIONAL THERAPY, PHYSIOTHERAPY and SPEECH AND LANGUAGE THERAPY. CLINICAL PSYCHOLOGY may also be involved. See Gilroy and Holliday (1982); Kolb and Wishaw (1990); Kaye (1991).

HeadMaster a mouse emulator system allowing those unable to use their hands to operate a computer. It does this by taking the place of the mouse. As the clients move their heads, HeadMaster measures the rotation of their head and moves the cursor on the screen. Activating the puff switch or single switch makes a selection. On-screen keyboards such as WiViK allow for hands-free typing and other keyboard functions. HeadMaster can be used with an IBM PC or compatible in Windows environment or mouse driven software or an Apple Mac. The same HeadMaster can be used for all computers and as a Remote HeadMaster by changing the configuration of three switches on the side of the control unit. The system comprises a control unit, a headset, a cable to link the control unit to the serial socket on the computer and another cable to link the headset to the control unit. A charging unit has to be attached to the control box at all times. The Remote HeadMaster allows the client to operate the computer without the cable linking the headset to the control unit, but it operates in the same way as the ordinary HeadMaster. See Appendix IV.

HeadMouse a mouse emulator system allowing those unable to use their hands to operate a computer. There is no headset or cables required, only a small reuseable sticker placed on the forehead, glasses, chin, finger or foot etc.; the optical sensor tracks the person's head movements. It is used with an Apple Macintosh computer. See Appendix IV.

hearing aid a device given to those who have a hearing loss. It works by taking in the sound vibrations from the air and converting them into electrical signals. These signals are amplified and converted back to sound waves which are sent via the earmould to the ear. To allow this to happen, the hearing aid consists of a microphone (for picking up the sound and converting it to electrical signals), amplifier (makes the signal stronger), receiver (receives the signal and converts it back to a sound signal, sending it through the tubing to the earmould in the auditory canal), battery (to power the aid) and the earmould (to make sure sound gets into ear). If the earmould does not fit in the canal correctly, sound leaks out causing feedback (a whistling sound). There are also buttons and dials used to control volume, switch it on/off (O = off, M = microphone (on), T = telecoil (to be used where there is a loop system)). There are different types of aid:

1. Body aids where the receiver is far from the microphone and amplifier. The sound signals are taken by a Y-cord to the earmoulds in each ear or

through a single cord to the ear-mould.

2. Ear level aids have the microphone at the top or bottom of the body of the aid facing forward. These are relatively inconspicuous but feedback is more common than with body aids.

3. In-the-ear aids are only suitable for low level losses. The components are built into a shell made from an impression of the client's ear.

4. CROS (contralateral routing of signals): hearing aids were originally used to pick up the sound in the deaf ear and send it to the good ear on the other side. This type of hearing aid is best suited for clients who have a rapidly falling audiogram of the 'ski-slope' type (*see* PURE-TONE AUDIOMETRY). This is because it cuts out the low frequencies it receives but produces good amplification in the higher frequencies. The signal is carried by a cord from one side of the head to the other. Nowadays, there are cordless CROS hearing aids, in which sound is picked up on one side and activates a small radio transmitter on that side. The radio waves pass through the head and are picked up by a small radio receiver on the other side. The sound waves are amplified and sent to the receiver and the open delivery tube in the ear canal.

5. BICROS (bilateral contralateral routing of signals): hearing aids are similar to CROS hearing aids but use two microphones, one on each side of the head. These are connected to the same amplifier with a single receiver coupled to the better but impaired ear, using a closed earmould to avoid feedback.

6. IROS (ipsilateral routing of signals): IROS hearing aids are standard hearing aids with an open earmould on the same side. It can be used with ear-level aids with the tubing entering the ear canal. It is a very useful type of aid for those who have a mild

to moderate, falling sensorineural loss and can be used binaurally. The only problem may be that feedback is more likely than with the CROS hearing aids.

See Miller (1972); Lysons (1978); Katz (1985).

hearing level the number of decibels above audiometric zero at which a client can hear sound. It is used in PURE-TONE AUDIOMETRY.

hearing loss a description of a person's hearing when the results of audiological assessment, e.g. PURE-TONE AUDIOMETRY, show that there is a varying degree of difficulty in receiving sound. There are several types of hearing loss such as CONDUCTIVE HEARING LOSS, SENSORINEURAL HEARING LOSS, mixed hearing loss, CENTRAL HEARING LOSS, CONGENITAL HEARING LOSS and ACQUIRED HEARING LOSS. *See* Katz (1985); Atkinson et al (1993); Plant (1993) (acquired hearing loss).

hearing threshold level (HTL) the smallest sound with a given frequency which someone can hear 50 per cent of the time.

heart the heart is divided into four areas – the right and left atria and the right and left ventricles. The heart pumps blood around the body. Blood enters the heart by the inferior and superior vena cavae into the right atrium which contracts and pushes the blood through the tricuspid valve to the right ventricle. The ventricle pushes the blood through the pulmonary valve into the pulmonary artery from where it goes to the lung; here it picks up oxygen, turns bright red and returns to the heart via the pulmonary veins, entering the left atrium. When it contracts, the blood is pushed through the mitral valve into the left ventricle which in turn pushes the blood through the aortic valve into the aorta. As it goes along this artery, it passes into other arteries of the body, arterioles (smaller arteries) and the capillaries where it loses oxygen and becomes dark blue. From these different areas of the body, the blood flows back to the heart. When the heart muscle contracts, it is a period of systole, when it relaxes, it is known as a period of diastole. *See* Tortora and Grabowski (1993).

Hector speech aid   an aid to help people who STAMMER to become more fluent speakers. It consists of a throat microphone placed against the LARYNX, a small amplifier and a control box which can be attached to a waist belt or put in a pocket. The microphone can be hidden under a high collar of a blouse, shirt or jumper. Its aim is to decrease the rate of the person's speech and hence allow the speaker to produce a type of PROLONGED SPEECH. If the speaker has a very fast rate of speech, it is picked up by the microphone and a tone is produced through the amplifier. The volume of the tone can be turned up or down so that it can blend into the background noise. It can be used for practice at home and during speech therapy sessions.

Helpmate   an early high tech means of communicating which has a display that can hold 40 characters actuated by a QWERTY keyboard. Each key has an associated word or phrase, so by touching the 'phrase key' followed by a letter, the preset word or phrase will appear on the screen. The memory can store a whole message of up to 250 characters in length. It has a rechargeable battery but can also work off the mains. It measures 350×199×100mm and weighs 2.7 kg without the battery and 3.6 kg with the battery. A clip-on finger guard is provided for those with motor difficulties.

hemiplegia   the result of trauma to the brain such as CEREBROVASCULAR ACCIDENT, HEAD INJURY or other trauma or disease which produces a focal lesion in the BRAIN. Two limbs are affected, usually the arm and leg on one side of the body. If the lesion occurs in the left cerebral hemisphere (*see* CEREBRAL HEMISPHERES), the hemiplegia will affect the person's right side. In such circumstances, ANASOGNOSIA can occur. PHYSIOTHERAPY is given to those with hemiplegia as well as OCCUPATIONAL THERAPY to increase upper limb function. *See* Kolb and Whishaw (1990).

herpes simplex   usually a simple virus infection of the skin which is self-healing but may be recurrent, producing cold sores. Rarely it may cause ENCEPHALITIS. Both children and adults are affected, with an equal sex ratio. The person presents symptoms similar to those of flu, e.g. headache, fever, followed by irritation to the MENINGES, and becomes disoriented in space. Later psychosis and memory problems can occur as well as APHASIA and monoparesis (one limb only is affected by weakness). The final stage is a coma. If a mother has this infection during pregnancy, it can cross the placenta and cause disorders to the fetus. It is part of the TORCH classification of infections which affect the fetus. *See* Gilroy and Holliday (1982).

hertz (Hz)   *see* ACOUSTIC PHONETICS.

hesitation   periods of silence or FILLED PAUSES while the speaker either thinks of more information or reiterates and amplifies what has been said. Certain positions have been found in an utterance where hesitation occurs. These are at certain appropriate places in the grammar of the utterance, after other constituents and at the beginning of an utterance before the speaker has decided finally how to continue the utterance. *See* Clark and Clark (1977).

hierarchy   a structure which starts with one unit at the top and has branches linking it to lower units. A TREE DIAGRAM is a type of hierarchical structure. The units above other units are called superordinate terms while the units below other units are subordinate terms. In the tree diagram, 'sentence' is superordinate to NOUN PHRASE and verb phrase (*see* CONSTITUENT ANALYSIS, while DETERMINER, ADJECTIVE, NOUN are subordinate to noun phrase. *See* Lyons (1968); Fromkin and Rodman (1993).

high a DISTINCTIVE FEATURE proposed by Chomsky and Halle to distinguish sounds produced with the tongue in a raised position of the mouth [+HIGH] from those produced with the tongue in a low position [–HIGH]. *See* Hyman (1975).

high frequency hearing loss the person who has this type of hearing loss is unable to perceive a high frequency such as some of the fricatives (*see* ARTICULATION).

high-level language in computer terms, the type of computer language used for writing a majority of computer programs. BASIC, FORTRAN, Pascal, etc. are examples of high-level languages. Such a language is independent of the type of machine used and it is easier to write application programs. High-level languages are made up from statements of English words, base ten numbers and mathematical notation. Each statement is specific to the task in question which makes it easier to find errors in the statement as well as write a program logically. *See* Bishop (1985).

hindbrain part of the brain which comprises the PONS, MEDULLA OBLONGATA and the CEREBELLUM. It is found below the MIDBRAIN. *See* Barr (1979); Kolb and Whishaw (1990).

histogram a type of graph used in DESCRIPTIVE STATISTICS to analyse the results of an experiment. It shows the frequency distribution of scores. It is also known as a bar chart. *See* Miller (1975).

hoarse voice a type of DYSPHONIA produced by the person straining to speak against the tension of the VOCAL FOLDS. Wilson (1979) described it as a 'combination of harshness and breathiness with harsh voice predominating in some cases and breathy elements in others.' *See* Fawcus (1991).

homeostasis the body has to keep in balance its intake and output of substances. Intake refers to what a person consumes while ouput refers to the working of the excretory pathways via the kidneys. *See* J.H. Green (1978); Atkinson et al (1993); Tortora and Grabowski (1993).

homonymy a phenomenon in SEMANTICS in which a lexical item can appear in different contexts with the same pronunciation but not necessarily the same spelling, and have at least two different meanings. Such words are homonyms. The form 'bear' has two meanings one of which is a noun referring to a type of animal, and the other a verb which is a synonym of 'carry'. *See* Palmer (1976); Fromkin and Rodman (1993).

homophony a phenomenon in semantic theory in which two words pronounced the same have a different meaning. Such words are called homophones. Examples are 'sun/son', 'boy/buoy', etc. *See* Palmer (1976); Fromkin and Rodman (1993).

homorganic a phenomenon where two articulations are made by the same articulators (*see* ARTICULATION). Thus, [p] and [b] can be described as homorganic sounds as they are both produced by two lips. *See* Ladefoged (1993).

hormones *see* ENDOCRINE SYSTEM.

host computer a computer from which data are sent to other computers being used as terminals. These terminals may have a direct link to the host computer or be linked by telegraph or telephone systems. *See* Bishop (1985).

HTL *see* HEARING THRESHOLD LEVEL.

Huntington's disease a rare autosomal dominant (*see* CHROMOSOMES) disease producing DEMENTIA. The onset of the disease occurs in middle age. The person's personality becomes psychopathic, violent and a dependence on alcohol begins. The person shows a tremor at distal parts of the muscles and athetotic (*see* CEREBRAL PALSY) movement begins. Although there is no treatment available for this condition, L-dopa (*see* LEVODOPA) is given to stop the tremor. It is caused by problems in the caudate nucleus and BASAL GANGLIA. *See* Stafford-Clark and Smith (1983); Kolb and Whishaw (1990); Atkinson et al (1993).

hydrocephalus a condition in which an abnormal volume of CSF is found in the skull. It can be caused by a tumour in close proximity to the FOURTH VENTRICLE with evidence of intracranial pressure increase. It can be treated by ventricular drainage. The incidence of infantile hydrocephalus is about 3-4 per 1000 and most children present with congenital abnormalities. The major clinical features in infants include: (1) FAILURE TO THRIVE; (2) Failure to achieve milestones; (3) Increased skull circumference; (4) Tense anterior fontanelle; (5) A cracked pot sound on skull when hit; (6) Being able to see through the skull when a strong light is held against it. In severe cases, there are also the following clinical features: (1) Impaired conscious level and vomiting; (2) 'Setting suns' appearance; (3) Thin scalp with dilated veins. The Arnold-Chiari malformation may also produce hydrocephalus. This malformation is produced by a disorder to the MEDULLA OBLONGATA and CEREBELLUM causing an obstruction for the CEREBROSPINAL FLUID. There are three types which differ mainly by severity. In adults, the major clinical features are headache, vomiting, papilloedema and deterioration of conscious state. *See* Gilroy and Holliday (1982); Kolb and Whishaw (1990); Kaye (1991); Tortora and Grabowski (1993).

hyoid bone *see* MUSCLES FOR SWALLOWING; Tortora and Grabowski (1993).

hyperkinetic dysarthria *see* DYSA-RTHRIA (1a).

hypernasality a condition caused by the failure of the soft palate (*see* MOUTH) to close when producing speech. This produces sounds which are both nasal

and oral. This can be caused by large ADENOIDS.

hyperplasia excessive growth of a tissue or of certain cells. *See* Tortora and Grabowski (1993).

hypertonia an abnormal amount of power in limbs. It refers to increased muscle tone and is expressed in terms of spasticity (*see* CEREBRAL PALSY). There is a stiffness in the muscles and increase in tendon reflexes and rigidity. Rigidity is an increase in muscle tone which does not affect the reflexes. *See* Tortora and Grabowski (1993).

hypochondriasis a NEUROSIS in which a person's life becomes tortured by fears of having contracted some serious disease. In most cases, such people have ordinary illnesses which can be as minor as an irregular heartbeat, sweating, minor cough, etc. Men tend to have this condition more than women. It is very difficult to reassure them that their illness is not as serious as they believe. The condition can be a symptom of depression. *See* Stafford-Clark and Smith (1983); Davison and Neale (1994).

hypoglossal nerve *see* INTRINSIC MUSCLES OF THE TONGUE; CRANIAL NERVES.

hypoglossus muscle *see* EXTRINSIC MUSCLES OF THE TONGUE.

hypokinetic dysarthria *see* DYSA-RTHRIA (1b).

hypoplasia a description of an anatomical structure which has not developed as fully as it should. *See* Tortora and Grabowski (1993).

hypothalamus a small structure in the DIENCEPHALON found below the THALAMUS forming the floor and part of the lateral walls of the THIRD VENTRICLE. It is important for regulating sleep, thirst, hunger and temperature within the body. It affects the AUTONOMIC NERVOUS SYSTEM. *See* Barr (1979); Kolb and Whishaw (1990); Atkinson et al (1993); Tortora and Grabowski (1993).

hypotonia a description of flaccidity found in muscles. *See* Draper (1980); Tortora and Grabowski (1993).

hysteria a NEUROSIS in which stress becomes so overwhelming that, unconsciously, the person presents, and may even experience, symptoms of physical illness. Stress can also be shown by severe mental illness, e.g. DEPRESSION, SCHIZOPHRENIA. Minor hysteria causes a loss in or interference with the person's normal or sensory function. Such problems take the form of blindness, deafness, anaesthesia, PARAPHASIA and paralysis or disturbance of motor activity. The symptoms must be primarily physical. Treatment involves the removal of the underlying stress and/or depression. PSYCHOTHERAPY or hypnosis have also been used successfully to remove such symptoms. *See* Stafford-Clark and Smith (1983); Davison and Neale (1994).

hysterical dysphonia *see* CONVERSION DYSPHONIA; Fawcus (1991).

Hz (hertz) *see* ACOUSTIC PHONETICS.

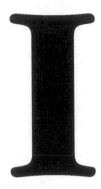

IA item and arrangement *see* MORPHOLOGY.

icon

1. There are arbitrary conventions in semiotics. However, icons are fixed signs such as onomatopoeic words 'splash', 'crack' and 'bang'. The form of these words can never change. *See* Robins (1971).
2. A symbol on a display. Instead of using the keyboard to operate the computer, icon programs can now be used for this purpose. When icons are called up, they appear in windows and the operator has to use a pointer to choose the appropriate icons. In some programs, the cursor keys can be used, others may require the use of a mouse, touchscreen or light pen. Icon programs are also known as icon software.
3. Symbols used on high-tech electronic devices using MINSPEAK such as WALKER TALKERS, ALPHA TALKERS, TOUCH TALKERS, LIGHT TALKERS, DELTA TALKERS, INTRO TALKERS and the LIBERATOR COMMUNICATION AID.

ICP *see* INTRACRANIAL PRESSURE.

ID *see* PERSONALITY.

ideal self *see* PHENOMENOLOGICAL APPROACH.

idiolect a term used for the individual linguistic system of a particular speaker – his or her dialect. There are regional dialects which have different variations of the spoken language. However, there are also differences of dialect between people in that they have particular ways of producing utterances which are different from other people. Idiolect continues to develop after a child has fully acquired language as the child picks up modifications from the language of his family. Haas (1963) writes of a child's phonological disorder as being 'a language of his own or idiolect'. In an important passage, he writes why speech therapists need to know about idiolect: 'It would seem speech therapy stands to gain in efficiency, if, to a greater extent than has been usual, it could take account of the underlying and interfering "idiolect" of the treated child' (Haas, 1963, p. 246). *See* Trudgill (1974); Fromkin and Rodman (1993).

idiom a phrase whose meaning is not given by analysing its constituent parts, e.g. 'kick the bucket', 'play the field'. *See* Lyons (1968); Fromkin and Rodman (1993).

idiopathic a disease which has no known cause.

IEP+ *see* INTERACTION, EDUCATION AND PLAY.

ill-formed a description of sentences which are ungrammatical in terms of a particular set of grammatical rules, i.e. they cannot be generated by the rule. It is found in discussions concerning

GENERATIVE GRAMMAR. If a sentence cannot be generated, it is ill-formed. *See* Huddleston (1976).

Illinois Test of Psycholinguistic Abilities (ITPA) a formal, standarised assessment devised by Kirk in 1969. It can be used with children aged 2–10 years old, although it is less useful for children below the chronological age of 4 years. It has twelve subtests: auditory reception; visual reception; visual sequential memory; auditory association; auditory sequential memory; visual association; visual closure; verbal expression; grammatical closure; manual expression; auditory closure; and sound blending. The raw score from these subtests together produce a psycholinguistic age or separate scaled scores. These scores can be drawn on a graph to show each child's psycholinguistic abilities. *See* Kirk et al (1969) in Appendix I; Paraskevopoulus, and Kirk (1985) in Appendix I; Beech et al (1993).

illocution a term used in speech act theories to denote the way in which a speaker intends his utterance to be taken. Examples are promising, requesting and regretting. In some types of language disorder, speakers are not able to convey their intention accurately. *See* Fromkin and Rodman (1993).

imitation

1. A process which has been proposed to explain the child's language acquisition as the imitation of sounds, words and sentences used by adults in his immediate environment. The realisation that children produced 'errors' never heard in their language environment, e.g. goed, camed, casts immediate doubt on the validity of imitation as a complete explanation. Imitation, however, is often used in language remediation by speech and language therapists. *See* Clark and Clark (1977); Fromkin and Rodman (1993).

2. A form of therapy given to those who have poor social skills. It is a difficult form of therapy as the instructor has to provide almost impeccable social skills for the person to try and copy exactly. *See* Trower et al (1978); Atkinson et al (1993).

IMPACT: Implementing Augmentative Communication Training a training programme to help those who work with communication aid users to implement the devices more successfully. There are many factors which work together to develop Augmented Communication skills. If any of these fail or the significant others helping the user of the device fail to realise something is wrong with the way they are trying to implement the Augmented System, the system itself may fail and the user or the device will be blamed. This programme tries to bring to the attention of those working with the device, what these factors are, how they may fail, and how they can put them right based on the experience of the author and his colleagues. The programme is divided into two parts – the first is a series of cartoons featuring the many situations in which devices may fail while the second part has notes on each topic presented by the cartoons. There is also an extensive bibliography of over 1000 references on AAC. *See* Jones (1995a).

impairment a disease or injury which causes people certain difficulties in functioning. For example, if a lesion in the BRAIN affects the motor coordination of the speech mechanism producing DYSARTHRIA, the person is said to have an impairment in the affected part of the brain.

impedance the opposition offered by an object to the transmission of sound or some acoustic energy. The greater the impedance, the less sound will be transmitted. It is opposed to COMPLIANCE.

impedance audiometry there are three types of impedance measures:

1. Static impedance which is measured when the pressure in the external auditory canal equals the atmospheric pressure and the muscles of the middle ear (*see* EAR) are at rest.

2. Dynamic impedance is measured when the tympanic membrane (*see* EAR) is moved suddenly from its position at rest by the contraction of the stapedius (*see* EAR) muscle, i.e. it shows the amount of reflected energy as a function of change in the position of and stiffness of the tympanic membrane.

3. Tympanometry measures changes to impedance with variations of pressure in the external auditory canal (*see* EAR).

The impedance bridge or impedance audiometer comprises three small rubber tubes which are attached to a small metal probe. One is attached to a miniature microphone which picks up the sound in the canal, another to a loudspeaker which puts a pure tone (*see* PURE-TONE AUDIOMETRY) of 220 Hz into the ear, and the third is attached to an air pump which creates either a positive or a negative pressure in the canal. An air-tight seal is created when the probe is placed in the canal. The results from static compliance are not particularly useful for making a diagnosis while the results from dynamic impedance are important. If there is a stapedius reflex, it indicates hearing is normal, the middle ear is functioning normally (if obtained at normal HL), or there is a sensory hearing loss (if obtained at a low SL). If there is no stapedius reflex this indicates a facial nerve (*see* CRANIAL NERVE VII) lesion is present on the side of the tested ear, there is a problem with the ossicles (*see* EAR), a CONDUCTIVE HEARING LOSS on the side of earphone (i.e. sound is not loud enough in the ear to elicit reflex), or a severe to profound SENSORINEURAL

HEARING LOSS in the earphone ear. The results from tympanometry are in the form of diagrams. Jerger found five types:

1. Type A – indicated normal middle ear function.

2. Type As (shallow) – indicates normal middle ear pressure and a partially immobilised stapes (possible OTOSCLEROSIS).

3. Type Ad (deep) – indicates malfunctioning of the ossicles (*see* EAR) producing high compliance;

4. Type B – indicates that the middle ear is filled with fluid, which makes it impossible to find a point of maximum compliance.

5. Type C – indicates negative pressure in the middle ear produced by a blockage in the eustachian tube (*see* EAR) causing serous otitis media (*see* OTITIS MEDIA (3)).

implosive a glottalic ingressive voiced stop. It is very difficult to produce voice with an ejective stop, while devoicing may be difficult with implosives. The sequence of movements for producing an implosive is:

1. Close the glottis.

2. Make a closure of the lips (e.g. [ɓ]).

3. Move the larynx downward (compare taking a gulp).

4. Release the closure.

5. A voiced implosive [ɓ] is produced.

See Catford (1977).

imprinting a learning process usually referring to the type of learning used by young birds to form an attachment to their parents. It takes place at a critical period just after birth and ends when a parent model is learned. *See* Atkinson et al (1993).

INCH *see* INTERACTION CHECKLIST FOR AUGMENTATIVE COMMUNICATION.

independent group design an experimental design which uses two groups, each randomly selected. One group is a control group while the other is the experimental group. *See* Miller (1975).

indirect object the term traditionally used for the syntactic relation obtaining between the verb and either a prepositional phrase (to Nara) as in (1) or the first noun phrase (Nara), as in (2), with verbs like 'give' in English:

(1) Joyce gave the book to Nara.
(2) Joyce gave Nara the book.

See Lyons (1968).

industrial hearing loss *see* NOISE-INDUCED HEARING LOSS.

infantile autism *see* AUTISM.

infantile swallowing pattern a persisting immature pattern of swallowing involving anterior tongue thrust. It may be associated with dental malocclusion and with articulatory disorder.

inferential statistics a study of statistics in which statistical tests are used to show whether or not a significant difference exists between the control and experimental groups. It also allows the experimenter to generalise the result of one small group to other groups of people. The tests which can be used are divided into parametric and non-parametric tests (*see* PARAMETRIC TESTS). *See* Miller (1975).

informal assessments assessments which do not have a fixed format. They are evolved by the therapist to assess a person's difficulties, if the person is unable to cope with a formal assessment, or used during therapy to assess the efficacy of a therapy programme. Such tests allow more latitude which may, by giving cues, discover how much and what kind of help the person requires to succeed. Material used in such tests must be different from the material used in formal assessments so as not to invalidate the results used later in therapy.

information processing a model of language in which there are three main components involved – a receiver, whereby information is taken in, i.e. the sensory channels in the case of language; an integrator which is responsible for perception of the incoming stimuli and for their storage in memory and a response system.

infra- a description of the area below the structure to which the prefix is attached.

infraglottic a description of the whole area including the structures below the glottis.

ingressive *see* AIRSTREAMS.

inhalation *see* OESOPHAGEAL VOICE.

initial interview the first session that a therapist or any other professional has with a client. This session is important for setting up a rapport with the client and any accompanying relatives and for taking a sufficient case history. The initial interview normally has six stages:

1. Introduction: often called 'meeting, greeting and seating' (Nelson-Jones 1982). It is important to make the client feel as comfortable as possible at this stage since therapy of any kind can be seen as a threat. There can also be a stigma attached to coming for therapy. On the other hand, some clients may have their hopes raised too high and expect therapists to be miracle workers.

2. Assessment of the presenting disorder: this can be either a formal assessment or an informal assessment (*see* ASSESSMENTS) to find out what the client can or cannot do. This should be explained to the client as some of the subtests can be very easy while others may be more difficult.

3. Exploration of presenting disorder: this is really the case history, finding out how the disorder occurred and how it affects family life and the relationships within the home.

4. Reconnaissance: the therapist tries to find out how the client views him/herself since the onset of the disorder and examines the history of the disorder.

5. Contracting: takes place when the therapist and client come to an agree-

ment on the type of therapy which the client will begin to receive regularly.

6. Termination: the final stage where the therapist clears up any confusions which may have arisen from this initial interview and, most importantly, another appointment is made.

During these six stages, the therapist should have in mind the following four interrelated objectives:

1. Creating a 'working alliance', i.e. a good rapport with the client.
2. Forming a 'working model' of the client, i.e. client's feeling concerning change in lifestyle and aspirations for the future.
3. Forming 'working goals', i.e. treatment programme.
4. Deciding which therapy method to use.

See Nelson-Jones (1982).

injection *see* OESOPHAGEAL SPEECH.

innateness a theory to explain how people learn. Noam Chomsky used this theory to explain the language ACQUISITION of children. He believes humans are born with several different areas in their brains for specific functions. Language is one of these areas. This innate knowledge of language has become known as the LANGUAGE ACQUISITION DEVICE. It is LAD which sparks off the hypothetical language area in the child's brain. *See* Steinberg (1982); Atkinson et al (1993)

input devices various means for the operator to communicate commands to the computer. These include a MOUSE, LIGHT PEN, CONCEPT KEYBOARD, TOUCH SCREEN and speech recognition systems such as MICROVOICE. Such devices are used if the operator has a physical handicap and finds it difficult to operate a normal QWERTY keyboard. *See* Brookshear (1991); Beukelman and Mirenda (1992).

insufflation *see* OESOPHAGEAL VOICE.

INTECOM devised by Jones in 1989, it is a programme to help develop the communication skills of clients with learning difficulties. It maximises functional communication, optimising a person's existing skills and communication opportunities. It is in two parts:

1. Programme planning package: it contains a rapid communication checklist, so that the therapist can plan a communication opportunities programme for each client.
2. Training package: speech and language therapists and psychologists can use this package to train carers and teachers how to develop communication skills through the use of the Communication Checklist and Programme Planner.

The programme planning package contains ten communication checklists and a manual, while the training package contains training notes and other necessary materials to run training courses in basic communication theory. *See* Jones (1989) in Appendix I.

intelligence the ability to learn skills necessary for normal living. Sternberg (1981, 1982) put forward four components which go to make up intelligence:

1. Ability to learn and profit from experience.
2. Ability to reason or think abstractly.
3. Ability to adapt to the vagaries of a changing and uncertain world.
4. Ability to motivate oneself to accomplish expeditiously the tasks one needs to accomplish.

See Atkinson et al (1993); Davison and Neale (1994).

intelligence quotient (IQ) the score obtained from carrying out an intelligence test. It is calculated by using the formula:

$$IQ = MA/CA \times 100$$

This reads 'the client's IQ is his mental age (MA) divided by his chronological age (CA) multiplied by 100 and rounded to bring the result to a whole number'. *See* Kolb and Whishaw (1990); Atkinson et al (1993).

intelligence tests psychological tests are aimed at finding out the ability of the child or adult to carry out various tasks presented to him usually without reference to previous learned material. Psychological testing tends to be controversial but there are safeguards built into most tests to make as sure as possible that the scores obtained are reliable and valid (*see* VALIDITY). The controversy surrounding the tests arises from a number of misconceptions. Some believe intelligence tests measure innate intelligence and that IQs are fixed and cannot be changed; they measure all one needs to know about the client's intelligence. IQs obtained from several tests are interchangeable and a battery of tests tells the psychologists all they need to know to enable them to make judgements about a person's competence. All such beliefs can be countered by arguing that test results should not be taken at face value but that any interpretation put on them must take into account other factors such as case history information as well as any behaviour disorder which the client may have, his temperament, e.g. fatigue, language disorders, etc., at the time of testing. In certain parts of the country, it will be necessary to take into account the child's cultural background. It is, therefore, important to note the time of testing and the appropriateness of the test used. Intelligence tests which are most frequently used include: (1) STANFORD-BINET INTELLIGENCE SCALE; (2) BRITISH ABILITY SCALES; (3) WECHSLER INTELLIGENCE SCALE FOR CHILDREN (REVISED) (WISC-R); (4) WECHSLER ADULT INTELLIGENCE SCALES (WAIS); (5) MERRILL-PALMER PRE-SCHOOL PERFORMANCE SCALE; (6) RAVEN'S PROGRESSIVE MATRICES and vocabulary scales. *See* Atkinson et al (1993); Davison and Neale (1994).

intention tremor a tremor caused by a disorder to the CEREBELLUM. The person's limb produces an observable tremor when specific movements are made. *See* Gilroy and Holliday (1982).

Interaction Checklist for Augmentative Communication (INCH) a checklist devised in 1984 by Bolton and Dashiell so that a therapist can decide on the most important needs for communication aid users to communicate to their caregivers and friends and relations. It looks at strategies used in a communicative exchange. It distinguishes four types of strategy: initiation, facilitation, regulation and termination. INCH also examines the modes or means by which messages are communicated. It looks at five major types of modes using verbal and non-verbal communication: linguistic, paralinguistic, kinesic (non-verbal communication such as facial expression and body movement including eye contact, etc.), proxemic (distance between those communicating) and chronemic (timing of responses and rate at which communication takes place). Finally, INCH analyses the contexts in which a communication aid will be used, i.e. those who will use it (both user and receiver) as well as the situations in which it will be used, e.g. at school, at home, in a restaurant or in hospital, etc. The authors have divided participants into four classes depending on the degree of familiarity or unfamiliarity with the user and on their competency with the user's communication aid. The four classes are: familiar-trained, familiar-untrained, unfamiliar-trained, unfamiliar-untrained. In general, by administering INCH, the authors hope to provide a 'systematic observation of interaction between augmentative system users and their receivers' (Bolton and Dashiell, 1984 p. 14). *See* Bolton and Dashiell (1984) in Appendix I.

Interaction, Education and Play (IEP+) devised by Bruno in 1988 and revised in 1990 (IEP+), it is a MINSPEAK APPLICA-

TION PROGRAM (MAP) for children with a mental age of 3;6–9;0. The icon set and prestored vocabulary need to reflect the user's abilities, needs, experiences, interests and goals. The user must be able to use a 128-location overlay with a cognitive/language performance at the 3;6 year level. The prestored vocabulary takes into account the following speech acts: (1) greeting and social exchanges; (2) protests and negative comments; (3) requests and clarification; (4) information; (5) requests. All these speech acts can be accessed by not more than two icon actuations. A single word lexicon is also available. A simple vocabulary can be accessed by using two icons. Commonly used words can be accessed so that the user can produce grammatically correct messages. A group of words can be accessed for classroom use. The system can also be used in play, accessing story books, rhymes amd songs as well as high interest vocabulary items. *See* Bruno (1989).

interdental *see* ARTICULATION.

interface the attachment of a central processor to various peripheral units. For example, when a printer or disk drive (*see* DISK) is linked to a computer, they are said to interface with the computer. This type of interface is sometimes called a master/slave interface because one machine, e.g. computer, has control over one or more machines, e.g. disk drive and printer. *See* Bishop (1985).

internal carotid artery *see* CAROTID ARTERY.

International Phonetic Alphabet (IPA) a system of symbols used in transcribing a person's speech. It was devised by the International Phonetic Association which was inaugurated in 1886 by a small group of language teachers in France who found phonetics useful in their work. The Association produced the IPA chart (1951, revised 1979 and 1989) which

divides up the sounds into place and manner of articulation (*see* ARTICULATION) for consonants. It also shows the CARDINAL VOWEL SYSTEM as well as a list of the DIACRITICS which can be used in narrow transcriptions (*see* TRANSCRIPTION SYSTEMS). *See* Appendix III; Abercrombie (1967); Duckworth (1990); Fromkin and Rodman (1993).

intervocalic a consonantal sound which appears between two vowels, e.g. /t/ in 'butter' where the /t/ sound is intervocalic.

intonation *see* SUPRASEGMENTAL PHONOLOGY.

intracranial pressure (ICP) pressure within the cranium produced by the amount of CEREBROSPINAL FLUID, blood and size of brain. If the pressure varies slightly in one area, another area can compensate. Large lesions to a particular area may be so significant that no compensation can take place and the pressure is increased with resultant damage to other structures. *See* Hosking (1982); Kaye (1991).

intraoral a description of structures or disorders which appear in the mouth itself.

intraoral pressure the build-up of pressure in the MOUTH to allow a person to produce the sounds for speech. For those who have a CLEFT PALATE, this pressure is usually lacking.

intrinsic muscles of the tongue the TONGUE has three intrinsic muscles which, with the three extrinsic muscles (*see* EXTRINSIC MUSCLES OF THE TONGUE), control its movement. The intrinsic muscles are named longitudinal, transverse and vertical. They are supplied by the hypoglossal nerve (*see* CRANIAL NERVE XII). The vertical muscle fibres pull the sides of the tongue down while the transverse muscle fibres help lengthen the tongue. *See* Tortora and Grabowski (1993).

Intro Talker a high-tech communication aid with digitised speech output. It uses MINSPEAK to organise vocabulary to store into the device. The Intro Talker uses an 8- or 32-location overlay with Minspeak icons which can be used in sequences to produce the required utterances. It has a memory of one minute standard speech and two minutes extended speech. The Intro Talker has a rechargeable battery which should be recharged regularly. If the battery becomes low, the machine will produce its own message 'battery low' and the LED lamp will flash on and off. The machine remains on when programmed for a particular client. If it is switched off (the main on/off switch is inside the machine), the contents in the memory will be lost. See Appendix IV. There are two models of Intro Talker, POINT AND SCAN INTRO TALKER and REMOTE-SWITCH INTRO TALKER.

Intro Talker IEP+ devised by Cross in 1991, it is a MINSPEAK APPLICATION PROGRAM (MAP) for use originally with the INTRO TALKER but can also be used with the ALPHA TALKER. It comprises a 32-location overlay with IEP+ icons which represent the interactive sentences from INTERACTION, EDUCATION AND PLAY. All the vocabulary can be stored into the Intro Talker without any extra memory modules if the device is switched into 'extended' speech. See Cross (1991).

introversion the process of turning in on oneself, becoming preoccupied with one's own thoughts and feelings. This can be 'normal' but when it becomes extreme it produces maladaptive behaviour, e.g. AUTISM. See Atkinson et al (1993).

intrusion sounds which do not appear in the written form of a language but do appear in some accents. A very common intrusive sound in English is the intrusive /r/ as in such phrases as /lɔr æn ɔrdə/. The first /r/ is intrusive as it does not appear when 'law and order' is written. See Cruttenden (1994).

intuition linguists use the native-speaker's intuition as to which sentences are acceptable or unacceptable as a guide to the validity of the set of rules they devise to generate the sentences of a language. Intuition thus becomes an important source of data in GENERATIVE GRAMMAR. See Lyons (1968).

inventory a gathering together of data concerning the sounds people use in different situations. There is no structure to this list. When an inventory, for example, of sounds has been collected, it is called that person's sound inventory.

IP (item and process) see MORPHOLOGY.

IPA see INTERNATIONAL PHONETIC ALPHABET.

ipsilateral a description of structures and nerves, etc. which are on the same side of the body. It is opposed to contralateral. See Tortora and Grabowski (1993).

IQ see INTELLIGENCE QUOTIENT.

irregular the form of words, phrase and sentences which do not follow the normal rules for these constructions. A very common example can be found in the use of plurals in English. The regular allomorphs (see MORPHOLOGY) used to show plurality in English are /s/, /z/, /ɪz/, e.g. 'dogs', 'trees', 'buses', while there are irregular plural forms in such plurals as 'mice', 'children', 'oxen', etc. See Matthews (1974).

isthmus of fauces see MOUTH.

item the different forms used in a language.

item and arrangement (IA) see MORPHOLOGY.

item and process (IP) see MORPHOLOGY.

ITPA see ILLINOIS TEST OF PSYCHOLINGUISTIC ABILITIES.

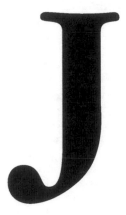

jack a place for fitting in a plug often found at the back of a computer or on a tape recorder or similar machine. It is also called a socket.

Jacksonian seizure a tonic/clonic-type seizure (*see* EPILEPSY) which gradually spreads throughout the body, involving ipsilateral structures. The focal lesion is in the precentral gyrus of the brain. *See* Gilroy and Holliday (1982).

Jackson's syndrome first described by Hughlings Jackson. A condition in which there is unilateral paralysis of the soft palate and LARYNX and a hemiatrophy of the tongue leading to a peripheral dysarthria (*see* DYSARTHRIAS (3)).

Jakob-Creutzfeldt disease (also known as Creutzfeldt-Jakob disease) a spongiform encephalopathy affecting the CENTRAL NERVOUS SYSTEM. It progresses slowly throughout the CNS and produces dementia. It affects people between the ages of 35 and 63 years of age and is found worldwide. It lasts for about 6 months to 3 years. The symptoms include a loss of short-term memory (*see* MEMORY), APHASIA and hallucinations. The person may also have cortical blindness, ataxia (*see* CEREBRAL PALSY) and myoclonus. There is a fast decline to DEMENTIA. There is no effective treatment. *See* Gilroy and Holliday (1982); Kolb and Whishaw (1990).

jargon aphasia Butterworth described jargon as a 'rare and spectacular manifestation of a dysphasic condition'. There are four types of jargon aphasia:

1. Undifferentiated jargon: a disorder of language where the person uses phonemically possible words, i.e. the structure of the words follows the rules for word formation in English. However, they do not come out as real words.
2. Phonemic jargon: the person does produce real words but sometimes substitutes non-words which are related phonologically to the target word.
3. Asemantic jargon: the person uses real words in possible syntactic contexts but the sequences produced do not make sense.
4. Neologistic jargon: the person uses non-words (unrelated to the target) placed in possible syntactic structures.

People who produce jargon are unaware they are not communicating satisfactorily. Jargon does not contain the hesitations, word-finding difficulties and self-corrections, etc. found with those who have APHASIA. *See* Butterworth (1984); Simmons and Buckingham (1992).

Jelly Bean Switch a single plate switch for operating toys, communication

113

aids or switch access software for computers. It can be mounted on table tops or wheelchairs using the SLIM ARMSTRONG MOUNT or the UNIVERSAL MOUNT. *See* Appendix IV.

joystick an input device used with a computer especially in arcade games for moving objects around the screen. It may also be used with icon software (*see* ICON). A joystick is also referred to as a games paddle. A joystick can also be used to access a high-tech communication aid which has a scanning system. *See* Bishop (1985); Beukelman and Mirenda (1992).

jugular vein there are two veins – the internal and external veins. They drain the veinous blood from the internal and external tissues of head and neck. *See* Tortora and Grabowski (1993).

juncture the phonetic or syntactic boundaries between words, phrases and sentences. These boundaries are often marked by silence although they can also be marked by changes in intonation and stress patterns. *See* Clark and Clark (1977).

Jung Carl Gustav Jung (1875-1961) disagreed with Freud's emphasis on libido and examined the interpretation of symbols and dreams. *See* Atkinson et al (1993).

justification the positioning of text in such a way that both right and left margins are equal. This occurs in word processing.

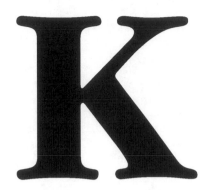

K an abbreviation for kilobytes and stands for the amount of memory which a computer contains. When used in this way, K is 1024. So, a computer with a 2K byte memory will have 2048 bytes of storage. *See* Bishop (1985); Brookshear (1991).

Kendal Toy Test a hearing test used with children from 2;6. Objects are placed on the table in front of the child. The tester checks that all the toys are known, then stands behind the child and names an object. The child must point to it. The test requires no verbal response from the child. The tester looks at the pattern of errors. For example, a confusion between 'duck' and 'bus', may indicate a high frequency hearing loss, as the high frequency sounds are missed. The tests consists of three sets of 15 toys.

Ke:nx an interface for the Apple Macintosh allowing those with physical or cognitive impairments to access their computers. The system has a hardware and software components. Ke:nx (pronounced 'connects') allows for switches and other input systems to be linked up to the Mac. These include a touch screen, various communication aids such as the Touch and Light Talkers, Liberator Communication Aid, Dynavox and other dedicated communication aids, an alternative keyboard which allows for squares or groups of squares to act like keys, mouse commands or voices. *See* Appendix IV.

keyboard the usual type of keyboard on a computer or communication aid is a QWERTY KEYBOARD. However, some people with a physical disability require an expanded keyboard which has larger keys and may or may not be in the ordinary QWERTY layout. Two examples are the Tash PC Mini Keyboard and the Tash PC King Keyboard where, in the latter, the most often used keys are in the centre of the keyboard and are laid out so that the common words are easily spelt. *See* Appendix IV.

KeyEmu software which allows Minspeak communication aids such as ALPHA TALKERS, DELTA TALKERS, TOUCH TALKERS, LIGHT TALKERS and the LIBERATOR COMMUNICATION AID to be used as keyboard emulators for the Archimedes ranges of computers and allows for stored vocabulary or MINSPEAK APP-LICATION PROGRAMS to be stored ontoa computer disk or loaded into any of the above devices from an Archimedes.

keypad it is similar to a keyboard but smaller as it may contain only number keys or function keys. *See* Chandor et al (1985).

kinaesthesia awareness of movement and position. In relation to speech – the position of the articulators. *See* Tortora and Grabowski (1993).

Klinefelter's syndrome one of the most common sex chromosome (*see* CHROMOSOMES) abnormalities, it was first described by Klinefelter and his colleagues in 1942. It affects about 1:500 males. Although not severe, it may be associated with LEARNING DISABILITY. Those who have this syndrome often have delayed speech and language development which may include degrees of anomia. Some may have an INTENTION TREMOR which may be severe enough to make drinking a glass of water difficult. There may also be behavioural problems. It is caused by the presence of two X chromosomes along with the Y chromosome. Males who are affected are eunuchoid, have gynaecomata, are infertile and are tall and thin with long legs and arms and small genitalia. *See* Salmon (1978); Smith (1985); Tortora and Grabowski (1993).

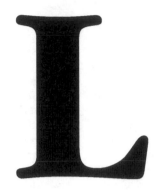

L-dopa *see* LEVODOPA.

label the name given to constituents in a CONSTITUENT ANALYSIS when represented by a TREE DIAGRAM or by BRACKETING. This occurs in GENERATIVE GRAMMAR. *See* Lyons (1968).

labial a description of where some sounds are made, as long as either one lip or both lips are moved to form the sound. Sounds in which one lip is moved are labio-dental (*see* ARTICULATION) while sounds in which both lips are moved are bilabial (*see* ARTICULATION). *See* Catford (1977).

LAD *See* LANGUAGE ACQUISITION DEVICE.

laddergram the graphic form of results obtained from tests of loudness balance such as the ALTERNATE BINAURAL LOUDNESS BALANCE.

laddering *see* PERSONAL CONSTRUCT THERAPY.

laminal a description of sounds made with the blade or lamina of the tongue. These include the alveolar (*see* ARTICULATION) sounds [t, d, s, z]. *See* Catford (1977).

Landau-Kleffner syndrome a possible symptom of those children who have a specific developmental language disorder. Such children have severe problems in comprehension, it is not just delayed. The errors they make are usually consistent and not found in unaffected children of the same age. These comprehension problems do not only occur with auditory stim-uli but also with written and signed stimuli. Thus, it does not matter how the sentence is presented to them, they have equal difficulty. Their problem in comprehension could be because they fail to understand the hierarchy of structures used to form the utterances presented to them. The TEST FOR RECEPTION OF GRAMMAR has been used with such children as the hierarchy of structures is presented in progressively more difficult sub-tests. *See* Bishop (1982); Byers Brown and Edwards (1989); Vance (1991).

language a term with several different senses. It can refer to a system of linguistic units, which, when put in the correct order provide spoken or written utterances. This is the performance or parole aspect of language. The underlying knowledge of a language is often referred to as the native's competence or langue. Dialects are regional variations of an established language while an idiolect is a personal variation of language. *See* Lyons (1968); Kolb and Whishaw (1990); Fromkin and Rodman (1993).

language acquisition *see* ACQUISITION and Appendix II.

language acquisition device (LAD) a psycholinguistic theory proposed by Noam Chomsky (*see* CHOMSKYAN LINGUIS-

117

TICS) to explain how children acquire language. He believes children's language acquisition is an innate process. Chomsky believes humans to be born with several areas in their brains which allow them to develop various skills. Language is one such skill and it is LAD which sparks off this hypothetical language area in the child's mind. *See* Steinberg (1982).

Language Assessment, Remediation and Screening Procedure (LARSP) a procedure devised by David Crystal in 1976 (revised 1989) to analyse the results of informal-type assessments to find out how well the child has developed expressive language. It shows how the child organises language, the main stages of language acquisition reached by the child as well as the way the child interacts with the therapist. There are no rules for carrying out the assessment. The procedure is to have a 30-minute taped play session, discussion, picture description, free conversation or a combination of all these. The tape is analysed and the grammatical structures summarised in a single profile chart. Any delay in grammatical development of the child can be discovered and the missing structures can be taught to the child. A computerised version of LARSP has been produced by Dorothy Bishop for both the BBC and Apple microcomputers. The program has been written so that the child's utterances can be analysed into the word, phrase and clause structures of the original profile. Each part of the program runs automatically from one stage to another. A summary sheet is printed out following the same format as the non-computerised profile chart with all the calculations carried out by the computer. *See* Bishop (1984); Crystal et al (1989).

language delay a condition in which the child's language level reflects that of a chronologically younger child. It will be less mature than is appropriate for his age compared with that of his peers. The child produces language of a much younger child, i.e. below his chronological age. The therapist uses assessments such as RDLS or DLS to find out how significant the delay is. Language delay may be associated with the following: (1) hearing loss; (2) mental handicap; (3) visual impairment; (4) severe emotional disorders; (5) gross neurological problems; (6) environmental deprivation. This differentiates children who have SDLD who would not have any of the six causes given above.

language deviance this does not fit into a normal developmental sequence. There may be abnormal sound structure, syntactic and or semantic manifestations. Gross deviance is frequently associated with pathology, it can also occur without any discernible cause. *See* Byers Brown (1976).

Language Imitation Test devised by Berry and Mittler in 1981. It assesses the expressive language of learning disabled children of 2;6-4;0, using six subtests: (1) sound imitation; (2) word imitation; (3,4) syntactic control (two subtests are used); (5) word organisation control; (6) sentence completion. The child has to repeat words and sentences after the therapist has said them. The child's production is scored so that a numerical score can be obtained or a score which will reveal the child's strengths and weaknesses in this area of expressive language. *See* Berry and Mittler (1981) in Appendix I.

Language, Learning and Living (LLL) a MINSPEAK APPLICATION PROGRAM (MAP) devised by Jones, it is designed for adolescent and adult individuals with developmental disabilities and associated learning difficulties. It uses a single word/phrase vocabulary with 11 parts of speech represented, including 57 classses of noun. As with all MINSPEAK programs, it uses Minspeak icons to represent different parts of grammar as well as functions. Spelling can also be used to increase literacy skills.

In 1995, Tony Jones devised a 'beginners' vocabulary called 'Pathways' which uses the 128-location overlay but uses single word and sentence formats. There are six pathways to the full LLL program. Pathway 1 has 128 single-key-activated sentences which relate to the sentences and words in LLL; Pathway 2 has 128 single-key-activated words which relate to LLL; Pathway 3 combines the first two pathways with single-key-activated words and sentences started with the 'judge' icon as in LLL; Pathway 4 allows the user to activate the sentences as in Pathway 3 but all the single hit words of Pathway 2 start with the 'name' icon; Pathway 5 introduces sentence types where statements begin with the 'judge' icon, questions with 'witch' icon, 'negations' with 'knot' icon, past tenses with 'biged' icon and amusing, rude or emphatic sentences with 'bottom' icon. The individual words used in Pathway 2 beginning with the 'name' icon are still available; Pathway 6 is a variation of Pathway 5. The words from Pathway 2 are available as a single activation except where the icon is used as a category icon in Pathway 5 ('witch', 'biged', 'knot', 'bottom' and 'name'). In these instances, the word can be obtained by a double hit on the icon. The majority of words, therefore, are available as a single hit but all other forms require a two-icon activation. *See* Jones (1989, 1991, 1992, 1995b).

Language Master a machine which can be used in a similar fashion to a tape recorder. It uses different sizes of cards with a two-track magnetic tape running along the length at the bottom of the cards. The cards can have sounds, words, phrases or pictures on them with the auditory stimulus on one of the two tracks spoken by the therapist for the person to imitate on the second track of the tape. The person can find out by listening carefully the difference between the way the stimuli are said as compared to the correct version by the therapist. *See* Code and Müller (1989).

langue the grammatical system which each person has in his or her mind after having learned the language. It was proposed by de Saussure and is opposed to parole. *See* Saussure (1916); Lyons (1968); Culler (1986).

LARSP *see* LANGUAGE ASSESSMENT, REMEDIATION AND SCREENING PROCEDURE.

laryngeal nerve palsies neuropathologies can produce a paralysis of one or both VOCAL FOLDS. Both the abduction and the adduction of the folds can be affected and paralysis can occur unilaterlally or bilaterally. There are several types of laryngeal nerve palsies:

1. Unilateral adductor paralysis is caused by a disorder in the arytenoids which bring the vocal folds together.
2. Bilateral adductor paralysis, where both the vocal folds take up a paramedial position and remain open and cannot be closed.
3. Unilateral abductor paralysis produces temporary hoarseness as the affected fold is held in the midline of the LARYNX. A teflon injection (*see* TEFLON INJECTION) is given to the vocal fold.
4. Bilateral abductor paralysis is perhaps the most serious condition as both folds remain closed at the midline of the glottis and cannot be opened. These patients require a tracheotomy to allow them to breathe. The person may also have to undergo an arytenoidectomy in which the arytenoids are removed.
5. Right recurrent laryngeal palsy is caused by a carcinoma in the oesophagus, thickening of the pleurae at the apex of the right lung, aneurysm of the right subclavian artery or pneumonectomy, i.e. part of the lung removed. Symptoms include a very weak, breathy voice. Straining it to produce voice will make the person hoarse.

119

6. Left recurrent laryngeal palsy, commonly caused by an aortic aneurysm with similar symptoms as with the right recurrent laryngeal palsy.

See Fawcus (1991).

laryngeal web most frequently a congenital condition in which a band of mucous membrane is stretched across the anterior part of the VOCAL FOLDS. It may produce hoarseness and a high pitched voice due to limited movement of the vocal folds. In severe cases, there will be inspiratory stridor, and surgical intervention will be necessary. The acquired type can occur following trauma or infective illnesses like diphtheria or tuberculosis.

laryngectomy it may be partial or complete.

1. Partial:
   (a) Hemilaryngectomy: this is a surgical procedure in which a vertical half of the LARYNX is resected. This usually involves removal of one VOCAL FOLD (CORDECTOMY), one of the false vocal folds and parts of the thyroid cartilage. Soft tissue is then rotated to provide a site against which the remaining vocal fold can vibrate. The resulting voice is hoarse and weak. Swallowing may also present a problem.
   (b) Supraglottic laryngectomy: this involves removal of the EPIGLOTTIS, aryepiglottic fold and the false vocal folds and the hyoid bone. The larynx is then raised and anchored to the base of the tongue to preserve a patent airway and to assist swallowing. Swallowing does present severe problems as a completely new swallowing pattern has to be learned. Voice may well be hoarse despite the fact that the true vocal folds remain intact.
2. Total laryngectomy: this procedure is carried out when the malignancy is extensive. Depending on the size of the tumour, resection may include the hyoid, the whole of the larynx,

part of the pharynx and trachea. The remaining part of the trachea is then sutured to an external stoma at the base of the neck anteriorly. Following surgery an alternative method of speech has to be acquired. This will be either by means of oesophageal (alaryngeal) production or through the use of an ARTIFICIAL LARYNX.

See Edels (1983).

laryngitis a cause of DYSPHONIA (*see* ACUTE LARYNGITIS and CHRONIC NON-SPECIFIC LARYNGITIS). *See* Tortora and Grabowski (1993).

laryngofissure the removal of one VOCAL FOLD which allows the other to compensate completely. *See* Fawcus (1991).

laryngoscopy there are three types of laryngoscopy:

1. Indirect laryngoscopy: the first examination using a palatal mirror to view the relevant parts of the larynx. If there appears to be a growth, a direct laryngoscopy will be undertaken.
2. Direct laryngoscopy: after anaesthesia is administered, a rigid laryngoscope is placed along the floor of the mouth and down the back of the person's throat. A light system shows up the subglottic and supraglottic areas of the larynx. If any tumours are found, tissue can be taken for further analysis by using long-handled biopsy forceps.
3. Microlaryngoscopy: the process of removing small growths from the vocal folds without damaging the folds. It is carried out by looking through an operating microscope.

See Edels (1983); Beech et al (1993).

larynx the organ of the voice. It contains the VOCAL FOLDS which produce voice. It extends from the back of the TONGUE to the TRACHEA. It is 4.5 cm long, 4 cm in transverse section and 3.5 cm from front to back. It is smaller in the female than in the male after puberty. It comprises cartilage held together by membrane and ligament. The hyoid bone (*see* MUSCLES FOR SWALLOWING) is at the top, the thyroid cartilage in the middle and the cricoid cartilage at the bottom. The thyroid cartilage is made up of two quadrilateral structures joined in the midline at the laryngeal prominence to which the vocal ligament is attached. The cricoid cartilage is like a ring. The arytenoid cartilage (*see* ARYTENOIDS) is attached to the lamina of the cricoid and has an apex and three roughly triangular surfaces. The larynx is controlled by the following muscles:

1. Cricothyroid muscle is formed by vertical and oblique fibres. The muscle tilts the cricoid up or thyroid down and tightens the vocal folds.
2. Arytenoid muscle: the transverse and oblique arytenoid muscles control the arytenoid cartilages and go up either side of the aryepiglottic folds.
3. Posterior cricoarytenoid muscle runs up to attach to the muscular process of the arytenoid. When it contracts, it abducts the vocal folds by rotating the arytenoid cartilage; when it pulls the arytenoid cartilages backwards, the vocal fold tenses.
4. Lateral cricoarytenoid muscle is attached to the superior border of the cricoid cartilage passing upwards and backwards and attached to the muscular process of the arytenoids. When it contracts, it adducts the vocal folds by rotating the arytenoid cartilage inwards.
5. Thyroarytenoid muscle is attached to the front of the inner surface of the laryngeal prominence. It passes backwards and upwards and becomes attached to the anterolateral surface of the arytenoid cartilage and its muscular process.
6. Vocalis muscle: part of the muscle is attached to the lateral aspect of the vocal ligament and some of its fibres run up to the aryepiglottic fold. When it contracts, the arytenoid cartilages rotate medially to adduct the vocal folds, while in pulling the arytenoid cartilage forward the vocal folds relax.
7. Thyrohyoid muscle leaves the thyroid cartilage and attaches to the greater cornu of the hyoid bone. It raises the thyroid cartilage and pushes down the hyoid bone.

See Tortora and Grabowski (1993).

latency   *see* PSYCHOSEXUAL STAGES OF DEVELOPMENT.

lax   a DISTINCTIVE FEATURE proposed by Jakobson and Halle to distinguish sounds made with little muscular effort [+LAX] from those which are produced with a stronger muscular effort [–LAX]. It is opposed to tense. *See* Hyman (1975).

learnability   a term used in language acquisition to refer to problem areas for learners. A general problem for the normal acquisition of language is assumed to be the absence of negative evidence. Negative evidence would be explicit information from mature language users that a particular form used by the learner, e.g. over-regularised past tense, was not grammatical in the language being learned. Retreating from incorrect hypotheses about the structure of the language being learned, on the basis of positive evidence only (the 'correct' forms of his language environment) is a learnability problem for the child learning his language.

learning   *see* CLASSICAL CONDITIONING; OPERANT CONDITIONING; INNATENESS.

learning disability   the politically correct term used in the United Kingdom for 'mental handicap' defined as 'a condition of arrested or incomplete development of mind which is especially characterised by subnormality of intelligence' (World Health Organization, 1967). Those children and adults who have a learning disability can have difficulty in learning tasks, in communication, with motor skills and with sensory input. Such problems can be helped by different types of therapy such as occupational therapy, speech and language therapy, physiotherapy and clinical or educational psychology. Whatever therapy is required by the client, the respective programmes must be planned carefully and take into account the specific learning difficulties found in such clients. Research has found these difficulties are complicated by additional handicaps such as:

1. Attention problems.
2. Inability to learn incidentally, so the client requires long and frequent exposure to the stimulus.
3. Reacting badly under pressure.
4. Auditory information processed better than visual information.
5. Memory improved by using more than one modality.
6. Clang associations produce confusion.
7. Difficulty in generalising what has been learnt.
8. Concrete stimuli should be used as these are learnt better than abstract stimuli.
9. Verbalising helps to improve memory during the task.

Clients who have a learning disability require a structured approach so that they can have a better chance of learning material as those without a learning disability. *See* Clarke and Clarke (1974); Shakespeare (1975); Kolb and Whishaw (1990); van der Gaag and Dormandy (1993); Davison and Neale (1994).

LED *see* LIGHT EMITTING DIODE.

Leiter International Performance Scale a non-verbal cognitive assessment, designed by Leiter in 1969, which is particularly well adapted to the needs of hearing- or language-impaired children. It involves a series of progressively complex matching tasks. The age range for administration is 2;0 years upwards. *See* Leiter (1969) in Appendix I.

length the period of time used to produce a sound or syllable. Length modifies the articulation and makes a difference between sounds. It is also known as duration and quality. *See* Catford (1977).

lenis a sound which has little air pressure in the airstream to produce the sound. There is also a reduction in muscle power required. It is opposed to fortis. *See* Cruttenden (1994).

lesser horn of hyoid *see* PHARYNX.

Let's Talk – Developing Prosocial Communication Skills a therapeutic programme for children and adolescents with a LEARNING DISABILITY, LANGUAGE DISORDER or HEARING LOSS or with those who are shy and find it difficult to communicate in social situations. *See* Wiig (1982a) in Appendix I.

Let's Talk – For Children a programme to involve children in real life interaction, by using hundreds of activities divided into four communication functions – ritualising, informing, controlling and feeling. The 41 different skills are sequenced developmentally and organised in learning steps. *See* Wiig (1983) in Appendix I.

Let's Talk – Intermediate Level a therapeutic programme for adolescents and young adults with developmental delays or acquired language disorders as well as those with literacy problems. The teaching activities provide real-life situations for adolescents. *See* Wiig (1984) in Appendix I.

Let's Talk – Inventory for Adolescents an assessment for adolescents and pre-adolescents consisting of 40 items in a picture manual. The adolescent is given a short description of the context of the picture and is asked what the adolescent in the picture might say in the given situation. The assessment pinpoints communication problems. The results can show where therapy begins using the Let's Talk Intervention Programmes for Adolescents, Let's Talk – Developing Prosocial Communication Skills and Let's Talk – Intermediate Level. *See* Wiig (1982b) in Appendix I.

Let's Talk – Inventory for Children based on the Inventory for Adults, this assessment gives a standardised method of assessing speech acts within the communication functions of ritualising, informing, controlling and feeling. The 34 pictures give a different situation involving peer or adult interactions. *See* Wiig (1987) in Appendix I.

letter-by-letter reader *see* ACQUIRED DYSLEXIA.

levator anguli labii superioris *see* MUSCLES OF FACIAL EXPRESSION.

levodopa (L-dopa) a drug which provides dopamine to those who have an insufficiency of dopamine in the brain. It can be used with those who have PARKINSON'S DISEASE as it has a significant effect on bradykinesia (*see* PARKINSON'S DISEASE). However, it can produce nausea, depression and dyskinesia (*see* CEREBRAL PALSY). *See* Gilroy and Holliday (1982); Kolb and Whishaw (1990); Kaye (1991).

lexical syntactic deficit a term used by Rapin and Allen (1987), to describe a subtype of language disorder. The predominant difficulty is one of word finding. There appear to be two groups: those who have a sparsity of language with difficulty in retrieving lexical items and those with similar word-finding difficulties but who use a number of word fillers and circumlocutions in an effort to retrieve words. *See* Byers Brown and Edwards (1989).

Liberator Communication Aid a high-tech communication aid with synthetic voice output (DECTALK). It uses MINSPEAK to organise vocabulary to store into the device. It has a memory of 512K and can be accessed using direct manual selection, infra-red headpointing, single, dual or two-switch scanning as well as joystick or multi-switch. Scanning and direct selection can be used on the same keyboard at the same time. It can be set up to use 8-, 32- or 128-location overlays. Other features include icon prediction, which shows by illuminating a light on a symbol which symbols have messages stored under them, predictive selection, which makes symbols with nothing stored under them inoperative when being used with direct manual selection or infra-red headpointing, while with scanning, the scanning light jumps the unused symbols. The Liberator Communication Aid also uses auditory prompts. This allows a user to hear the names of the symbols before they are activated. This feature can be used either with direct manual selection, infra-red headpointing or with switch access. The memory can be backed up on a computer. It can also be used for computer emulation and can be linked to the DIRECTOR, an environmental control. Other features include Notebooks which allows large amounts of text to be stored and spoken or printed out on the Liberator's internal printer. These may include songs, essays, different educational subjects and so on. A maximum of four unique programmes can be loaded into one device simultaneously. Maths problems can be solved using either the Maths Scratch Pad or the four-function calculator. *See* Appendix IV.

light emitting diode (LED) a light which illuminates when a machine is switched on to show that it is functioning. It is usually placed on control panels or the machine's surface. *See* Chandor et al (1985).

light for dates a light birth weight is a third of the normal birth weight. The child is born near to full term. This condition is caused by placental insufficiency produced by toxaemia, multiple pregnancy or smoking, intrauterine infections, e.g. TORCH and chromosomal abnormalities (*see* CHROMOSOMES). The babies are very alert, thin, wasted and have wrinkled skin and a poor response rate. There is fetal distress in labour and the baby passes meconium after the first day of delivery. If the child inhales meconium in the juices around it and starts poor breathing, producing meconium aspiration syndrome, this can cause brain damage and can lead to death. *See* Illingworth (1987).

light pen an input device to operate a computer instead of using the keyboard. The device looks like a pen but has a light-sensitive end. An example of such a pen is the 'Robin Light Pen' which can be used with the BBC Micro/Master series computers. *See* Bishop (1985).

Light Talker a high-tech communication aid with synthetic voice output (*see* DECTALK). It uses MINSPEAK to organise vocabulary to store into the device. It has about 40K of memory. It can only be accessed by optical headpointing, single, dual or two-switch scanning as well as joystick or multi-switch. The Light Talker has 25 different selection techniques which can be divided into 3 groups: 'direct selection' when using the optical headpointer or the Direct Selection Sensor for programming the device, 'switch scanning' either row/column scanning in 32 and 128 locations or circular, linear or count when in 8 locations and 'joystick' or 'multi-switch'. The device can be set into 8, 32 or 128 locations and, if the Light Talker uses the ENHANCED MINSPEAK OPERATING SYSTEM (EMOS), it can also be set into the 'alternative' overlay. The memory can be backed up on a computer. It can also be used for computer emulation and can be linked to the DIRECTOR, an environmental control. *See* Appendix IV.

Lightwriter a high-tech communication aid with optional synthetic speech (*see* DECTALK). It has a double screen and a QWERTY or alphabetic keyboard. The message is typed onto the screens, one screen facing the client and the other facing the 'listener'. Model SL4a has a word store and a phrase store with 40 memories. It has a rechargeable battery which, when fully charged, lasts for a continuous six

hours operation. A printing facility and speech synthesiser are also available. The SL1 and SL3 were the first of the smaller models. The latest models follow from these earlier ones. The SL5 has 2K memory with 36 memories while the SL30 is the same but allows for speech, a printout and 5K memory. The SL35 has three types of speech output: 'articulate', 'EuroTalk' (British speech) and 'DECtalk'. It has a memory of 32K with 2K of high-security memory as standard. It can be linked up to printers, remote displays, a giant keyboard, a remote control telephone and a plug-in scan module. It has an 8-function calculator among other functions. The SL55 is the same as SL5 with two keyboards while the SL56 is the same as the SL55 with all the options of the SL35. The SL8 and SL80 can be accessed by scanning. The SL8 allows for a row-column scan while the SL80 allows for an linear scan and an enlarged character for clear use. The SL81 and SL82 are similar to the SL8 and SL80 respectively but have a separate bright screen. *See* Appendix IV.

lingual tonsil a structure formed by some lymphoid tissue at the back of the TONGUE. *See* Tortora and Grabowski (1993).

linguistic profiles assessment procedures proposed by Crystal in 1982. There are profiles of phonology (PROPH), prosody (PROP) and semantics (PRISM). LARSP is included as one of these procedures. The analyses are derived from a sample of speech obtained in free conversation, play sessions and picture description. *See* Crystal (1992).

linguistic variation *see* ACCENT; DIALECT; IDIOLECT.

linking a sound which appears in the spoken language but does not appear in the orthographic form of the language. An example is the intrusive /r/. *See* Cruttenden (1994).

lip reading a form of communication used with people who have a hearing loss. The person concentrates on lip movement alone to try to understand what is being said. However, only about one-third of sounds produced can be clearly seen, e.g. bilabials, labiodentals, interdentals, some alveolars (*see* ARTICULATION) and vowels (*see* CARDINAL VOWEL SYSTEM). Another difficulty is that many of these sounds can look the same such as [p,b,m]. Speech reading is now preferred where the person takes into account not only lip movement but also facial expression and gesture, etc.

liquid a description of sounds such as [l] and [r]. *See* Ladefoged (1993).

LIS *see* LOCKED-IN-SYNDROME.

literal paraphasia although the person's articulation is unaffected, syllables can be produced in the wrong order or wrong sounds are placed in a word producing confusion. *See* Goodglass and Kaplan (1983).

lithium a drug treatment technique used in manic-depression. The level of the drug rises in the body as it is only effective in this manner; it will take a few days after therapy begins for it to take effect. It is used mainly for the maintenance of recovery from manic-depression. *See* Stafford-Clark and Smith (1983); Atkinson et al (1993); Davison and Neale (1994).

liveware those people who work with computers such as programmers, operators and so on. It is opposed to hardware and software. *See* Chandor et al (1985).

Living Language a remedial package, devised by Locke, for children who have a LANGUAGE DELAY, which can be used from pre-school to 16 years of age. It is designed to help children to develop their use of expressive language normally. The package is divided into three parts: 'Before Words'; 'First Words' and 'Putting Words Together'. 'Before Words' is used with children who have no use or comprehension of language. In this part of Living Language, the child is taught the basic skills required to acquire language, such as social-emotional development, play, listening and expressive language skills. The norms for such development are given in the manual. 'First Words' is used with children who are using single words but the level of vocabulary is not up to the child's age level and they do not have sufficient words to put two words together. This part of the programme contains 100 words which children first respond to or use – 58 nouns (e.g. toys, clothes, food, etc.), 30 verbs (e.g. describing concrete, easily identifiable actions, etc.) and 12 other words (e.g. early prepositions and adjectives). Picture cards are presented to the child by the teacher or therapist to assess the child's expressive language. 'Putting Words Together' is used with children who have a basic vocabulary and are beginning to put words together to form simple sentences. It comprises three parts: (1) a vocabulary of objects and events, including over 600 of the most familiar nouns and verbs; (2) a vocabulary of properties and relationships, including 200 adjectives, adverbs and prepositions used to describe objects and their relationships to each other, together with basic number words and more abstract vocabulary; and (3) a selection of syntactic features, including more than 200 grammatical constructions which children need to know to benefit from traditional teaching. Each of these three parts is divided into levels placed in developmental order. *See* Locke (1985).

LLL *see* LANGUAGE, LEARNING AND LIVING.

locationist theory proposed by a group of aphasiologists known as the BOSTON SCHOOL. The theory itself dates from the 1860s when Paul Broca and Karl Wernicke and their contemporaries proposed groups of language disorders produced by lesions in certain parts of the brain producing specific aphasic characteristics (*see* APHSIA). *See* Eisenson (1984).

locked-in-syndrome (LIS) a condition in which damage to parts of the BRAIN-STEM restricts the motor pathways to such an extent that in the complete state vertical movement of the eyes is the only one possible. Sensory and cognitive function may be retained. Incomplete LIS allows some movement of the limbs but communication is anarthric and therefore restricted to almost unintelligible vocalisations.

logogen the British psychologist John Morton introduced this term to refer to a hypothetical memory unit which links together various aspects of a word such as its semantic, auditory, visual and pictorial properties. Morton suggested that individual 'logogens' (his name for word recognition units in the visual input lexicon) have variable thresholds. 'A logogen's threshold determines the amount of activity that must be present within it before it will 'fire' and cause a word to be recognised' (Ellis 1993, p. 28). *See* Reber (1985); Ellis (1993).

logopaedics a name given to speech and language pathology in other parts of Europe.

Logotron Logo software developed for use by children. It is designed to allow the child to operate a computer rather than allow the computer to control the child. Thus, it follows Piaget's beliefs that a child learns from experience. When the child enters the Logo program, he will find a small triangle on the screen called a turtle. By using a simple computer language, the child finds he can move the turtle forwards, backwards, sideways, diagonally, draw a white line, draw a coloured line or not draw a line at all. Thus, the child learns a form of language for moving the turtle. The graphics which the child produces in this way are called turtle graphics. It has been designed for the Apple computers in the USA and for the BBC computers in the UK. *See* Bishop (1985).

longitudinal method a research procedure using several subjects over a period of time.

longitudinal muscle *see* INTRINSIC MUSCLES OF THE TONGUE.

loop a process found in a computer program which allows instructions given to the computer to be repeated until a particular condition is satisfied. The types of loops may differ from computer to computer. The loops most often found in BASIC are for...next and repeat...until. *See* Bishop (1985).

loudness *see* AUDITORY PHONETICS.

low a DISTINCTIVE FEATURE proposed by Chomsky and Halle to distinguish sounds made by lowering the TONGUE in the MOUTH [+LOW] to produce open vowels (*see* CARDINAL VOWEL SYSTEM) from those made with the tongue raised in the mouth [–LOW]. It is opposed to high. *See* Hyman (1975).

low-level language a computer language, e.g. assembly language, which is closer to the type of language which a computer can understand without translation as it is close to machine code. It is opposed to high-level languages such as BASIC. *See* Bishop (1985).

lumbar puncture a technique for diagnosing such infections as MENINGITIS. A certain quantity, usually about 1 ml, of CEREBROSPINAL FLUID is drawn off the MENINGES to check for infection. If the fluid is clouded by the presence of organisms and white cells, this may indicate the presence of meningitis. The pressure is also increased and the sugar decreased. Normal CSF fluid is clear. *See* Gilroy and Holliday (1982); Kaye (1991).

lungs there are two lungs in the thoracic cavity covered by a pleural lining. Air reaches the lungs by the TRACHEA and the BRONCHI which branch into the right and left lung. The right lung is divided into three lobes by an oblique fissure and transverse fissure. The left lung is divided into two lobes by an oblique fissure. Each lobe is supplied by a bronchus, an artery and a vein. They are necessary for respiration. The microscopic structure of the lungs is seen as a series of passageways. The bronchi divide into bronchioles which become respiratory bronchioles. These bronchioles divide into alveolar ducts, subdividing into alveolar saccules which produce alveoli at their ends. *See* Tortora and Grabowksi (1993).

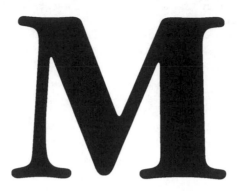

MA *see* MENTAL AGE.

Macaw a high-tech communication aid which uses digitised speech producing natural sounding speech to produce messages. The Macaw is set to be used with a 32-cell overlay although the keyboard can be divided into sections of 2, 4 or 8 keys. Pictures or symbols are placed on the cells of the keyboard. The appropriate picture or symbol is chosen and the message recorded through the internal microphone. The Macaw has three modes:

1. String mode: a series of keys is selected, the 'talk key' is actuated and the messages are produced in the correct order.
2. Levels mode: there are eight levels which expands the number of messages which can be produced although the restriction of 64 seconds for recording speech is still a constraint on how much is placed in the Macaw.
3. Keylink mode: messages are produced by sequencing two to three cells.

See Appendix IV.

machine code the internal language of the computer in which all its instructions are coded and stored. The computer can execute instructions in this form. Instructions in a high-level language such as BASIC must be translated into machine code form before the computer can execute them. It is this translation which slows down the processing time of the computer. It is possible to write programs directly in machine code which allows the same program in machine code to be processed much faster than the one in BASIC. *See* Bishop (1985); Brookshear (1991).

machine language the language for writing in machine code. It takes the form of binary notation. *See* Bishop (1985); Brookshear (1991).

macrocephaly an abnormally large head caused by an increased amount of tissue or fluid in the BRAIN. It is opposed to MICROCEPHALY.

macroglossia an abnormally large TONGUE. The condition may be congenital. It has been proposed that children who have DOWN'S SYNDROME have a longer tongue than those children who do not have this syndrome. However, the tongue may just seem very large because the child has a particularly small upper or lower jaw. Surgery can be used to reduce its size. Articulation disorders can occur. *See* Travis (1971).

magnetic resonance imaging (MRI) also known as nuclear magnetic resonance imaging. The patient is exposed to a uniform magnetic field which orientates some of the atomic nuclei in the body. This is especially true of water, i.e. containing protons. When placed in a magnetic field some absorb this energy and move from a low to a high energy state, i.e. resonance effect. The images resemble CT scans and can be presented in colour or two- or three-dimensional images. MRI can be used as the guidance system for biopsy tumours. It can also assess mental disorders, show changes in the brain in PARKINSON'S DISEASE as well as show the causes of CEREBROVASCULAR ACCIDENTS, i.e. haematomas and infarction. *See* Kolb and Whishaw (1990); Kaye (1991); Tortora and Grabowski (1993).

main program the principal part of a computer program which may branch into SUBROUTINES. *See* Bishop (1985).

mainframe computers a central processor or host computer with various terminals linked up to it. It is often used to distinguish between large computers and microcomputers, although the latter can now perform the same function as mainframe computers. Networks are set up linking terminals to the mainframe computers in businesses so that several employees can use the mainframe at the same time. *See* Bishop (1985).

maintenance *see* CARRY-OVER.

major class feature a major grouping of Chomsky and Halle's DISTINCTIVE FEATURES. This group distinguishes sounds which are made with different degrees of openness in the VOCAL TRACT. This produces the distinctive features of sonorant/non-sonorant, vocalic/non-vocalic and consonantal/non-consonantal. *See* Ladefoged (1993).

major depression *see* DEPRESSION.

Makaton a sign vocabulary system devised by Margaret Walker in 1977 for adults who were deaf and had severe learning difficulties. It contains about 350 words in nine developmental stages, and is the only sign system which follows closely the normal acquisition of vocabulary. Learning Makaton can increase the child's eye contact, attention, sociability, vocalisation and EXPRESSIVE LANGUAGE. Far from interfering with the child's ACQUISITION of speech and language, it can encourage it. It is sometimes used in therapeutic programmes for various communication disorders including those with LEARNING DISABILITY and those with APHASIA who have WORD-FINDING DIFFICULTIES. By producing the sign, the person may find it easier to produce the word verbally. Makaton symbols, pictorial representations of the signs, have been developed so that it will be easier for children to use and understand the original sounds. Computer programs have also been written for use with Makaton. *See* Kiernan et al (1982); Peter and Barnes (1982); Grove and Walker (1990).

Makaton symbols *see* MAKATON.

maladaptive behaviour *see* ABNORMAL BEHAVIOUR.

malignant a description of a tumour which can grow within different parts of the body destroying any neighbouring tissue. It is opposed to benign. See Tortora and Grabowski (1993).

malleus *see* EAR.

malocclusion *see* ORTHODONTICS.

Maltron keyboard a keyboard that has been designed to be more suitable for use because of its comfort and accuracy. The keyboard has been divided into two parts with two groupings of 26 switches on each side. The thumbs are left to operate 'SPACE', 'RETURN', 'E', '&' and full stop. The way the two groupings are set up takes away the strain on the wrists and keeps them straight. The Maltron keyboard can be attached to the normal BBC keyboard. There is a single-handed keyboard for those who have a physical handicap and cannot use even the standard Maltron. Again it has been specially manufactured for comfort and accuracy. Maltron have also produced a keyboard which can be mounted on a stand and operated by a head or mouth stick if the patient cannot use any other limbs for operating the computer. All the keyboards have been designed for use with the BBC microcomputer. Similar keyboards are also available for other types of computers such as Apple Macintosh computers.

management includes all the decisions which a therapist makes concerning the patient, from the taking of a CASE HISTORY through to decisions concerning the best method of ASSESSMENT, the DIAGNOSIS, TREATMENT PROGRAMME and possible PROGNOSIS. *See* Byers Brown (1981).

mandible the lower jaw. It is used in the act of chewing or mastication. It has four muscles attached to various parts of its body – temporalis muscle, lateral pterygoid, medial pterygoid and masseter muscles (*see* MUSCLES OF MASTICATION). *See* Tortora and Grabowski (1993).

mandibular nerve the mandibular branch of the trigeminal nerve (*see* CRANIAL NERVE V). To distinguish this nerve from the other two which form the trigeminal nerve, the mandibular nerve is denoted as Viii. The sensory part of the nerve supplies the posterior two-thirds of the TONGUE, the MANDIBLE and lower teeth, and the mucous membrane of the floor of the mouth. See Tortora and Grabowski (1993).

manic-depression mania nearly always appears with DEPRESSION to create a bipolar disorder compared with depression itself which is a unipolar disorder. Those who have attacks of mania appear in a happy and euphoric mood. While in this mood, people become overtalkative, overactive, suffer from sleeplessness, become very distractible, have sudden flights of ideas and can begin punning and rhyming. A severe case of mania causes physical collapse, incoherent thought processes and superficial

moods. The treatment is by trycyclic antidepressant drugs (*see* ANTIDEPRESSANTS), MONOAMINE OXIDASE INHIBITORS, LITHIUM, chlorpromazine (*see* PHENOTHIAZINES) and three to four sessions of ELECTROCONVULSIVE THERAPY. *See* Stafford-Clark and Smith (1983); Davison and Neale (1994).

Mann-Whitney test a non-parametric test (*see* PARAMETRIC TESTS) used in INFERENTIAL STATISTICS. It is used in experiments using the INDEPENDENT GROUP DESIGN and has its equivalent parametric test, the independent *t*-test (*see* T-TESTS). It is used for data which are arranged on a scale which makes no assumptions concerning the shape of the population distribution, e.g. two independent groups of subjects who are taught to read by different methods and subsequently rated on a scale of reading fluency from 1 to 10. The ratings are put on an ordinal scale, so the results of the experiment in this example could be ranked in order of fluency. Such scales do not allow for the calculations of mean score and so the Mann-Whitney test cannot show differences of means between subjects. 'By finding the sum of the ranks of one of the samples, this test allows the tester to determine the probability that a given difference between the ranks of the two samples could have arisen by chance.' (Miller, 1975, p. 82). *See* Miller (1975).

manner of articulation *see* ARTICULATION.

manual approach *see* EDUCATION OF HEARING-IMPAIRED CHILDREN.

MAOI *see* MONOAMINE OXIDASE INHIBITORS.

masking during audiometric tests such as PURE-TONE AUDIOMETRY, there is a possibility that the results will be contaminated by CROSS-HEARING. On such occasions, masking is necessary. Masking should be used when air conduction (*see* PURE-TONE AUDIOMETRY) thresholds in the test ear measure 40 dB or are poorer than bone conduction (*see* PURE-TONE AUDIOMETRY) in the non-test ear because sound is then loud enough to set the skull in vibration and stimulate the cochlea (*see* EAR) of the non-test ear. In bone-conduction testing, if the thresholds are better than air-conduction thresholds, masking should be used.

mass noun a noun which is not countable. An example of such a noun is 'butter' because 'one butter', 'two butters' cannot occur. *See* Palmer (1976).

masseter muscle *see* MUSCLES OF MASTICATION.

mastoid process *see* EAR.

matched subjects design a design used in preparing to carry out an experiment, so that the results will be reliable. In this approach, there are two groups, but, unlike the INDEPENDENT GROUP DESIGN, they have different people in each group. The subjects are matched according to their similarity in relation to the variables that will be the subject of the experiment. *See* Miller (1975).

matrix sentence the sentence that exists before embedding takes place or after the embedded sentences have been removed.

(1)   The car which the man bought was a Rolls Royce.

In (1), the matrix sentence is 'the car was a Rolls Royce' while the embedded sentence is 'which the man bought'. *See* Allerton (1979).

maxilla the upper jaw. It is formed by the fusion of the palatal shelves during intrauterine growth. The maxilla comprises the hard palate (*see* MOUTH), the floor and sides of the nasal cavities, the floor of the orbits and the part of the nasolacrimal canal. The teeth in the top dentition are rooted in the maxilla. *See* Tortora and Grabowski (1993).

maxillary nerve a sensory nerve that supplies some of the skin of the scalp, part of the face, the lower eyelid, part of the inside cheek, the mucous membrane of the nasal cavity, palate and maxillary sinus, the upper teeth and gum. It is part of the trigeminal nerve (*see* CRANIAL NERVE V). To distinguish the maxillary nerve from the other two parts of the nerve, the maxillary nerve is denoted as Vii. *See* Tortora and Grabowski (1993).

mean *see* CENTRAL TENDENCY.

mean length of utterance (MLU) a theory used in language acquisition, proposed by Brown, which compares the child's age to the length of utterances measured in morphemes. They give a more precise idea of the complexity of the utterance than counting words. Brown put forward five stages of development of MLU:

Stage	MLU	Age (years)
I	1.75	1;6–2;3
II	2.25	1;9–2;6
III	2.75	1;11–3;1
IV	3.50	2;2–3;8
V	4.00	2;3–4;0

Age is not a good guide to development, as the rate of acquisition is so variable among children. However, MLU is a good guide to grammatical development especially until stage V. With children who have a language disorder, the MLU can show up mismatches between the child's language acquisition and the normal order. Age plus MLU is important as they can give indicators to the size of the delay which a child has. *See* Cruttenden (1979).

meconium aspiration syndrome *see* LIGHT FOR DATES.

medial pterygoid muscle *see* MUSCLES OF MASTICATION.

median *see* CENTRAL TENDENCY.

medulla oblongata part of the BRAINSTEM. It is about 3 cm long. The SPINAL CORD ends in the medulla. There are several tracts which it has in common with the PONS and MIDBRAIN. *See* Barr (1979); Tortora and Grabowski (1993).

megalencephaly a condition found in children who have an oversized head and overweight brain without neurological disorders. When these children are born, they have an abnormally large head and big bodies. Anatomical megalencephaly is inheritable as an autosomal dominant trait (*see* CHROMOSOMES) and can be familial. In a study in 1972, out of 18 children the incidence was 4:1 in favour of males and half of the children were familial cases. *See* De Meyer (1972).

mellow a DISTINCTIVE FEATURE proposed by Jakobson and Halle to distinguish sounds which are made with a low frequency such as plosives and nasals (*see* ARTICULATION) [+MELLOW] from those made with a high frequency such as fricatives (*see* ARTICULATION) [−MELLOW]. It is opposed to STRIDENT. *See* Hyman (1975).

melodic intonation therapy (MIT) devised by Sparks, Helm and Albert (1974), Sparks and Holland (1976) and revised by Sparks (1981), it is a therapeutic technique originally devised for aphasic patients. It is based on a theory of right hemisphere dominance for music. The person is required to learn to intone propositional sentences in a manner which replicates their natural prosody and thus to facilitate verbal output. Some success is reported on its use with apraxic subjects. *See* Eisenson (1984).

membrane a layer or sheet of tissue that can surround cells, structures, line canals and separate structures. *See* Leeson et al (1985); Tortora and Grabowski (1993).

memory.

1. There are two types of memory: short-term memory (STM) and long-term memory (LTM). This is known as the dual memory theory. It is believed that these two areas of memory are linked. When STM receives input, it is rehearsed so that it will be remembered and can be transferred to the LTM area. When information is displaced from memory, it never reaches LTM but leaves STM. STM has a storage capacity of 7 ± 2 chunks of information whereas the storage capacity of LTM is limitless. When information is retrieved from STM, there are few errors, while it is more likely errors will occur in information retrieved from LTM. At one time, it was thought that these types of memory were used for storing all the contents of memory but research has shown this to be a false assumption. In particular, there seems to be different types of LTM for storing facts, e.g. the name of the Prime Minister, storing skills, e.g. how to play tennis, storing general facts about the world, e.g. April comes after March, and storing of personal facts, e.g. a person's likes and dislikes. *See* Atkinson et al (1993).

2. The part of the computer in which a computer program is stored when the computer is executing that program. It also holds text for word processors until it is sent to the disk drive (*see* DISK) or printed out and other data which the executing program may store and use. It is important to remember that programs and text can be edited when in memory, but if being saved on disk, the edited text or program must be resaved or the old program/piece of text will remain, as it will not have been changed. The memory consists of cells in which information is stored. In most microcomputers, each cell stores 1 byte of information. Each cell in memory is identified by its ADDRESS. The address of the cell and its contents are held in binary. The memory capacity is measured in kilobytes. *See* Bishop (1985); Brookshear (1991).

memory trace *see* CLASSICAL CONDITIONING.

Memowriter a high-tech communication aid with a QWERTY keyboard covered by a keyguard allowing the person to place his hand on top of the machine without activating the sensitive membrane keys. Other keys on the keyboard include on/off, write memo, read memo, list memo, cursor keys, return, print and paper feed. There are 26 programmable memories (55 characters each) which can be recalled by depressing two keys. The client places a message in the memory, deciding which key to code it under. To recall the message, he depresses 'read memo' and the letter code. The Memowriter has a 24-character liquid crystal display and has a buffer memory for 240 characters. It is rechargeable.

meninges a membranous covering of the brain and the spinal cord. If it becomes infected, meningitis occurs. *See* Barr (1979); Tortora and Grabowski (1993).

meningiomas *see* TUMOURS OF THE CENTRAL NERVOUS SYSTEM.

meningitis an infection of the lining membranes of the BRAIN and SPINAL CORD. Viruses are the most common cause. The symptoms are headaches, neck stiffness, fever and vomiting. Diagnosis has to be made from the CEREBROSPINAL FLUID which looks milky. The CSF is extracted by LUMBAR PUNCTURE. Treatment depends on the type of infection. There is no specific treatment for virus infections but antibiotics are used in bacterial infections. *See* Gilroy and Holliday (1982); Tortora and Grabowski (1993).

meningothelial meningiomas a type of meningioma (*see* TUMOURS OF THE CENTRAL NERVOUS SYSTEM) coming from the arachnoid cap cells, consisting of sheets of cells which contain large, vascular nuclei. *See* Gilroy and Holliday (1982).

mental age (MA) an age-equivalent score which is obtained from INTELLIGENCE TESTS. It is used to calculate the IQ score by comparing it to the chronological age to find out if the child is below or above average compared with children of the same age. *See* Atkinson et al (1993).

mental handicap *see* LEARNING DISABILITY.

menu in computer terms, a list of options from which an operator can choose a particular function or part of a program to use. These may be a selection of games or operations in a business package. The option is automatically booted into the computer's memory. *See* Chandor et al (1985).

Merrill-Palmer Pre-School Intelligence Test an assessment to find out the learning abilities among children between the ages of 1;6 and 5;0 years. Devised in 1931, the scale has 19 verbal and performance subtests which test motor and language skills, manual dexterity and matching skills. Most of these subtests take the form of games so that children readily pay attention to them. The raw scores which are obtained can be converted to MENTAL AGE, intelligence quotients, percentile ranks and standard deviations. *See* Stutsman (1926-1931) in Appendix I.

MessageMate a high-tech communication aid with digitised speech. It can be hand-held. There are several models all of which have similar features. Single keys can be made into larger keys. It can be accessed by direct manual selection or by linear and column-row scanning using one or two switches. The memory differs from model to model. It starts with the 20-20 model of 20 seconds up to the 20-120 model with 120 seconds. The MeesageMate40 starts with the 40-60 model with 60 seconds and increases to the 40-240 model with 240 seconds. *See* Appendix IV.

metalinguistics the study of knowledge of language. The way in which one thinks and knows about its properties.

Metaphon Resource Pack devised by Dean and her colleagues in 1985 (revised 1989) and published in 1990, it is a complete assessment and therapy programme for children with phonological disorders. It is most effective with children up to 5;0 years but can be used for children of 7;0 years. The thrust of Metaphon is developing the child's knowledge of sounds and organisation of sound processing. It has four stages:

1. Screening: the child is asked to name pictures. The screening test assesses 13 systemic and structural simplifying processes in the child's phonological system, identifying areas for which the therapist should not expect the child to produce processes because of the age of the child.
2. Probing: a more in-depth assessment of the problem areas identified in the screening test. Responses are recorded on a quantitative and qualitative record form.
3. Intervention: the results of the probes will lead to appropriate strategies for treatment detailed in the manual.
4. Monitoring: the monitoring procedure happens regularly to assess the effectiveness of the treatment strategies.

See Dean et al (1990) in Appendix I; Beech et al (1993).

metastasis a malignant seedling of tumour which has come from a distant primary. Many tumours form metastases in the brain especially bronchial carcinomas. They develop in the CEREBRAL HEMISPHERES and can push the contents of the hemispheres across the midline. This is shown up on COMPUTED TOMOGRAPHY. The symptoms are headache and partial or generalised fits. Treatment is by corticosteroids with a possibility of radiotherapy for multiple tumours. *See* Gilroy and Holliday (1982); Kaye (1991); Tortora and Grabowski (1993).

microcephaly a condition marked by an abnormally small head and small BRAIN and low levels of intelligence. Microcephaly can be divided into primary microcephaly and secondary microcephaly. The former is inherited as an autosomal recessive trait (*see* CHROMOSOMES). It can occur as part of other conditions associated with chromosomal and non-chromosomal deficiencies such as Roberts' syndrome, Williams' syndrome and de Lange syndrome. Secondary microcephaly is produced by infection or other problems which may arise in the PERINATAL period. See Hosking (1982); Smith (1985).

microcomputer the smallest type of computer which comprises one unit. Microcomputers, like the BBC series (*see* ACORN COMPUTERS), have one unit which contains circuitry with a microprocessor chip and groups of chips which provide the memory for the microcomputer while others deal with operating the keyboard, sending data to the screen, printer and disk drive. The single unit has the keyboard on it to input data. This is attached to a monitor, disk drive, and a printer and any other peripheral unit which can be added. *See* Bishop (1985).

microglossia an abnormally small tongue. The condition is relatively rare and is caused by the failure of the anterior two-thirds of the tongue to grow normally. It occurs in the prenatal stage. The person's speech can sound muffled. *See* Travis (1971).

micrognathia the failure of the mandible to develop normally.

Micromike an input device for the BBC Micro/Master series (*see* ACORN COMPUTERS). It comprises a hand-held or lapel microphone which is attached to a small control box. It fits into the analog port of the computer. The control box also controls the sound threshold and has a button to operate some parts of the software. The person has to use voice to make things happen on screen, e.g. helicopter rescuing a drowning man, a boat moving among islands in a river and so on. It encourages a young child to use vocal play and his voice.

Micronose a device which can be attached to a BBC computer to show a child how much nasality (*see* RESONANCE) there is in his speech. A flat switch is placed between the mouth and the nose. When the computer program is run, a graphic of a face appears. If the child has hypernasality, the nose on the face becomes bigger, whereas if the child is hyponasal, the mouth becomes bigger. A graph appears at the bottom of the screen which shows the amount of nasality the child produces. The teacher or therapist can give a pattern for the child to copy and it can be superimposed on top of the child's graph to show more easily the difference between the two graphs.

Microscribe a small, portable word processor. It has a QWERTY keyboard and an 80-character display in which the person can write, edit, send, receive or delete text. The memory has a capacity of 8000 characters which can be put onto 9 documents plus a 10-message memory capable of holding 80 characters. It can be used as a word processor with a voice synthesiser or can be linked to a microcomputer. It is battery operated with a rechargeable battery.

Microvoice an input device for the BBC Micro/Master series. It comprises a control box, a ROM, a microphone and demonstration disks. The unit plugs into the 1Mhz bus port. It can only distinguish ten words at a time but blocks of ten words can be loaded as required. These words are stored on a template. The one major problem, a problem which most voice recognition systems have, is that it can only recognise the voice of the speaker and the word must be spoken in the same way for it to be accepted.

Microwriter a machine with six keys which, when pressed in different combinations, produce a letter. The operator has to learn these combinations. It is said that someone can learn these in one hour and become proficient in the use of the Microwriter after a few weeks. Its memory holds five pages of text which is held in memory even when the machine is switched off. It is portable and can be linked up to a speech synthesiser, printer or television.

midbrain part of the brain which is found above the PONS. It is the smallest of the three parts of the BRAIN – HINDBRAIN, forebrain (*see* DIENCEPHALON) and midbrain. It is about 12.5 cm long, 2.5 cm wide and 2 cm thick. There are ascending and descending tracts of cranial nerves III and IV (*see* CRANIAL NERVES). The floor of the THIRD VENTRICLE is formed at the front between the cerebral peduncles. The substantia nigra is situated in the midbrain. See Barr (1979); Kolb and Whishaw (1990).

minimal pairs two words are said to have a different meaning if they differ by one sound in the same environment of the word. For example, 'pin' and 'bin' are minimal pairs because they differ by one sound, i.e. /p/ vs /b/, and thus the meaning is changed. A minimal pair can only exist if there is one difference in the sounds which occur in the same place in either word. This is also known as variation in sound. Minimal pairs have an important role in speech and language therapy, since they mark the fundamental difference between treatment programmes for phonological or articulation delay or disorder. In the former, the therapist teaches the child sound oppositions such as the difference between /tutər/ and /kukər/, while in the latter, the therapist teaches the child how to make particular sounds which the child has previously been incapable of making. *See* Grunwell (1987) .

135

Minnesota Test for the Differential Diagnosis of Aphasia (MTDDA) devised by Schuell in 1965 and revised in 1973, this is a formal assessment for testing the severity of a language disorder affecting those with APHASIA. Five modalities are tested: (1) auditory disturbance; (2) visual-reading; (3) speech/language; (4) visuomotor/ graphic; (5) numeric/arithmetic functions. The 47 subtests in each section are arranged in ascending order of difficulty. There are 'easy' tests for examining residual skills in those who have a severe aphasia and 'hard' tests for those who have a mild aphasic impairment. The person's performance in the tests between these extremes allows the therapist to determine the level of breakdown in each language modality. The test is American but in some of the subtests British amendments have been made so it is possible to use the test more reliably in Britain. There are two rating scales to establish the functional ability of the person and the severity of his condition. The severity scale is from 0 (no impairment) to 4 (severe impairment). The five types of communicative behaviour are rated on a severity scale of 0–6. It has a prognostic potential. *See* Eisenson (1984); Beech et al (1993).

Minspeak the software system which operates WALKER TALKERS, ALPHA TALKERS, INTRO TALKERS, DELTA TALKERS, TOUCH TALKERS, LIGHT TALKERS and the LIBERATOR COMMUNICATION AID. It means 'minimum effort speech'. It uses multi-meaning icons to access messages programmed into one of these devices. Bruce Baker, who developed Minspeak, started from the basis of semantic compaction in which one or two icons can have different meanings depending on the semantic context in which they are used. Thus, the icon of the 'sun' can mean 'sun', 'hot', 'fire', 'face', 'happy', 'orange', and the user

may think of many more. When used in conjunction with another icon the meanings increase. Semantic compaction also allows for a smaller number of graphics to represent a large number of semantic concepts, especially when the icons are combined together to produce messages. These messages can be accessed by fewer key actuations. Icons have three characteristics:

1. Transparent: the icons should be easily recognisable.
2. Multi-meaning: the icons should be able to represent several meanings.
3. Combinational potential: the icons should be able to be combined easily with other icons to produce new messages.

Although the icons produced by Bruce Baker are known as Minsymbols, they do not have to be used as any set of symbols can be used such as REBUS, BLISSYMBOLS or Makaton symbols (*see* MAKATON). Minspeak is the way the symbols interact with each other as long as they have the characteristics already given. Minspeak is reported to provide fast, effective communication in that as many characters as the user wishes can be represented by just two icons. It allows for routine, frequent needs to be communicated using themes (*see* TOUCH TALKER) as well as emergency needs. It allows for conversational control for entering, initiating and controlling the conversation while the user can make formal presentations in class, at home or conferences. *See* Baker (1982).

Minspeak Application Programs (MAPs) these programs have been designed by authors who are experts with a particular client-group. The programs apply the MINSPEAK principles for various client-groups. The aim is to produce fast, effective communication allowing the client to:

1. Communicate everyday needs.

2. Communicate needs in an emergency.
3. Enter and control a conversation.
4. Produce spontaneous and interactive dialogue.
5. Give lectures or speeches at conferences or social events, etc.

The Minspeak applications that have been designed recently are: POWER IN PLAY; STORIES AND STRATEGIES FOR COMMUNICATION; TOPICS TO LEARN COMMUNICATION; INTERACTION, EDUCATION AND PLAY; LANGUAGE, LEARNING AND LIVING; WORDS STRATEGY; and UNITY/128. There is also a MAP which combines Blissymbols and Words Strategy known as Blissymbol Minspeak Words Strategy (BMW). These programs can be loaded into the DELTA TALKER, TOUCH TALKER, LIGHT TALKER or LIBERATOR COMMUNICATION AID. Each program can be customised for individual users. Rumble and Robertson, two speech and language therapists, have written a set of lesson plans for the MAPS Language, Learning and Living and Words Strategy. The starter module has 21 levels which, it is hoped, will produce a 400-word core vocabulary. Every fifth lesson there is a practice level to revise what the person has learnt in the previous four levels. Following this Starter Module, there are 40 topic modules covering a broad range of interests and communication needs such as food/drink, going on holiday, making telephone calls, art and sports and leisure and religion. Each of these modules will have five levels in the same format as the Starter Module. *See* Baker (1989); Rumble and Robertson (1995).

MIT *see* MELODIC INTONATION THERAPY.

mixed transcortical aphasia a particular syndrome used in the classification of APHASIA. The symptoms are non-fluent language, impaired comprehension and naming while repetition remains intact. *See* Eisenson (1984).

MLU *see* MEAN LENGTH OF UTTERANCE.

Möbius syndrome a CONGENITAL DISORDER which produces weakness of the facial muscles and the bilateral failure of the eyes to abduct. The syndrome may be caused by a congenital abnormality in the sixth and seventh cranial nerve nuclei in the BRAIN-STEM. It is an IDIOPATHIC condition which can run in families. Other associated symptoms are syndactyly, club feet and LEARNING DISABILITY. *See* Gilroy and Holliday (1982).

mode *see* CENTRAL TENDENCY.

Model 1600 Voice Analyzer the voice analyser can be used in the clinic, home, hospital or school. It is designed to pick up fundamental frequency (Fo) and intensity level at the same time on the monitor. There are two lines which can be compared, the top one with the therapist's mode; and the lower one for the patient's attempts. Both can be superimposed on the other for an easy comparison. The machine can be linked up to a printer so that the therapist can keep accurate records of assessments and progress during therapy.

modelling a therapeutic approach to BEHAVIOUR THERAPY devised by Bandura in 1969. It is known also as vicarious conditioning since its aim is to provide a model participating successfully in the person's feared situation while being watched by the person. After each stage the person is encouraged to copy this behaviour. *See* Atkinson et al (1993).

modem a device for transmitting data over the telephone system from a computer. It stands for MOdulator/ DEModulator. There are many on the market. They can be connected to the operator's telephone system, so that data can be transmitted over long distances to another computer. *See* Bishop (1985); Brookshear (1991).

modification the aim in therapy to bring about a change in behaviour. Also a term used in BEHAVIOUR THERAPY.

monoamine oxidase inhibitors (MAOI) a form of drug treatment used with those who have DEPRESSION. The three main MAOI drugs are phenelzine, isocarboxazid and tranylcypromine. The evidence of efficacy of these drugs on depression is poor but they can act as a mild anti-anxiety drug. There is also a possibility that they are effective in cases where phobias and irrational anxiety are prominent. Dizziness, dry mouth and fatigue are common side effects in the first few weeks of starting the drugs. These drugs interact with certain foods, e.g. cheese, broad beans, yeast, producing unbearable headaches and a swing to low blood pressure. They should not be mixed with tricyclic antidepressant drugs (*see* ANTIDEPRESSANTS) or ELECTROCONVULSIVE THERAPY. *See* Stafford-Clark and Smith (1983); Davison and Neale (1994).

monozygotic twins identical twins who develop from a single fertilised egg, having the same heredity. *See* Atkinson et al (1993).

Monterey Fluency Programme devised by Ryan and Kirk in 1978 and based on the ideas of those who follow the SPEAK MORE FLUENTLY approach to the treatment of those who have a STAMMER, it is a highly structured behaviour modification programme following the principles of OPERANT CONDITIONING. Its main aim is to establish complete fluency; an ACCEPTABLE STAMMER is not regarded as success. It begins with a fluency interview lasting 30 minutes during which the patient is put into as many communication situations as possible. The next stage is a criterion test in which the person is asked to perform for five minutes in three modes – reading, monologue and conversation. If the stuttering rate is less than 0.5 stuttered words per minute in any of the three modes, the person is put through an establishment programme in a particular mode using two techniques GILCU or DAF. Another criterion test follows; if the person stutters

more than 0.5 stuttered words per minute, he progresses to the transfer programme while if he produces less than 0.5 stuttered words per minute, the person is recycled through the establishment programme. The third criterion test follows the transfer programme with similar requirements to the previous one. If the person succeeds, he is placed on a maintenance programme which can last several months. If the person maintains fluency over a period of 22 months, he can be discharged. *See* Dalton (1983).

morbid jealousy also known as delusional jealousy, the person becomes so jealous, he becomes fanatically preoccupied at finding out if his beliefs have any truth. For example, the person has a delusion that his wife is having an affair. He begins to follow her everywhere and may assault anyone with whom she stops to speak. If the wife gives a false admission about any man she knows, it could lead to murder. *See* Stafford-Clark and Smith (1983); Davison and Neale (1994).

morphology the part of linguistics that deals with the formation of words. Morphology recognises processes of inflection and derivation in the construction of words. Inflection relates to regular, rule-governed grammatical processes such as plural or past tense in English. Derivation refers to semi- or partially productive processes of word-formation such as suffixation of -ness on to adjectives in English to provide nouns, e.g. happiness, sadness. These affixes are called morphemes – the smallest meaningful unit in any language. The realisation of morphemes, e.g. /s/, /z/, /ɪz/ for the plural morpheme is called an allomorph. Each individual unit, i.e. each of the allomorphs in the last example, is called a morph. There are two types of morpheme:

1. A bound morpheme is an affix which can be attached to a word to represent number and tense, etc.

2. A free morpheme is a whole word which stands on its own without affixes.

An example of both of these types of morpheme is the word:

anti - dis - establish - ment - arian - ism .

The bound morphemes are 'anti, dis, ment, arian, ism' while 'establish' is the free morpheme. There a three models discussed in morphology:

1. Item and arrangement (IA): this examines word structure and syntactic structures which follow particular, logical sequences in a linear way:
(1) The men played cricket .
The example in (1) is analysed in the form:

det + MAN + plural + PLAY + past + CRICKET .

Difficulties in explaining some morphological phenomena occur, such as 'mice' in the form 'MOUSE + plural'.
2. Item and process (IP): a process is a derivational procedure which accounts for the form 'mice' as a vowel change from 'mouse'.
3. Word and paradigm (WP): a morphological model which takes the root of a word and fits it into a paradigm. The resulting words and structures are formed by rules such as Latin verb declensions, e.g. amo, amas, amat, amamus, amatis, amant.

See Matthews (1974); Fromkin and Rodman (1993).

morphophonology refers to the study of the phonological effects or consequences of morphological processes. In the regular plural in English, the exact form of a plural noun is affected by the phonological form of the final segment of that noun. If the noun ends in a voiced segment (except /z/), the plural form is /z/; if the noun ends in a voiceless segment (except /s/), the plural form is /s/; if the noun ends in /s/ or /z/, e.g. bus, haze, the plural form is /ɪz/. *See* Matthews (1974); Fromkin and Rodman (1993).

mother's depression abnormal moods which a mother has which may affect her child. These moods are associated with low self-esteem, loss of energy, poor sleep, poor appetite or compensatory overeating, anxiety, obsessional symptoms, increased use of drugs and alcohol and a loss of sexual desire and pleasure. Maternal depression can double the chance of disturbance in the child from 15 to 30 per cent. The moods have specific effects on the child. The mother's apathy produces decreased interaction and stimulation which causes speech and language delay and attention-seeking behaviour in the child. If the mother's use of discipline and management is inconsistent, this may produce behaviour problems of all sorts (e.g. temper tantrums, eating and sleeping problems). If the family is socially isolated, there may be a lack of peer contact for the child which could produce a failure to develop social skills and, possibly, speech and language problems. A mother's resentment and threats of abandonment can produce fearfulness and SEPARATION ANXIETY. Irritability in the mother may make her use excessive physical punishment against the child which produces fearfulness and/or aggressiveness between the child and his peers. The child's difficult behaviour in turn can worsen the mother's depression. When the mother comes to the clinic, she will probably present psychosomatic complaints or anxiety about the child. She may not openly admit she has depression. Depression affects 5 per cent of women and 2 per cent of men. It affects 30–50 per cent of women in the lower social classes. PSYCHOTHERAPY can be used in treating such conditions. *See* Rutter (1975).

motor aphasia *see* APHASIA (1).

motor area *see* BRAIN.

motor equivalence the general pattern of planning of a configuration of movement necessary to achieve a target. In relation to speech, it is the determination of the sequence of movement throughout the entire vocal tract which is necessary to deliver the message.

motor neuron disease also known as amyotrophic lateral sclerosis, this is a progressive disease which causes failure in the motor neurons in the SPINAL CORD, loss of motor neurons in the BRAIN-STEM and a loss of Betz cells in the cerebral CORTEX. Only motor cells are affected. The cause is uncertain. There is complete loss of motor control which produces DYSARTHRIA, i.e. progressive deterioration in speech, as well as the onset of DYSPHAGIA, loss of hand function and mobility. There is neither sensory loss nor DEMENTIA. Treatment is aimed at making the patient's life as comfortable as possible since the disease progresses steadily until death. Speech therapy for these patients consists of maintaining the intelligibility of speech for as long as possible. When speech worsens significantly, some form of ALTERNATIVE AUGMENTATIVE COMMUNICATION will have to be found. Treatment is also given for the patient's swallow. There can be remission but this may be just for a few weeks or months. *See* Gilroy and Holliday (1982); Beukelman and Mirenda (1992) (amyotrophic lateral sclerosis and AAC).

mouse an INPUT DEVICE which can move the cursor about a screen. It can be used with icon software in which windows are produced on the screen with menus of one or more item. The mouse is used to move an arrow around the menus to choose which option the operator wishes to use. It can be held under the hand and requires the touch of only two or three buttons and lateral movement over a flat surface. *See* Bishop (1985); Brookshear (1991).

mouth often called the oral cavity. The mouth has a roof which is formed by the hard palate and soft palate towards the posterior of the mouth. This part of the mouth is supplied by the greater palatine and nasopalatine nerves, the fibres of which travel in the MAXILLARY NERVE. The floor of the mouth is formed by the tongue which is supplied by the lingual nerve (*see* TONGUE) while the walls of the mouth, i.e. the cheeks, are supplied by the buccal nerve; both of these are branches of the MANDIBULAR NERVE. In the posterior wall of the mouth is the fauces (fauces are arches) which is also known as the oropharyngeal passage. Between the arches, the uvula hangs. Behind the uvula is the palatine tonsil or true tonsil. The palatopharyngeus muscle (*see* MUSCLES FOR SWALLOWING) runs to the palate behind this tonsil. The front wall is formed by the teeth which are set in the upper and lower dentitions or dental arches. The alveolar ridge is the bony ridge behind the upper dentition. *See* Tortora and Grabowski (1993).

mouth breathing a symptom of adenoidal problems. The child's mouth is affected as he will have a high arched maxilla. He will also have narrow nostrils and the pharyngeal tonsils will be enlarged. This will produce the typical 'look', i.e. ADENOIDAL FACIES, of a child who has adenoidal problems. The sense of smell will be affected and he will lose taste, thus providing a possible reduction in the child's appetite. There could also be a CONDUCTIVE HEARING LOSS. *See* Travis (1971).

MRI *see* MAGNETIC RESONANCE IMAGING.

MTDDA *see* MINNESOTA TEST FOR THE DIFFERENTIAL DIAGNOSIS OF APHASIA.

mucous membrane a sheet of EPITHELIUM which is supported by a basal lamina made of CONNECTIVE TISSUE. It lines a cavity in the body which reaches the exterior, e.g. the respiratory tract. The layer of epithelium secretes mucus which keeps the cavities moist. The connective tissue binds the epithelial layer to the underlying structures. It keeps the blood vessels in place and protects muscles. *See* Tortora and Grabowski (1993).

multi-infarct dementia a type of dementia which may occur in people who have hypertension and diabetes in whose CEREBRAL HEMISPHERES and BRAIN-STEM small lacunar infarcts appear. The development of these infarcts is irregular and so the progression of the dementia is irregular. Such people produce a gradual deterioration in intellectual functioning, including impairment in judgement and lack of insight; memory is impaired while there is also lability of mood and sudden crying associated with DEPRESSION. Associated problems which have gradual onset include DYSARTHRIA, DYSPHAGIA, HEMIPLEGIA, ataxia of gait and the type of loss of emotional control associated with those who have pseudobulbar palsy. *See* Gilroy and Holliday (1982); Stafford-Clark and Smith (1983); Davison and Neale (1994).

multiple sclerosis a disease of unknown aetiology, the features of which are due to multiple areas of demyelination of the BRAIN and SPINAL CORD. It affects all the areas, especially around the ventricles, spinal cord and BRAIN-STEM. The symptoms are optic neuritis, double vision, DYSARTHRIA, ataxia, spastic gait (*see* CEREBRAL PALSY), HEMIPLEGIA and, occasionally, DEMENTIA. The diagnosis is made following tests such as visual evoked responses and an examination of CEREBROSPINAL FLUID which should show evidence of lymphocyte infiltration. It can follow a remission-relapse course and is a progressive disease which produces dysarthria. The main dysarthric symptoms are poor volume, harsh voice and poor articulation. *See* Darley et al (1975); Gilroy and Holliday (1982); Beukelman and Mirenda (1992).

multisensory approaches *see* EDUCATION OF HEARING-IMPAIRED CHILDREN.

Munchausen syndrome named after Baron Munchausen who told very tall stories concerning how good a cavalry officer he was, this is a form of DEMENTIA. An example of someone who had this syndrome concerns the person who likes hospital operations so much, that he will be admitted, followed by discharge. The person goes to another hospital and a similar procedure ensues. A person who had this syndrome requested speech therapy a few years ago. He complained his speech was dysarthric as most consonants were substituted by glottal stops and, although he claimed to suffer from multiple sclerosis, his speech had none of the typical characteristics associated with MS. It seemed his speech disorder was functional. He was put on a treatment programme of having his speech taped followed by his listening to it. Having listened to it, he began using normal speech quickly. His response to such therapy was very similar to the response of those with functional dysphonia. *See* Kallen et al (1986).

muscles for swallowing four muscles are used for swallowing:

1. Mylohyoid muscle: stretching along the mylohyoid line of the mandible. It originates from the inner surface of the mandible and inserts into the body of the hyoid bone. It is supplied by the mandibular branch of the trigeminal nerve and elevates both the hyoid bone and floor of the mouth and depresses the mandible.

2. Digastric muscle has two parts:
   (a) posterior belly originates from the mastoid process of the temporal bone and is supplied by the facial nerve VII;
   (b) anterior belly originates from the inner side of the lower border of the mandible and is supplied by

141

the mandibular nerve. Both parts insert into the body of the hyoid bone through an intermediate tendon. The digastric muscle elevates the hyoid bone and lowers the jaw as in opening the mouth.

3. Stylopharyngeus muscle: originating from the base of the styloid process, its fibres insert into the lateral aspects of the pharynx and thyroid cartilage. This muscle lifts up the larynx and expands the pharynx to allow the food bolus to descend to the oesophagus.

4. Palatopharyngeus muscle: originating at the soft palate, its fibres insert into the back of the thyroid cartilage and the side and back wall of the pharynx. It is supplied by the pharyngeal plexus. It lifts up both the larynx and the pharynx and closes the nasopharynx during the swallowing process.

Other muscles associated with the process of swallowing are described in the discussion concerning the PHARYNX. *See* Tortora and Grabowski (1993).

muscles of facial expression these muscles are supplied by cranial nerve VII (*see* CRANIAL NERVES). There are two type of muscle:

1. Sphincters which close off openings.
2. Dilators causing structures to open.

They modify the expression of the face and/or meaning to what is being said. The orbicularis oculi surrounds each eye and can be used to screw up the eyes. The orbicularis oris muscle allows pouting of lips. The muscle is supplied by the buccal and mandibular branches of the facial nerve. The buccinator allows the person to smile while the levator anguli labii superioris and depressor anguli labii inferioris allow the person to elevate and lower the lips respectively. All these facial muscles are derived from the second pharyngeal arch. *See* Tortora and Grabowski (1993).

muscles of mastication four muscles control the function of chewing or mastication:

1. Temporalis muscle: fan-shape muscle, the fibres of which reach a tendon that is inserted on the coronoid process. The anterior and superior fibres raise the mandible. The muscle is supplied by the deep temporal nerves which are branches of the anterior division of mandibular nerve.

2. Masseter muscle: originating at the ZYGOMATIC ARCH, the fibres go downwards and backwards and are attached to the lateral aspects of the ramus of the mandible. It is supplied by the mandibular nerve. Its function is to lift the mandible, covering the teeth during the process of chewing.

3. Medial pterygoid muscle: originating at the middle of the lateral pterygoid plate, its fibres go downwards, backwards and laterally and end in the middle of the angle of the mandible. It is supplied by the mandibular nerve and assists in raising the mandible.

4. Lateral pterygoid muscle: originating from two places – one being the infratemporal surface of the greater wing of sphenoid and the second being the surface of the lateral pterygoid plate. Fibres reach the front of the mandible neck and articular disc of the temperomandibular joint. It is supplied by the mandibular nerve. Its function is to pull forward the neck of the mandible by the articular disc as the mouth opens. It also causes the rotating action of chewing.

See Tortora and Grabowski (1993).

mutism an inability to speak or phonate. It may be organic as in profound deafness or non-organic as an extreme example of conversion behaviour. *See* Fay (1993).

'My Turn to Speak' designed as a package to help those working with people using a communication aid to develop a consistent and cohesive team approach to their training in school and at home. It comprises five 90-minute sessions which cover the main factors affecting the communication of those using any augmentative communication system, including positions in and accessing of the device, methods of communication, functions of communication and communication breakdown. The workshop also concentrates on the child's current skills and setting long term aims. The workshop can be organised by speech and language therapists, occupational therapists, physiotherapists and teachers with a special interest in AAC. It can be used with teachers, classroom assistants, parents, management and therapists. The pack consists of a Tutor's Manual, Participant's Manual and a video. *See* Pennington et al (1993).

myasthenia gravis a neuromuscular disorder. It is an autoimmune condition in which the person has a progressive muscle weakness during exertion but recovers after rest. There is a reduction in the number of acetycholine receptors in the neuromuscular joint. Thus, repetitive stimulation will result in the decrease of muscle fibres as there is receptor insufficiency in each neuromuscular joint. This is evidenced by progressive weakness. It is a rare disease with a prevalence of about 1 in 10 000. It is more common in females than in males by 2:1. The mean age of onset is 26 years of age in females and 31 years of age in males. There is no significant familial occurrence. It can produce DYSARTHRIA which worsens as the amount of speech increases. The muscles used for speech become tired, hypernasality increases, articulation becomes worse and dysphonia sets in with the voice becoming quieter. *See* Darley et al (1975); Gilroy and Holliday (1982); Kolb and Whishaw (1990); Tortora and Grabowski (1993).

myelography a diagnostic test to locate a lesion on or near to the SPINAL CORD. In this test, a radio-opaque material is instilled into the spinal cord and its movement up the canal is recorded by serial X-rays. *See* Kaye (1991); Tortora and Grabowski (1993).

myelomeningocele a form of SPINA BIFIDA. There is a flaccid paralysis of the legs as well as of the bladder and bowel. Abnormalities to the skin, SPINAL CORD, vertebrae and MENINGES also occur. It is often associated with HYDROCEPHALUS. *See* Hosking (1982); Kaye (1991).

mylohyoid muscle *see* MUSCLES FOR SWALLOWING.

myoclonus a movement disorder characterised by sudden jerks. It can occur in the normal population while asleep but it becomes a disorder when associated with EPILEPSY. It is a symptom of acquired BRAIN-STEM diseases such as JAKOB-CREUTZFELDT DISEASE which causes degeneration of the BASAL GANGLIA, hypoxic brain damage or drug dependency. *See* Gilroy and Holliday (1982); Kaye (1991).

MyVoice a high-tech battery-operated communication aid. The machine can be customised to each user's individual needs. It produces messages by digitised speech recorded through a microphone. These programmed words or phrases can be accessed using the keypad with the appropriate overlay. The keypad has 40 cells which can be divided into as few as two areas to make it easier to access. The concept keyboard or a switch-operated scanning system can also be attached. The overlays can be made to the requirements of the user with either symbols, pictures or words. The messages can be preprogrammed into different levels to expand the number of phrases although it can only accept two minutes of speech.

myxoedema a metabolic disorder which results from under-secretion of the thyroid gland. There is a congenital form which if not diagnosed and treated at an early stage may lead to CRETINISM. Onset may also occur later in child-

143

hood as juvenile myxoedema. It is also sometimes a feature of senescence. In all cases, the predominating feature is change of pitch and voice quality. The voice becomes hoarse and pitch drops owing to thickening of the VOCAL FOLDS. *See* Greene and Mathieson (1989); Tortora and Grabowski (1993).

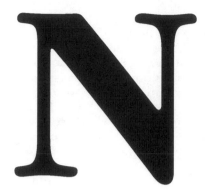

N-indicator a machine to help people who have speech problems due to hyper/hyponasality. It operates by working out how much vibration exists at the end of the NOSE by having the person place a contact microphone on this part of the nose; the amount of vibration is shown by the deflection of the needle on the display unit. A green and red light shows if the pointer is less or greater than 50 per cent deflection. The indicator should be adjusted for each person. It may also be possible to show the degree of PHONATION.

naming a language function which is assessed and treated in those who have APHASIA. There are four stages of naming:

1. Picture recognition.
2. Retrieval of the semantic relation corresponding to the picture.
3. Accessing a phonological form using the semantic relation.
4. Producing the spoken word to name the picture.

If the person has an aphasia compounded either by AGNOSIA or by a difficulty in retrieving SEMANTICS, naming will be even more difficult. *See* Benson (1979); Rosenbek et al (1989).

narrow transcription *see* TRANSCRIPTION SYSTEMS (2).

nasal

1. A description of sounds which are produced by using the resonating nasal cavities. These sounds are /n,m,ŋ/. *See* Ladefoged (1993).
2. A description of any structure or disorder related to the NOSE. *See* Tortora and Grabowski (1993).

nasalisation a condition in which there is excessive nasal resonance throughout speech.

nasopalatine nerve *see* MOUTH.

nasopharynx *see* PHARYNX.

natural phonology a phonological theory proposed by David Stampe in the late 1970s. In essence, he believes a child will simplify sounds which cause difficulty. These simplifications are called PHONOLOGICAL PROCESSES. The thrust of his theory is that as these processes are INNATE, those sounds which are found difficult by the child will automatically be simplified by young children as they acquire speech and language. Thus, natural phonology becomes a suitable means for analysing children's speech as it is based on simplifying sound systems (*see* PHONOLOGY). By treating the child's simplifications the therapist is showing the complexity of sound production to the child and the sounds for which he is aiming. *See* Grunwell (1987).

natural process analysis devised by Shriberg and Kwiatowski in 1980 to obtain a sample of SPONTANEOUS SPEECH for the therapist to discover which PHONOLOGICAL PROCESSES are used by the child when he produces sound changes. The elicited words are transcribed and then coded into stops, nasals/glides, fricatives/affricates (*see* ARTICULATION) and the information can be summarised. *See* Grunwell (1987).

negation the process of denial of the whole or part of an utterance. It is represented in English by the negative units 'no, n't and not'. Negative affixes such as 'un-' and 'non-' can also be used. *See* Huddleston (1976).

neologisms *see* APHASIA.

neologistic jargon *see* JARGON APHASIA (4).

network a series of computers all linked together so that information can be transferred among them. This could be used in business such as the Stock Exchange where all the terminals will have the relevant data supplied from the main computer so that several stockbrokers can have the same information ready at hand. *See* Brookshear (1991).

neurilemmoma a benign tumour which affects cranial nerve VIII (*see* CRANIAL NERVES), the acoustic nerve. It produces TINNITUS, progressive HEARING LOSS and episodic vertigo. As it increases in size, it involves the other cranial nerves and structures of the BRAIN such as the CEREBELLUM. Such interference can produce cerebellar ataxia (*see* CEREBRAL PALSY). Treatment is by surgery. *See* Gilroy and Holliday (1982).

neurofibroma *see* TUMOURS OF THE CENTRAL NERVOUS SYSTEM (3).

neurolinguistics the study of neurological programming for the comprehension and production of language and reasons for the breakdown in language or articulation. Research has come from clinical linguistics, to try to construct models to explain language breakdown in APHASIA, stammering (*see* STAMMER), DYSARTHRIA, etc., and hypotheses can be found to show how the brain can organise language. *See* Clark and Clark (1977).

neuron the cell which is responsible for passing nerve impulses to muscles. Motor neurons receive information which makes movement possible. *See* Tortora and Grabowski (1993).

neuropsychological assessment there are several goals for making assessments in clinical neuropsychology including finding evidence of cortical damage or dysfunction and its location; facilitating rehabilitation and patient care; showing mild disturbances where other test results may be equivocal and identify unusual brain organisation which may produce behavioural rather than organic problems. *See* Kolb and Whishaw (1990).

neurosis neurotic disorders are those which affect emotional and intellectual functioning without losing reality. Such disorders include ANXIETY, STRESS, OBSESSIVE–COMPULSIVE DISORDERS, DEPRESSION and MANIC-DEPRESSION. *See* Stafford-Clark and Smith (1983); Davison and Neale (1994).

neutral a vowel sound which is described as being produced not at the front or back of the mouth or high or low but in a central position. This is shown clearly in the diagram of the CARDINAL VOWEL SYSTEM. The vowel in question is known as SCHWA or shwa /ə/. *See* Cruttenden (1994).

neutralisation a phenomenon which describes sounds which can be interchangeable in certain contexts with other sounds because they lose their distinction. For example, /p,t,k/ and /b,d,g/ can be distinguished from each other by the opposition of voicing (*see* ARTICULATION) and ASPIRATION. In the former set of sounds, aspiration is present, e.g. 'pin/bin', 'pit/bit', etc., while in the second set of sounds there is no aspiration present. However, when they follow /s/, e.g.

146

'skate', 'spate', 'steak', they do not require the distinction because /b,d,g/ in similar positions do not exist, e.g. *sgate, *sbate, *sdeak. Thus, the distinction between these two sets of phonemes (*see* PHONOLOGY) is lost in the context following /s/, i.e. s_V where 'V' = vowel. *See* Cruttenden (1994); Fromkin and Rodman (1993).

NMR nuclear magnetic resonance *see* MAGNETIC RESONANCE IMAGING.

noise-induced hearing loss when exposed to a loud noise for any length of time, a person may eventually have a noise-induced hearing loss which is sensorineural (*see* SENSORINEURAL HEARING LOSS) in character. The degree of loss depends on how long the person has been exposed to the sound and its intensity. If a depressed threshold goes back to normal after a few hours, it is called temporary threshold shift (TTS) but if the exposure is for a longer time, it can become a permanent threshold shift (PTS). This form of hearing loss is also known as industrial hearing loss. PTS can also occur if there is a sudden burst of noise – known as acoustic trauma and found on an audiogram (*see* PURE-TONE AUDIOMETRY) by a dip at 4000 Hz and a recovery at 8000 Hz. The loss is sensorineural. *See* Katz (1985).

non-fluent aphasia *see* APHASIA (1).

non-word *see* NONSENSE WORD.

nonsense word a word that follows the PHONOTACTIC structure of a true word in English but does not have any meaning, e.g. dup, sep, mib, etc. *See* Fromkin and Rodman (1993).

norm describes what is regarded as normal. *See* Atkinson et al (1993); Davison and Neale (1994).

normal distribution a statistical analysis of scores which are analysed by CENTRAL TENDENCY. It can be drawn in graph form as a normal distribution curve. *See* Miller (1975).

normal pressure hydrocephalus a condition which can produce DEMENTIA. The features are a clumsy gait, urgency of micturition and eventual incontinence. The person's unsteadiness is due to a mixture of ataxia, spasticity (*see* CEREBRAL PALSY) and dyspraxia of gait. It can be reversed by placing a shunt in the ventricles of the brain to drain the excess CEREBROSPINAL FLUID. *See* Stafford-Clark and Smith (1983); Davison and Neale (1994).

Northwestern Syntax Screening Test devised by Lee in 1969, it is a SCREENING TEST which can measure independently levels of verbal comprehension and expressive language in children between the ages of 3;0 and 7;0 years. The comprehension section requires a picture-pointing response to verbally presented stimulus sentences and the expressive section involves sentence repetition. *See* Lee (1969) in Appendix I.

nose the front part of the nose has two U-shaped cartilages forming the nostrils. At the posterior of the nose, there is an opening to the nasopharynx (*see* PHARYNX). The nasal cavity is formed by a roof, floor and wall. The floor is the top surface of the hard palate and the roof is divided into three parts – the anterior part is the slope or bridge of the nose, the middle part is the ethmoid or cribriform plate, while the posterior part is formed by the anterior and inferior surfaces of the cribriform plate. The cavity is divided by the nasal septum. The lateral walls are formed by the superior, middle and inferior conchae or folds. Between these folds are the superior, middle and inferior meati. Around the middle meatus, there are four openings of the frontal sinus, the anterior ethmoid sinus, the maxillary sinus and the middle ethmoid sinus. At the lower edge of the cavity, just above the floor, is the naso-lacrimal duct. This structure draws tears from the eyes down the nose through a flap in the nose. When

147

the nose is blown, it stops material being blown upwards. If the flap does not shut and the nose is blown, bubbles may appear at the side of the eyes. Blood supply is by the ophthalmic, maxillary and facial arteries while the nerve supply comes from the ophthalmic, maxillary and facial nerves. *See* Tortora and Grabowski (1993).

noun in traditional grammar, a noun was said to be the name of a person, place or object. However, this definition was inappropriate for modern linguists, who preferred to define nouns and other grammatical categories in terms of their formal syntactic behaviour. Nouns, then, are elements which can only be placed in particular positions in the sentence and to which plural affixes can be attached. *See* Lyons (1968); Fromkin and Rodman (1993).

noun phrase a noun phrase is a constituent (*see* CONSTITUENT ANALYSIS) in GENERATIVE GRAMMAR and is generated by a head noun with optional premodification and/or postmodification. *See* Lyons (1968); Fromkin and Rodman (1993).

nuclear magnetic imaging *see* MAGNETIC RESONANCE IMAGING.

nucleus *see* SUPRASEGMENTAL PHON-OLOGY.

Nuffield Dyspraxia Programme devised by Connery and colleagues, it is a complete programme comprising an assessment and a detailed therapeutic programme. The required therapy is based on the scores of the assessment which assesses oral-motor skills and sound-sequencing abilities of speech in isolation, single words with differing phonotactic structures and sentences using picture material and imitation. It concentrates on improvement of speed and accuracy of articulatory movement. *See* Connery et al (1985) in Appendix I.

null hypothesis this hypothesis must be disproved by statistical analysis. It states there is no significant difference between the distributions of scores. All researchers start off with the null hypothesis which, if their experiment is worth while, will be rejected. If they fail to reject it, there must have been something wrong with the experiment either methodologically, e.g. the wrong design was used, or theoretically, e.g. the assumptions made about the experiment were wrong, or else there was too great a variation in the variables present in the environment in which the experiment was to be carried out. If researchers have doubts about the possibility of rejecting the null hypothesis, they may use a more rigorous level of significance than 0.5 and may use 0.01 or 0.001. This could result in a type 2 error where a significant difference is said to exist but does not exist. *See* Miller (1975).

numeric keypad a grouping of numbered keys usually 0–9 on a keyboard although they can form their own unit. Many computer keyboards have such a grouping with arithmetical functions on a separate section of the keyboard.

nystagmus an involuntary rhythmical movement of the eyes which can occur at rest or during eye movement. It can happen to both eyes or just to one and is caused by a disorder of the CEREBELLUM. The involuntary movement of the eyes can be horizontal, vertical, oblique or circular. They can also be swinging or jerky. *See* Gilroy and Holliday (1982); Kolb and Whishaw (1990); Tortora and Grabowski (1993).

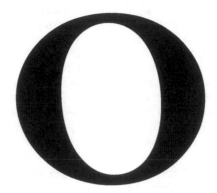

object *see* DIRECT OBJECT; INDIRECT OBJECT.

object permanence a theory developed by Piaget on the cognitive development of children. Piaget argued that if a child is presented with a toy which he is allowed to play with or handle, and it is then hidden under a box or cloth, the child will not make any effort to find or look for it. This stage is present until 5–6 months of age. According to Piaget, this shows the child's egocentricity (*see* PRE-OPERATIONAL STAGE), i.e. the child is only concerned with his own world and ignores external stimuli. The critics put forward the argument that it was how the object was hidden which was important. Thus, if the object was hidden gradually, the child might try and find it but, if hidden suddenly, then the child would not try to look for it. *See* Donaldson (1987); Atkinson et al (1993); Boden (1994).

observation an informal technique for assessing the person's behaviour. It is important for the therapist to decide the target behaviour to be aimed for and the stages through which the person has to pass to reach this behaviour. It is possible by observation to see changes in behaviour patterns from a baseline (found in initial assessment). If two therapists are observing the one person, they must have a common language which they can use to express their findings. This language must be objective so that the biases and wishes of the therapists are not reflected in their reported findings. There are two main types of observation:

1. Direct observation: the researcher watches the types of behaviour presented by a client in particular environments or in a laboratory.

2. Indirect observation: the researcher uses interviews or questionnaires to find out how people feel about particular issues such as political affiliations, preferences for particular products, etc. The researchers have to be trained to use the questionnaire, the questionnaire itself has to be carefully assessed before use, a sample of people has to be chosen and appropriate methods of data analysis have to be used to make sure the results are interpreted correctly. *See* Atkinson et al (1993).

obsessive–compulsive disorder a neurosis present in 0.5 per cent of the population at any one time. Those who have obsessions or compulsions about something, e.g. keeping clean, will spend their life carrying out such activities as are required to fulfil their obsession. For example, if a person has a compulsion concerning cleanliness, there could be extensive hand-washing, washing utensils several times before using them, washing sink surrounds before using them to wash in, as well as keeping soap, cloths and towels in receptacles for cleanliness. Compulsive rituals are carried out a certain number of times which becomes a magical figure. If the ritual is repeated more often than the magical number of times the ritual starts all over again. Repetitive, unwelcomed and resisted thoughts become strengthened, i.e. ruminations. People's lives can be ruined by this disorder. PSYCHOTHERAPY such as BEHAVIOUR or PSYCHOANALYSIS can be used successfully. See Stafford-Clark and Smith (1983); Davison and Neale (1994).

obstruent a sound which is produced by an obstruction in the mouth made by the articulators such as plosives, fricatives, affricates (see ARTICULATION). It is also a DISTINCTIVE FEATURE proposed by Chomsky and Halle to distinguish such sounds from those produced without such an obstruction. It is opposed to SONORANT. See Fromkin and Rodman (1993); Ladefoged (1993).

obturator in relation to speech, a palatal device used to improve resonance and intraoral pressure as, for example, in the case of cleft palate where there is a residual fissure.

occlusion in relation to articulation:

1. The degree of closure necessary for the production of different consonants.
2. The relationship between the maxilla and mandible.

A malocclusion may contribute to articulatory defects. Angle's classification delineates the different types of occlusion (see ORTHODONTICS). See Tortora and Grabowski (1993).

occupational therapy an occupational therapist works with people who have difficulty in coping at home on their own due to physical handicap resulting from neurological incidents, e.g. CVA, head injury, progressive degenerative diseases, orthopaedic operations or problems with their upper limbs, especially hands. The therapist may have to help the person with dressing, eye/hand coordination and general cognitive skills. They will carry out home visits before the person is discharged from hospital to find out if the person will require particular adaptations for the house such as hand rails, an extra bannister, widening of doors if the person uses a wheelchair and even hoists to allow the person to get in and out of a bath. They use assessments such as the COTNAB to assess the person's abilities. Treatment consists of using microcomputers, making objects in a workshop and working in the kitchen. The latter allows the therapist to assess the person's independence in the kitchen and gives the person help to cope in that environment. All these types of treatment have the aims of improving the person's performance in communication skills, initiative and decision-making, concentration, confidence and self-esteem. As with most therapies, motivating the person to capitalise on their strengths and compensate for their weaknesses is paramount. See Hopkins and Smith (1993).

Oedipus complex the very young child forms a close bond to his mother or a substitute, e.g. foster mother. This bonding is produced by an emotional tie between the child and the mother. Thus, the child finds difficulties in life when separated from his mother (see SEPARATION ANXIETY). The child faces another problem when he sees his father as a rival for the affection of his mother. The child is faced with a terrible dilemma: on the one hand he is jealous of his father as a rival, while on the other hand he knows he depends on his father emotionally in the family circle. Such frustrations lead to feelings of aggression against the father which the child has to suppress because of the love and respect he has for his father. As the child is so young, he cannot speak about these feelings towards his father. He is in conflict over his emotional feelings towards his father. The Oedipus complex was first proposed by Freud, who suggested it was a possible cause of various neuroses which some people have. *See* Stafford-Clark and Smith (1983); Atkinson et al (1993); Davison and Neale (1994).

oesophageal voice alaryngeal phonation. A method whereby, following a complete LARYNGECTOMY, PHONATION is achieved by intake of air through the mouth which, by combined compression of the pharyngo-oesophageal sphincter and intraorally, is driven into the OESOPHAGUS. There are three methods of sound production – by injection of air, by inhalation of air and by swallowing air. The last method is not generally recommended. *See* Edels (1983).

oesophagus a structure that is 25 cm long, and starts at the level of the sixth cervical vertebra and ends about the thoracic level of the eleventh vertebra where it enters the stomach. It narrows at the PHARYNX, where it passes through the diaphragm and at the bottom of the thorax. It has an inner circular layer of muscles and an outer longitudinal layer of muscles. The top part of the oesophagus is covered with STRIATED MUSCLE while the bottom is covered with SMOOTH MUSCLE. It is possible to use the upper part for producing oesophageal voice as it has striated muscle. It runs behind the TRACHEA. *See* Tortora and Grabowski (1993).

off-/on-glide a description of movements of articulators (*see* ARTICULATION) which occur in the production of contiguous sounds. An off-glide occurs after the production of one sound and the articulators are beginning to take up the

position of the next sound, while an on-glide occurs as the articulators are taking up the position for the intended sound from a previous sound or from rest. *See* Cruttenden (1994).

olfaction the sense of smell. The receptors are found in the epithelium in the roof of the NOSE on either side of the nasal septum. The free end of each olfactory cell contains a dendrite which ends in the olfactory vesicle from which six to eight microscopic hairs extend. These hairs react to the odours in the air, which then stimulate the olfactory cells, producing an olfactory reaction. *See* Kolb and Whishaw (1990); Atkinson et al (1993); Tortora and Grabowski (1993).

olfactory *see* CRANIAL NERVES.

oligodendrogliomas *see* TUMOURS OF THE CENTRAL NERVOUS SYSTEM.

on/off phenomenon *see* PARKINSON'S DISEASE.

one-tail test a statistical interpretation of any parametric or non-parametric test (*see* PARAMETRIC TESTS). Assumptions are made about the experiment before it is carried out. It is a rule that one or two assumptions are made. The assumption for a one-tail test is that the difference between the two distributions will be significant at five per cent. This is the normal level of significance for all tests. If the experimenter is uncertain about the result being significant, then he must use a two-tail test so there is only a 1 in 2.5 per cent chance of the result being significant. The tails refer to the ends of a normal distribution curve. In a one-tail test only the positive tail is used, while with a two-tail test both tails of the curve are used. *See* Miller (1975); Clarke and Cooke (1992).

open bite an orthodontic condition in which the upper anterior teeth do not align with the lower teeth leaving a gap. Sometimes associated with tongue thrust and with an immature swallowing pattern.

open class word *see* PIVOT GRAMMAR.

open syllable a syllable ending in a vowel. In speech pathology, this refers to incomplete articulation of a word by omission of the final consonant. Also known as final syllable deletion. *See* Renfrew (1966).

open vowel see CARDINAL VOWEL SYSTEM.

operant conditioning a learning theory used in BEHAVIOUR THERAPY. It is also known as radical behaviourism and was put forward by B.F. Skinner. He developed these principles by experimenting with rats in boxes known as Skinner boxes. These boxes had a bar in them which, when pressed, released a pellet of food. Thus, the rats were conditioned to press the bar because they learnt they would receive food. Those who undertake such behaviour modification believe that the reaction of a person to his environment causes the person's maladaptive behaviour. Such therapists see all maladaptive behaviour as a learned response received through environmental reinforcement. To combat this, a suitable reinforcement conditioning programme has to be evolved. First of all, a functional analysis is developed to provide a set of possible sources in the environment of the reinforcement of the present maladaptive behaviour. Sometimes such behaviour can be caused by the acceptance of it by others thus allowing the person to continue living in a comforting situation and so they give the person an indirect reward. The functional analysis must detail the maladaptive behaviours of the individual, showing the number of occurrences and the particular environments in which these behaviours take place. A target behaviour pattern is then developed and various interventions decided on to try and establish a more acceptable behaviour pattern. These treatment plans are specific to each individual person. Such therapeutic interventions are individual conditioning paradigms which attempt to identify the source of the reinforcement of the maladaptive behaviour and try to remove it either by physical removal or aversive reinforcement. TOKEN ECONOMIES are also used in this form of therapy. *See* Atkinson et al (1993); Davison and Neale (1994).

operating system the software which enables a computer to perform different functions within itself to operate other pieces of hardware, computer programs and data. These can be controlled manually from the keyboard or by use of software. *See* Bishop (1985); Brookshear (1991).

operating system commands the direct communication between operator and the computer. In APPLE Macintosh and IBM PC and compatible computers which use Windows environment as their operating systems, these commands are carried out automatically by operating a MOUSE while in computers such as IBM PC and compatibles using Microsoft DOS, special commands have to be given following a prompt on the monitor screen.

optic nerve *see* CRANIAL NERVES.

Orac a high-tech communication aid with digitised speech and synthetic voice (ORAtalk or DECTALK) systems which can be used independently of one another. It can be accessed by direct manual selection, single and two- switches, joysticks and concept keyboards. There can be various sizes of overlay from 2 to 128 squares. When using digitised speech over 7 minutes can be stored. Word prediction can also be used to increase spelling rate. Prestored items can be combined with spelling messages. There is a disk drive which allows for rapid saving and loading of information. It can be mounted onto a wheelchair. *See* Appendix IV.

oral approach *see* EDUCATION OF HEARING-IMPAIRED CHILDREN.

oral apraxia *see* APRAXIA.

oral sounds those sounds which have no nasal quality in their production. As suggested by the name, these sounds are produced in the oral cavity which produces the difference between them and nasal sounds made in the nasal cavities. *See* Ladefoged (1993).

oral stage *see* PSYCHOSEXUAL STAGES OF DEVELOPMENT.

orbicularis oculi *see* MUSCLES OF FACIAL EXPRESSION.

orbicularis oris *see* MUSCLES OF FACIAL EXPRESSION.

orthodontics the study of teeth formation and other structures in the MOUTH which require treatment by the placement of various prostheses (*see* PROSTHESIS) to realign the dental arches if they are deformed. There are three descriptions of teeth formation:

1. Class I: the teeth are well related to each other as are the two dental arches, i.e. top teeth at front cover one-third or half the bottom teeth when clenched.
2. Class II (division 1): top teeth are protruding away from the bottom teeth by more than 2–4mm.
   Class II (division 2): an increase in overbite where the lower incisors are completely covered.
3. Class III: lower teeth completely cover over the top teeth when clenched.

Classes II–III are known as malocclusion. Orthodontists can also be involved with the treatment of children with cleft palate as the teeth may be formed in a haphazard formation. *See* Edwards and Watson (1980).

ossicles *see* EAR.

otitis media a condition produced by an infection in the middle ear often found in children. There are different types:

1. Acute otitis media: often produced by respiratory infection entering the eustachian tube (*see* EAR). The resulting HEARING LOSS is usually of a conductive nature. The hearing loss will clear up when the middle ear is ventilated. Antibiotics may be required to clear the infection completely.

2. Chronic otitis media: there are different causes for this type of otitis media. It may be the stage following an unresolved otitis media where the organisms contained in the infection destroy the eardrum with a resulting perforation. It may also be the result of a long-lasting low-grade infection. The size and site of the perforation will determine the degree of hearing loss which the person has. If the perforation is small but above the round window, the hearing loss will be greater than with a larger perforation sited elsewhere. Perforations can be closed by a tympanoplasty. Incus necrosis and ossicular damage are other possible causes and are produced by subacute infection. Even with an unaffected eardrum, damage to the ossicles can cause a hearing loss up to 60 dB. The eardrum perforation can be small or perhaps repaired, but the client can still have a significant CONDUCTIVE HEARING LOSS produced by large cartilage-like masses of plaques grouping in the middle ear involving the ossicles. This is known as tympanosclerosis. An audiometric assessment will show an air–bone gap, low compliance and absent stapes reflexes on immitance measures.

3. Serous otitis media: one of the most common causes of conductive hearing loss in children. This form of otitis media is usually caused by an infection or allergy although there can be other causes. It is presumed the middle ear fails to function correctly because of some form of disorder in the eustachian tube. The pressure in the middle ear is thus negative, so the tympanic membrane is pressed inwards, reducing the efficacy of the conducting mechanism and producing a conductive hearing loss. This can be worse in the low frequencies. If this is not resolved, fluid can collect in the middle ear, producing a conductive loss in the high frequencies. To over-

come this problem, a myringotomy is undertaken in which a tube is inserted to ventilate the middle ear. This action should bring the child's hearing back to normal. On initial audiological assessment, the curve will show a greater loss in the low frequencies spreading to the high frequencies as time goes on. Tympanometry (*see* IMPEDANCE AUDIOMETRY) may show the presence of fluid in the middle ear even when it cannot be found under physical observation through oto-scopy.

See Pracy et al (1974); Ginsberg and White (1985); Tortora and Grabowski (1993); Williamson and Sheridan (1994) (a test of hearing reception in otitis media).

otorhinolaryngology a name used in the UK and other countries to refer to the study of the ear, nose and throat.

otosclerosis a disease which begins in the bony labyrinth of the inner ear (*see* EAR) and produces a bony growth in the inner ear. It has been found to occur twice as often in women as in men, with TINNITUS occurring approximately 50 per cent of the time whilst hearing loss is noticed at an average age of 36 years. If it reaches the middle ear, the footplate of the stapes (*see* EAR) becomes stuck to the oval window. The hearing loss progresses slowly and, in most cases, it is conductive. The audiogram shows a low-frequency conductive loss with an air–bone gap (*see* PURE-TONE AUDIOMETRY) during the early stages, followed by CARHART'S NOTCH, and in a later stage, a flat loss. The hearing loss may become sensorineural when the structures in the bony labyrinth are affected. Treatment takes the form of removing the stapes and replacing it with a piston-type structure which acts in its place. *See* Pracy et al (1974); Katz (1985).

output devices machines which will accept data or information from a computer. These include the various types of printer, disk drive (*see* DISK), VISUAL DISPLAY UNITS and MODEMS. *See* Bishop (1985).

oval window *see* EAR.

overextension at the two-word stage of language acquisition, overextensions may occur. A child learns a new word, but may only recognise some particular aspect of it, e.g. shape, movement, size, sound, texture and, sometimes, taste, so that every time he sees a similar object, he uses the same name. For example, the child may call all four-legged animals with a tail 'dog', as the first time he saw such an animal, it was a 'dog'. *See* Clark and Clark (1977).

overgeneralisation a stage of language acquisition. It occurs as a child learns how to use syntactic functions, e.g. past tense, singular vs plural, etc. The regular way to form the past tense is to add 'd' or 'ed'. However, there are irregular ways of making the past tense e.g. 'went', 'gone', 'ran', etc. Once the child has learnt how to use the regular form of the past tense, he may over-generalise its use to irregular forms, e.g. 'wented/goed', 'ranned/runned', etc. *See* Cruttenden (1979); Fromkin and Rodman (1993).

overlapping a description in phonology of sounds which are mutually exclusive. In other words, if the sound /k/ is to exist by itself and not be realised by /f/ from time to time, there must be certain contexts in which /k/ appears and not /f/ and vice versa. If this were not the case, the two sounds would overlap and lose their contrasting qualities. Such contrasts are sometimes lost in phonological delay/disorder and the making up of rules becomes almost impossible. *See* also NEUTRALISATION and MINIMAL PAIRS. *See* Grunwell (1987).

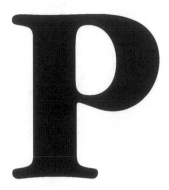

P

PAC (portable adaptable communication) *see* SPEECHPAC, EVALPAC, TOYPAC.

PACE *see* PROMOTING APHASICS' COMMUNICATIVE EFFECTIVENESS.

PACS *see* PHONOLOGICAL ASSESSMENT OF CHILD SPEECH.

PACS Pictures: Language Elicitation devised by Grunwell in 1987 for use with children with speech disorders. When the elicited speech is analysed, the therapist will have a complete description of the child's sound system (*see* PHONOLOGY) with several examples of each sound. It can be used as a screening test with a sample of 100 words including 41 words from the EAT while the basic assessment allows the same sample to be analysed with various techniques including PACS and the full assessment elicits a sample of 200 words allowing for more detailed phonological and grammatical analysis. *See* Grunwell (1987).

PACS Toys Screening Assessment devised by Grunwell and Harding in 1995, the PACS Toys Screening Assessment is a rapid screening procedure for assessing both speech and pre-speech vocalisation. It provides a descriptive and qualitative assessment using appropriate play items in a flexible and interactive way. Sixty words are targeted which can be elicited using any toys of any shape or colour as the test has not been standardised. It is suggested that this test can be used to monitor the phonetic development of young children between the ages of two and three years, to monitor the phonetic development in pre-verbal vocalisations, to screen children's speech patterns to determine if a more in-depth assessment is required using PACS PICTURES or PHONOLOGICAL ASSESSMENT OF CHILD SPEECH (PACS) or as an outcome measure. *See* Grunwell (1995) in Appendix I.

paddle an input device for moving objects around a monitor screen, usually used when playing arcade games. It can also be used to operate pieces of software which have been specially designed to be operated by this method. *See* Bishop (1985).

paediatric audiology part of audiology in which hearing tests are carried out on children to find out the severity and type of HEARING LOSS which a child may have. The audiologist has to counsel the child's parents as to the effects of a hearing loss both in the short term and the long term.

Paget-Gorman Sign System (PGSS) one of the earliest sign systems to have been developed. Designed by Paget in the 1930s and developed into the 1950s, by which time he and his colleagues had made up a 3000 word sign vocabulary. When Paget died, his work was carried on by Dr Pierre

DET	N	V	PREP	DET	N
His	mouse	lay	in	the	cage
That	dog	barked	from	his	kennel
My	friend	sat	on	the	seat

Gorman and Paget's widow. The original signs were revised and the system named 'A Systematic Sign Language'. In 1971, Lady Paget changed the name to 'The Paget-Gorman Sign System' in recognition of Gorman's help in its development. The sign system has one sign corresponding to one word and has a sign for each morphological ending in English, i.e. plurals, tense endings, etc. The system has 21 standard hand positions and 37 basic signs used in different combinations. The basic signs represent groups of words with a common concept, e.g. time, position, animal life, etc. One hand gives the concept, while the other hand is used to modify the concept to make the required communication clear. *See* Kiernan et al (1982).

PAL *see* PREDICTIVE ADAPTIVE LEXICON.

palatal lift *see* PROSTHESIS.

palatal shelves *see* PIERRE ROBIN SYNDROME.

palatalisation the process of raising the front of the tongue towards the hard palate, e.g. palatalised /ʎ/. It is an example of secondary articulation and occurs also in phonological delay/disorder when a child produces a non-palatal sound with a palatal quality.

palatine tonsil *see* MOUTH.

palatopharyngeus muscle *see* MUSCLES FOR SWALLOWING.

palilalia a type of acceleration rhythmic disorder. It takes the form of increasingly rapid reiteration of an utterance with diminisihing loudness and reduced intelligibility. It is associated with extra-pyramidal pathology.

PALPA *see* PSYCHOLINGUISTIC ASSESSMENTS OF LANGUAGE PROCESSING IN APHASIA.

Panje voice button made of silicon with two flanges, it is placed in the tracheo-oesophageal wall. The operation is reversible but the person for whom the voice button is suitable is limited by the diameter of the stoma, dexterity of the client and thickness of the tracheo-oesophageal wall. Placement is completed by out-patient surgery and no special instruments are required. The button is self-contained in the tracheo-stoma. *See* Edels (1983).

papillae *see* TONGUE.

papillomata benign neoplasms appearing on the VOCAL FOLDS, but they can appear in the TRACHEA which can produce dyspneoa, i.e. difficulty with breathing. They are little bunches of pinkish growths which are found in the airways. Juvenile papillomata are the most common laryngeal tumours in children, occurring most frequently between the ages of 4;0 and 6;0 years. They can be removed by various surgical techniques and also by drug therapy but there is a strong tendency for them to recur. *See* Greene and Mathieson (1989); Fawcus (1991).

paradigm a base form from which other forms are made by adding affixes. *See* Matthews (1974).

paradigmatic relationships between elements of a grammatical category. They refer to subgroups of linguistic units, the subgroups being determiners, adjectives, nouns, etc. For an example see the box at the top of this page.

The sentence analysed in this way is seen as a number of slots. Each slot can only be filled once by one of the units. A sentence such as that shown in the box at the foot of this page is

DET	N	V	PREP	DET	N
my the	book	is	on	the	table

unacceptable as there are two units in the determiner slot. A different sentence analysis examines the syntagmatic relationships of units in a sentence. *See* Lyons (1968).

paralanguage *see* SUPRASEGMENTAL PHONOLOGY.

parallel items of information dealt with simultaneously. It is opposed to serial.

parallel interface an interface where there is a parallel exchange of information between the central processor and other peripheral units. Most interfaces between computers and printers are parallel interfaces. It is opposed to serial interface.

parameter information which is written into a computer program, SUBROUTINE, LOOP, etc., the value of which can be changed each time it is encountered in the program.

parametric tests one of two types of test which are used in INFERENTIAL STATISTICS. Parametric tests are perhaps the most powerful tests from a statistical point of view and are very rigorous in their assumptions which are three in number:

1. the data must fall into a NORMAL DISTRIBUTION;
2. the STANDARD DEVIATION and variation must be relatively equal producing homogeneity of variation;
3. the data must be on an interval-ratio scale.

Two parametric tests used to a large extent in statistics are the independent *t*-test (*see* T-TESTS) using an INDEPENDENT GROUP DESIGN and the related *t*-test (*see* T-TESTS) with a REPEATED MEASURES DESIGN. These tests take account of all the data which are collected by the assessment or whichever method is used to gather it. If the data do not fall under a normal distribution curve, a non-parametric test must be used. These tests are less powerful and discard some of the data. Two such tests are the MANN-WHITNEY TEST for independent group design and the WILCOXON TEST for repeated measures design. These tests compare the results by ranking the results of both groups, and the experimenter can calculate if there is a significant difference in the results. Because of the ranking system of scores used in this type of test, much of the actual data are lost and thus they become less powerful than parametric tests. *See* Miller (1975); Clarke and Cooke (1992).

paraphasia an error usually found in the language of those with APHASIA, where they substitute a word, sound or morpheme for another in the spoken as well as the written form of language. This condition is produced in asphasic people by the degeneration of the BRAIN while with others these errors may be caused by stress, fatigue or lack of attention. In the subtests of the expressive language section of the BOSTON DIAGNOSTIC APHASIA EXAMINATION, it is possible to score the type of paraphasic error produced. *See* Eisenson (1984).

parasympathetic nervous system part of the AUTONOMIC NERVOUS SYSTEM which produces the opposite effect to the sympathetic nervous system. It operates at its maximum potential during sleep, slowing down the heart. It is used to innervate the muscles controlling the digestive system as well as defaecation and micturition. *See* J.H. Green (1978); Tortora and Grabowski (1993).

parental speech *see* BABY TALK.

Parkinson's disease caused by disorders to the BASAL GANGLIA. The main areas of the BRAIN affected are the caudate nucleus and the substantia nigra (*see* MIDBRAIN). The disease itself can be caused by viruses, e.g. encephalitis lethargica, drugs given for other diseases, e.g. chlorpromazine, and poisons, e.g. manganese, producing a neural loss in the basal ganglia, CEREBELLUM and substantia nigra. There are three main symptoms:

1. Tremor which is the least disabling but, perhaps, most embarrassing as it can produce pill rolling. It may disappear but, during anxiety, can become worse.
2. Rigidity of the so-called cog-wheel type. There is also loss of facial expression.
3. Bradykinesia produces a slowness in carrying out purposeful movements.

The typical posture is a hunched forward appearance with head down against the chest, shoulders pushed forward with the arms hanging loosely at the side. Forward movement produces a festinant gait, i.e. a faster and faster progression. Speech is also affected producing the following characteristics:

1. Monotonous pitch, reduced stress and monotone.
2. Imprecise articulation.
3. Inappropropriate silences and occasional repetitions of syllables and phonemes.
4. Speech is produced in short bursts with variable rate.
5. Breathy voice.

However, although this may seem like 'DYSARTHRIA', it is not strictly speaking a dysarthria but rather what Scott and Caird (1981 quoted in Scott et al, 1985, p.11) call a 'dysprosody'. The client also starts to produce micrographia i.e. very small writing.
The medical condition is treated with drugs such as LEVODOPA which is used to control the tremor as is bromocriptine. Speech problems are treated with exercises to maintain intelligible speech for as long as possible. If the voice becomes very weak so that it is almost impossible to hear what is being said, a PERSONAL SPEECH AMPLIFIER such as the Voicette, the Easitalk or Porta-amp may be recommended. If speech becomes significantly unintelligible, a form of ALTERNATIVE AUGMENTATIVE COMMUNICATION may be prescribed. *See* Darley et al (1975) (communication problem); Gilroy and Holliday (1982)(medical); Scott et al (1985) (communication problem); Le Dorze et al (1992) (effects of therapy); Beukelman and Mirenda (1992) (AAC); Adams and Lang (1992) (use of masking on speech); Davison and Neale (1994).

parole the act of using the internalised LANGUE which everyone has in their mind. It was proposed as a linguistic description by de SAUSSURE in 1913. He regarded parole as the way in which a speaker combines linguistic units to give meaning to their utterances and how the movements which are required to produce the utterance are made. *See* Saussure (1916); Culler (1986).

parotid duct/glands *see* SALIVARY GLANDS.

Parrot a high-tech communication aid which produces stored spoken messages produced by digitised speech. Its vocabulary is limited but can be highly functional. The memory can hold 16 single messages, so it can be used with users who have limited communication needs, to start users off with a small communication aid before being given a more advanced system or for immediate needs, e.g. in intensive care or during treatment. It gives 32 seconds of uninterrupted speech which can be extended to 64 seconds although the speech quality may be reduced. *See* Appendix IV.

passive usually contrasted with active, it refers to a grammatical construction in which the patient or theme of a verb is highlighted by appearing in subject position. This is accompanied by passive verb morphology and sometimes also by the appearance of the agent as a prepositional phrase following the verb. The 'short' or 'agentless' passive is illustrated in (1) and the 'agent' passive in (2):

(1) The man was killed.
(2) The man was killed by his neighbour.

See Lyons (1968); Fromkin and Rodman (1993).

Pausaid a small machine which makes the person's speech more intelligible. It has a throat microphone which will detect continuous phonation and prompt the client by an audible signal and make regular stops in speech. The therapist can alter phonation, length of pause and the machine's sensitivity level.

pausing *see* PROLONGED SPEECH.

Pavlov *see* CLASSICAL CONDITIONING.

PC abbreviation for PERSONAL COMPUTER, e.g. IBM PC. PCs are particularly manufactured by IBM, and IBM compatible computers are manufactured by other companies.

Peabody Picture Vocabulary Test (Revised) (PPVT-R) devised by Dunn (revised 1981), it is a formal standardised assessment to test the child's rate of vocabulary acquisition. It can be used with children between 2;6 and 18;0 years. The revised version has 175 pictorial plates, each with four pictures. The child has to choose the correct picture from the four at the request of the therapist. *See* Dunn (1969) in Appendix I; Aiken (1985).

peak experience *see* PHENOMENOLOGICAL APPROACH.

perceived self *see* PHENOMENOLOGICAL APPROACH.

percentile score a score or rank which shows how many subjects belonging to the norm will fall below the raw score in question. For example, if a person is given a percentile score of 79, this means there are 79 per cent of the norm group below the person's score with the same age range. *See* Aiken (1985).

Perceptions of Stuttering Inventory (PSI) devised by Wolff in 1967, it is a personality inventory used to discover situations in which those with a stammer expect to stammer, or produce struggling behaviour and which they try to avoid. There are five reasons for carrying out this inventory:

1. To describe what the stammerer does.
2. To give greater understanding of why the person stammers.
3. To give insight into the person's emotional state.
4. To give a check on progress.
5. To provide a profile for working out goals and expectations.

See Dalton and Hardcastle (1989).

performance the deployment of the speaker's competence in producing utterances. It is opposed to COMPETENCE. Both have been proposed by Chomsky. *See* Chomsky (1965); Lyons (1968).

performative specific speech acts in which the act is performed by the particular sentence uttered, with the verb in the sentence being crucial. For example:

1. I hereby name this ship HMS Fortress.
2. I promise to pay the bearer on demand.... (British £5 pound notes)
3. I apologise for the delay.
4. I congratulate you on your recent success.

All the verbs in (1)–(4) and other verbs which can be used in a similar way, e.g. advise, order, thank, announce, etc., are performative verbs. Huddleston writes: 'A performative verb identifies a particular kind of speech act that can be performed by virtue of uttering a sentence containing the verb...' (Huddleston, 1976, p.134). *See* Huddleston (1976); Clark and Clark (1977); Fromkin and Rodman (1993).

perinantal period the period from the 28th week of gestation to the 28th day after birth. At this time, there are several factors which can produce a delay in the child's future development. Among these are birth asphyxia, birth trauma, preterm babies and those who are LIGHT FOR DATES. *See* Illingworth (1987).

peripheral unit any device which can be connected to a computer and, hence, controlled by it. These include disk

159

drives, printers, visual display units, modems and all types of input, output and storage devices. *See* Bishop (1985).

peristalsis *see* SWALLOWING.

perlocution a term used in speech act theories to denote the effect that a speech act has on the hearer. Certain types of language disorder, in particular those where prosody is affected, may convey an interpretation different from that intended.

perseveration the persistence of an abnormal or incorrect response made by a brain-damaged or dysfluent (*see* DYSFLUENCY) person even when the stimulus which induced the initial response has been removed. It may take the form of continuous repetition or blocking, where the person makes repeated efforts to make a sound. *See* Eisenson (1984).

Persona an integrated system which can control the environment and a wheelchair and can be used as a small communicator. It has a large display screen with word or symbol representation and choice of text/symbol and up to 50 different selection screens. It can be accessed by switches using various scanning methods. As a communicator, it has five minutes of DIGITISED SPEECH, text to synthetic speech and word processing. *See* Appendix IV.

personal aid for communication an electronic box divided into squares with a light above each. Overlays are placed into the box and by pressing a switch, the client can switch on the light above the appropriate picture, word or phrase. The standard PAC unit can take eight stimuli while the PAC 6, which is operated in a similar fashion, can take six stimuli.

Personal Communication Plan devised by Hitchings and Spence in 1991, PCP aids in the assessment of communication skills of those over 16 years of age who have mild to severe learning disabilities. It involves all relevant people in the person's life, takes full account of the communication environment

and provides a practical framework for joint action planning. There are five parts which can be used interchangeably concerning: background information, speech and language profile, social communication skills, the person's environment, and shared action planning. *See* Hitchings and Spence (1991) in Appendix I.

personal computer (PC) a microcomputer which has sufficient memory to carry out business applications, word processing and spreadsheets. *See* Bishop (1985).

personal construct theory (PCT) a psychological theory proposed by Kelly in 1955. The Centre for Personal Construct Psychology in London practises PCT. The basis of the theory is put into the form of a fundamental postulate. According to Kelly, this refers to the way in which a person views the world and this depends on how much experience the person has of the world and what the experience has taught him. Human personality does not stand still but is an ongoing process which goes forward from construct to construct. Constructs are always being revised, validated, invalidated, discarded, added to and so on. It is anticipated that constructs will allow a person to foresee his own behaviour and the reactions of others. 'Yet constructs themselves undergo change. And it is in the transitions from theme to theme that most of life's puzzling problems arise ' (Kelly, 1955). In therapy, the therapist has to discover how clients view the world from their experience, i.e. what constructs they use. If the therapist deems that these constructs require revision, then therapy will be given. Assessment techniques used in PCT are REPERTORY GRIDS, laddering and SELF-CHARACTERISATION. *See* Dalton (1983, 1994).

personal speech amplifiers devices given to those who have a weak voice either as a result of a LARYNGECTOMY or a

160

medical condition such as PARKINSON'S DISEASE or MULTIPLE SCLEROSIS. There are different types:

1. Voicette: an amplifier which can be carried over the shoulder. The microphone is hand-held and attaches to the amplifier directly. It is particularly suited for teachers or others who have to speak to groups.
2. Porta-amp portable public address system: similar to the Voicette, the amplifier is in a case which can be placed on a flat surface or carried over the shoulder. A hand-held microphone attaches directly to the amplifier.
3. Easi-talk: an ear piece is placed behind the ear which allows an arm with the microphone to be placed in front of the mouth. The microphone is attached to an amplifier which can be clipped to a pocket or waistband. It can be operated by battery or recharged regularly. Since it has an ear attachment, users can use their hands while wearing it.
4. Jedcom speech amplifier: the system comprises a control box, a lightweight amplifier which can be carried in a jacket pocket, placed on a table top or hand-held, headset or throat microphone. The control box has an on/off switch and volume control.

personality Freud proposed PSYCHO-ANALYSIS to describe the development of personality. It consists of three parts – the id, ego, superego. The id is present at birth and works at the unconscious level. The child's personality at this stage requires immediate gratification. The overriding need is pleasure and is often known as a primary process. If the child is going to develop from this stage, the 'ego' must develop. Unlike the 'id', the 'ego' works at a conscious level. It produces the reality principle which makes children react to what is happening around them. Fantasies occur rarely as the child's personality is guided by the secondary process. Just

as the 'id' produces the biological self, the 'ego' produces the psychological self. The 'superego' operates on the social and moral functioning of the person. These three parts of the development of personality can be summed up as: 'The id seeks pleasure, the ego tests reality and the superego strives for perfection' (Atkinson et al, 1996). *See* Atkinson et al (1993).

personality profile *see* TRAIT APPROACH.

petit-mal epilepsy *see* EPILEPSY.

PGSS *see* PAGET-GORMAN SIGN SYSTEM.

phallic stage *see* PSYCHOSEXUAL STAGES OF DEVELOPMENT.

pharyngeal tonsil *see* TONSIL.

pharyngoplasty a surgical procedure in which the posterior wall of the PHARYNX is advanced so as to improve nasopharyngeal competency. Sometimes combined with the insertion of a pharyngeal flap in which the free end of a band of muscular tissue dissected from the pharynx is inserted into the upper (nasal) surface of the soft palate.

pharynx an anatomical structure which begins at the base of the skull and stretches downwards to the sixth cervical vertebra where it becomes continuous with the OESOPHAGUS. The pharynx is divided into three parts:

1. Nasopharynx: starts at the posterior openings of the nose and ends above the posterior opening of the MOUTH.
2. Oropharynx: continues from the end of the nasopharynx, passes the posterior opening of the mouth and ends close to the LARYNX.
3. Laryngopharynx: continues from the end of the oropharynx to the top of the oesophagus. The ADENOIDS are found in the nasopharynx while the tonsil can be found in the oropharynx.

The pharynx consists of three muscles:

1. Superior constrictor muscle: fibres leave the hamulus, pterygomandiblar ligament and, from the MANDIBLE, the

upper fibres end at the pharyngeal tubercle while the lower fibres mingle with the middle constrictor muscle and attach themselves to the posterior wall of the pharynx.

2. Middle constrictor muscle: fibres leave the stylohyoid ligament, the lesser and greater horns of hyoid and attach themselves to the posterior wall of the pharynx.

3. Inferior constrictor muscle: fibres leave the oblique line, the side of the cricoid cartilage (see LARYNX) and insert themselves into the posterior wall of the pharynx.

Cranial nerve IX (see CRANIAL NERVES) provides the sensory nerve input to the pharynx while cranial nerve X provides motor nerve input. The pharyngobasilar fascia is a membrane which runs down the vertebrae. As the person swallows, all these muscles lift up together. The salpingopharyngeus muscle leaves the auditory tube and inserts itself into some of the fibres of the palatopharyngeus muscle (see MUSCLES FOR SWALLOWING). This muscle raises the top part of the side wall of the pharynx and opens the auditory tube. See Tortora and Grabowski (1993).

phases of stuttering a description of how stuttering (see STAMMER) can develop from a mild problem to a very severe problem interfering in the person's daily life. Four phases were described by Bloodstein:

1. Mild repetitive stammering which becomes worse in communicative stress.

2. Stammering at school where the disorder becomes chronic and blocking behaviour becomes more common.

3. Continual blocking produces secondary symptoms.

4. Full-blown pattern of stammering found in adolescents and adults with the ensuing avoidance of speaking situations, e.g. speaking to boss, using the telephone, speaking in front of groups, etc.

See Dalton and Hardcastle (1989).

162

phenomenological approach an approach often considered to be a reaction against PSYCHOANALYSIS. It was developed by Carl Rogers. The personality is viewed as a conflict within the unconscious mind. However, it is the way in which the client perceives and interprets events which are important. Some theories within this approach are termed humanistic while others are theories of the self. An important part of Rogers' self theory is how people evaluate their self-image as this may have a bearing on how they perceive the world and events happening around them. This is often called perceived self. The person is also made to think of how he/she would like to be, compared with what they are. This is known as the ideal self. Self-actualisation occurs when a person chooses what they want to become and progresses to this goal rather than regresses from it. A peak experience occurs when people go through periods of self-actualisation. It is usually characterised by feelings of fulfilment and happiness because they have reached their goal. In general terms, this approach is subjective in that individuals must examine their own experiences of the world and their reaction to them. See Atkinson et al (1993).

phenothiazines the type of drugs used in treating SCHIZOPHRENIA. The parent drug is chlorpromazine (Largactil). It can be given orally, intramuscularly or intravenously. It does have some side effects which include drowsiness, hypotension, hypothermia, rare cholestatic jaundice (reversible when drug stopped), Parkinsonian symptoms and dyskinesias. Thioridazine (Melleril) is from the same family of drugs but, if given a high dosage, it can produce rare retinal damage. Trifluoperazine (Stelazine) tends to produce Parkinsonian symptoms rather than problems with blood pressure and jaundice. It produces alertness rather than drowsiness. See

Stafford-Clark and Smith (1983); Atkinson et al (1993).

phenylketonuria described by Mabry and colleagues in 1963, it is an autosomal recessive (*see* CHROMOSOMES) condition. It is an inborn error in the metabolism of phenylalanine as the gene lacks a certain chemical. An entirely preventable condition if detected by the GUTHRIE TEST. Children are put on a special diet low in phenylalanine for the rest of their lives. If it is untreated, LEARNING DISABILITY, MICROCEPHALY and seizures can result. The face is rounded with prominent glabella and epicanthal folds. Strabismus is frequent. *See* Hosking (1982); Smith (1985); Atkinson et al (1993); Tortora and Grabowski (1993); Davison and Neale (1994).

phenytoin SEE EPILEPSY.

phobias a neurosis and a possible cause of anxiety. A phobia is an irrational fear which will not be dissipated by any amount of logical discussion. Such a fear-provoking behaviour may happen only in particular situations. For example, someone who has a phobia of dogs will only show this irrational fear in the presence of dogs and will produce quite normal, rational reactions to other aspects of daily life. As the person approaches a feared situation, the irrational fear may produce an acute anxiety state. Some phobias, like the one just cited, may not affect the person's life significantly, while other social phobias such as agoraphobia, i.e. fear of crowds, enclosed spaces, etc., can cause isolation and loneliness to such a degree that the person's life-style can be altered significantly. Sixty per cent of all phobias are agoraphobic by nature with an incidence of 2:1 in favour of males; 8 per cent of phobias are social by nature with a similar incidence in favour of males; animal phobias account for 20 per cent of phobias with an equal sex incidence.

Behaviour therapy is often used for the treatment of phobias. *See* Stafford-Clark and Smith (1983); Davison and Neale (1994).

phonation the sound type that results from setting of the vocal and ventricular folds. The three main types of phonation are voice, breathy and creaky voice. Those who have DYSARTHRIA or DYSPHONIA can have problems with phonation. *See* Catford (1989).

phonemic jargon *see* JARGON APHASIA (2).

phonetics the study of the articulatory mechanism which produces sounds. Starting from the lungs, a pulmonic egressive airstream (*see* AIRSTREAMS) is produced and forces the air through the VOCAL TRACT into the mouth where the articulators (*see* ARTICULATION) move in particular sequences to produce the desired sound. The phonetician, who makes this study, describes consonants in terms of place and manner of articulation (*see* ARTICULATION) and voicing (*see* ARTICULATION) and vowels (*see* CARDINAL VOWEL SYSTEMS) in terms of openness and rounding of lips. Such descriptions of sounds can be used in describing all the languages of the world. The phonetician also studies the characteristics of sound waves and the way sounds are interpreted by the cochlea (*see* EAR) and CORTEX. There are three different types of phonetics which are studied: ARTICULATORY PHONETICS, ACOUSTIC PHONETICS and psycho phonetics (*see* AUDITORY PHONETICS). *See* Ladefoged (1993).

phonic ear VOIS there are three different models:

1. VOIS 130: a portable machine with 45 phonemes, 352 words and 19 phrases which can be programmed into four levels. By depressing word keys, sounds, words and phrases are produced by a speech synthesiser. There is also an overlay for BLISSYMBOLICS.

2. VOIS 135: the memory allows 5000 entries. The pre-programmed memory holds 46 words, 45 phonemes, 12 morphemes, and 10 commonly used phrases. There is a light touch-sensitive display area with nine selectable functions. Speech can be edited by the use of the 'review' command and by combining the use of words, phonemes, morphemes and letters. The available vocabulary is unlimited. A keyguard can be placed over the touch-sensitive keyboard.

3. VOIS 160: it has a similar keyboard to the VOIS 135 with an LED display. Below the display is a numberpad with various function keys.

Phonological Assessment of Child Speech (PACS) devised by Grunwell in 1985, it is a framework within which the therapist can assess and analyse the child's sound system (*see* PHONOLOGY). Two types of analysis are possible of the data obtained:

1. Contrastive analysis: comparisons are made between the child's phonetic inventory and the adult's sound system as well as with a developmental profile which shows which sounds the child should have learnt at a particular CHRONOLOGICAL AGE. This is the usual type of contrastive analysis. However, Grunwell goes further in PACS and has produced an assessment and analysis for CONSONANT CLUSTERS. Another addition to the Contrastive Analysis and Assessment used in PACS is a comprehensive analysis and assessment of phonotactic possibilities in the child's pronunciation patterns. Again, the information found is compared with the adult's syllabic and word formation in a matrix format. In describing this part of the PACS assessment and analysis, Grunwell writes: '.... PACS attempts to provide a comprehensive framework for analysis and assessment based, in the instances of the Contrastive Analysis and Assessment procedures, on the principles of phonological analysis....' (Grunwell 1987: 121).

2. Phonological process analysis: an analysis is made of spontaneous speech samples. The processes used to analyse these samples are described under PHONOLOGICAL PROCESSES. The number of times a particular process occurs is entered on a table as well as examples of the type of process. When the analysis is completed, the child's pronunciation patterns are compared with a developmental profile.

The characteristics of children's phonological disorders are discussed in the PACS manual, namely, persisting normal processes, chronological mismatch, unusual/idiosyncratic processes, variable use of processes and systematic sound preference. Thus, PACS provides a comprehensive assessment and analysis of the child's sound system taking account of developmental processes and how it may compare with the adult's sound system. *See* Grunwell (1985a, b) in Appendix I; Grunwell (1987); Beech et al (1993).

phonological delay this should not be confused with an ARTICULATION DELAY which is phonetically based. It is a delay in producing appropriate adult contrasts between phonemes, e.g. voice/voiceless, fronting/backing, etc. It is a delay because a child may produce /gɔgi/ for [dɔgi] at the age of 3;6–4;0 years when this substitution should have stopped between 2;0–3;0 years. *See* Grunwell (1987).

phonological disorder the severe form of phonological delay in which the child's sound system (*see* PHONOLOGY) is completely disordered. For example, the child may have no fricatives (*see* ARTICULATION) in their sound system or they may just have fricatives which do not belong in the spoken

English sound system e.g. [ɵ,β]. Such a system for children of 4;0–5;0 years would be described as a significant phonological disorder. *See* Grunwell (1987).

phonological dyslexia *see* ACQUIRED DYSLEXIA (1).

Phonological Process Analysis (PPA) devised by Weiner in 1979 for use with children between 2;0 and 5;0 to discover the PHONOLOGICAL PROCESSES used in their speech. Each process is tested in a set of four to eight words illustrated by line drawings. The test contains 136 pictures. The responses are recorded on sheets for each process. The processes are tested in a set of words in sequence. There are also control items to check if the child is producing assimilative or substitution processes. The developmental stages of process acquisition are not used. A phonetic inventory can be produced as well as the processes on the Process Profile Form. *See* Grunwell (1987).

phonological processes rules which are used in natural phonology to describe the simplifications made by a child. These processes include:

1. Weak syllable deletion: children omit one or more unstressed syllables
   'banana'' ['nɑnə]
   'pyjamas' ['dɑməd]
2. Final consonant deletion: children produce open syllables by omitting the final consonant of the word
   'pen'   [pɛ]
   'cold'   [ko]
   'bib'   [bɪ]
   'zip'   [zɪ]
   'bath'   [bɑ]
   'cat'   [kɑ]
3. Reduplication: children repeat the first syllable in the position of the second syllable
   'mummy'   [mʌmʌ]
   'kitten'   [kɪkɪ]
4. Consonant harmony: children make consonants in the word phonetically similar. The place of articulation (*see* ARTICULATION) changes but the voicing (*see* ARTICULATION) distinction is maintained between the realisation and the target sound.
   'cup'   [pʌp]
   'table'   [pebʌ]
   'duck'   [kʌk]
   'kettle'   [kɛk]
   'goat'   [gok]
   'cat'   [kæk]
5. Cluster reduction: children reduce a group of consonants which begin words.
   'smoke'   [mok]
   'string'   [srɪŋ]
   'skid'   [kɪd]
   'splash'   [plæʃ]
   'christmas' [kɪsməs]
   'scratch' [skæt]
6. Stopping: children substitute a stop for a fricative or affricate (*see* ARTICULATION) and at the same place of articulation (*see* ARTICULATION).
   'fine'   [bain]
   'church'   [tʌt]
   'size'   [taid]
   'jump'   [dʌmp]
7. Fronting: children produce all velar sounds at the front of the mouth, usually, as alveolar sounds.
   'cat'   [tæt]
   'cake'   [tek]/[tet]
   'cow'   [taʌ]
   'key'   [ti]
8. Gliding: children produce the target liquid sounds /l,r/ as [w,j]
   'lunch'   [wʌn]
   'red'   [wɛd]
9. Context-sensitive voicing: children change the voicing of obstruents. Voiced obstruents become voiceless word-initially and word-medially while voiceless obstruents become voiced word-finally.
   'fat'   [væd]
   'cat'   [gæd]
   'sad'   [zæt]
   'bid'   [pɪt]

See Grunwell (1987).

165

phonology the study of the sound systems in any given language. A sound system reveals contrasts in sounds and how such contrasts account for different meanings in language. A phonologist undertakes such a study. These systems are made up of phonemes. The phoneme is represented in speech production by the phone. Variations of the phoneme are known as allophones, e.g. the phoneme /p/ can have the allophones /pʰ/ (aspiration), /pˡ/ (ejective), etc. When all the allophones are put together, they form a phoneme and the phonemes together within an accent form a phonemic system. In English, there are about 44 phonemes, depending on the accent. *See* Hyman (1975); Grunwell (1987); Carr (1993); Fromkin and Rodman (1993); Ladefoged (1993).

phonotactics rules that allow the possible combinations of sounds in any language. The most basic syllable in English is the vowel (V) with consonants added to each side. In English, a maximum number of three consonants can be added before the vowel while a maximum of four consonants can be added after the vowel as in the word 'strength'. Rules exist for the production of two place consonant clusters:

1. Where C1 is /s/, C2 must be one of the following /p,t,k,m,n,l,j,f/
2. where C2 is one of /w,r,l,j/, C2 may be one of a large number of consonants, predominately obstruents including /p,t,k,b,d,g,f/ etc. (Grunwell, 1987, p.14).

Phonotactics are useful in speech therapy as the therapist can show the sounds which are not contrasting and in which position of the word or cluster the errors occur:

C1		C2	
[p,b,t,d,f]		[ɹ]	
'pram'	[pɹam]	'queen'	[tɹin]
'bread'	[bɹ ɛd]	'glove'	[dɹ əv]
'swing'	[fɹ ɪŋg]	'straw'	[dɹɔ]

(from Grunwell, 1987, p.18)

In her Phonological Assessment of Child Speech (1985a) in Appendix I, Grunwell has incorporated an assessment and analysis of phonotactics. *See* Grunwell (1987); Fromkin and Rodman (1993).

photonic wand an input device to operate a BBC computer where the person cannot use a conventional keyboard. Sitting in front of the screen, the person places the wand on the head and points it at the screen to move the cursor. An invisible beam of light is emitted from the wand to move the cursor. Thus, it is possible to produce graphics, text or music depending on the type of software package used. The photonic wand attaches to the analog port at the back of the BBC Micro/Master computer.

phrase structure grammar a grammatical model discussed by Chomsky in 'Syntactic Structures' in 1957. The basis of the model is a CONSTITUENT ANALYSIS using rewrite rules. However, Chomsky did not believe it was powerful enough to explain the structure of all sentences in the language. *See* Chomsky (1957); Huddleston (1976); Fromkin and Rodman (1993).

physiology the study of how the body functions. While an anatomist studies structures of the body, a physiologist studies how these structures function. Thus, some of the subjects which interest a physiologist are the workings of the heart, the breathing system, the autonomic and central nervous systems and the digestive tract. *See* J.H. Green (1978); Tortora and Grabowski (1993).

physiotherapy the physiotherapist works with physically handicapped patients. The handicap may be congenital, e.g. CEREBRAL PALSY, or acquired, e.g. HEMIPLEGIA, due to a CEREBROVASCULAR ACCIDENT, HEAD INJURY, etc. Patients will also be shown how to transfer, e.g. moving from a chair into a wheelchair, or from wheelchair to a commode or toilet. If someone is admitted to hospital in a coma, the physiotherapist will make sure their airways are kept clear by suction, and will also use suction if the patient is dysphagic and aspirates when taking food if it goes down into the TRACHEA.

Piaget Jean Piaget (1896-1980), a Swiss psychologist, observed children's cognitive behaviour from birth to about 11 years of age. He included his own child, and as a result evolved a theory of cognitive development which proceeded through several distinct stages as the child grew: (1) SENSORIMOTOR STAGE; (2) PREOPERATIONAL STAGE; (3) CONCRETE OPERATIONS; (4) FORMAL OPERATIONS. Piaget's theory of language development is based on the empiricist view according to which a child is believed to be born with a 'tabula rasa' or an empty mind and develops language only by his own experience and experimenting with what he hears in the environment around him. This is opposed to Chomsky's theory of INNATENESS in language development and to the existence of a LANGUAGE ACQUISITION DEVICE. *See* Atkinson et al (1993); Boden (1994).

PICA *see* PORCH INDEX OF COMMUNICATIVE ABILITIES.

PICAC *see* PORCH INDEX OF COMMUNICATIVE ABILITIES IN CHILDREN.

Pick's disease a rare type of DEMENTIA caused by neuron degeneration in the frontal and temporal lobes of the BRAIN (*see* CEREBRAL HEMISPHERES). The neurons which survive have special characteristics and are known as Pick's cells. It is thought to be a familial disorder. A major characteristic is the change of personality in later life particularly in the person's moral standards. APHASIA can also appear. Treatment is similar to other forms of dementia such as ALZHEIMER'S DISEASE. The prognosis is not good as death can occur within 6–12 months, caused by chest problems. *See* Gilroy and Holliday (1982); Stafford-

Clark and Smith (1983); Kolb and Whishaw (1990).

Pierre Robin syndrome a syndrome caused by hypoplasia of the mandibular area during the seventh week of *in utero* growth, allowing the TONGUE to be positioned at the posterior of the mouth preventing the palatal shelves meeting in the midline. As the tongue is obstructing the airway, it may have to be sutured to the lower lip or the head placed forward on the chest. Thus the four main characteristics of this syndrome are cleft palate but not cleft lip, respiration problems, small mandible and glossoptosis (drooping of the tongue backwards). *See* Edwards and Watson (1980); Smith (1985).

pill rolling the manifestation of the tremor (*see* PARKINSON'S DISEASE) affecting those who have Parkinson's disease. It appears at the fingers which, with the thumb, produce a rolling motion similar to that of the old apothecaries when they were making pills. *See* Gilroy and Holliday (1982).

pitch *see* AUDITORY PHONETICS.

pivot grammar a grammatical system proposed by Braine in the 1960s. He found that, as children acquired language, they produced sentences containing repeated words in one position while other words were used less often. The former process was called a pivot while the latter was an open class word. The system was used to explain the two-word stage in language acquisition. *See* Cruttenden (1979).

pixel the smallest unit used for forming a computer graphic. When a computer is placed in the graphics mode, the screen becomes a 'grid' (although this is not seen on the screen) of small areas which can be illuminated in any of the available colours or white, or can be left dark. These areas are known as pixels. *See* Bishop (1985).

place of articulation *see* ARTICULATION.

placenta part of the chorion which attaches the fetus to the wall of the uterus. Its highly specialised functions allow transfer of nutrients and oxygen from mother to baby and excretion of metabolic products from the fetus. *See* Tortora and Grabowski (1993).

plain a DISTINCTIVE FEATURE proposed by Jakobson and Halle to distinguish sounds which are produced with the mouth open and a high frequency [+PLAIN] from those produced with the mouth more closed and a low frequency [−PLAIN]. It is opposed to flat. *See* Hyman (1975).

plantar response a response obtained by stimulating the sole of the foot with an object. If the response exists, the hallux will flex. If there is extension, this is an abnormal response and is recorded as an extensor plantar response. This indicates an upper motor neuron lesion. *See* Gilroy and Holliday (1982).

play a vital component in the child's development as it allows him to develop manipulative and social skills so that he can learn to cope with his total environment. It functions also as a bridge between the child's internal world of fantasy and the external world of his environment, thus the child plays out his anxieties and fears, his jealousies and feelings of aggression. Play is often used in psychotherapy for treating the child's emotional disorders and conduct disorders. It can also be used in speech therapy to produce a natural setting for children to develop their communication skills, especially with those who suffer from language delay. Garvey has described play happening 'in a period of dramatically expanding knowledge of self, the physical and social world, and systems of communication' (Garvey, 1977, p.7). *See* Garvey (1977); Wood (1981).

play audiometry *see* CONDITIONING TESTS.

play therapy the use of play in treating a child's emotional disorders, conduct disorders and also communication disorders. *See* Wood (1981); Davison and Neale (1994).

plosive *see* ARTICULATION.

Point and Scan Intro Talker a high-tech communication aid with digitised speech output. It uses MINSPEAK to organise vocabulary to store into the device. There are three modes in which the scanning system can be used with a single switch:

1. A 32-location row/column scanning in which the device first scans through the rows and then, once a row is selected, scans across the chosen row until the desired location is selected.

2. An 8-location circular scan, i.e. the device scans each location in a clockwise direction, and once the selection has been made the scan automatically continues.

3. An eight count in which each activation selects the next location in the scan. Once the desired location has been reached, it is automatically selected after an adjustable period of time.

An optical headpointer can also be used with the Point and Scan Intro Talker in either 8 or 32-locations. All other features are described in the description of the ordinary INTRO TALKER. *See* Appendix IV.

polyps organic growths which can appear in nasal cavities and VOCAL FOLDS. They occur on the latter unilaterally, they may be round, vascular, oedematous and inflammatory. A polyp may produce hoarse voice, coughing and perhaps even choking, interfering with the person's PHONATION. Therapy for DYSPHONIA includes voice rest and a complete ban on smoking. *See* Fawcus (1991).

pons a structure within the BRAIN. It is part of the HINDBRAIN, measures about 3.5 cm wide and 3 cm long, and is situated above the MEDULLA OBLONGATA. It comprises fibres which make up the middle cerebellar peduncles, while further into its centre, it is essentially a continuation of the medulla oblongata. It is associated with cranial nerves V, VI, VII and VIII (*see* CRANIAL NERVES). The CEREBELLUM is found above the pons. *See* Barr (1979); Kolb and Whishaw (1990); Tortora and Grabowski (1993).

population a grouping of people, objects or abstract material which is to be analysed statistically. On occasion, the population will be so large that it would be impossible to test every member of the population. In such cases, the tester has to pick a random sample and then project the scores of this sample onto the population. For example, the organisations such as Gallup, MORI, Marplan, etc. which test the public's opinion, usually on their political views, take a random sample of the population around the country, ask them questions and work out the results. By statistical analysis, they can work out the voting intentions of the population with varying accuracy. *See* Miller (1975).

Porch Index of Communicative Abilities (PICA) devised by Porch in 1967 (revised 1971), it is a formal assessment, which has been standardised, to test the language function of those with APHASIA. Porch changed the aim of aphasia testing. He wanted to find out which of the person's responses could be reliably and objectively quantified. The 16-point scoring system, unique to Porch, is based on four principles: (1) responsiveness of the patient; (2) accuracy of the patient; (3) promptness of the response; and (4) efficiency of response, i.e. evidence of motor delay. Such a test provides the therapist with an extremely detailed performance record for each patient. There are at least 18 test tasks in the form of four verbal tasks, eight gestural tasks and six picture tests. Ten objects are also used and have to be presented in the required order. The therapist must attend a 40-hour workshop to become a registered user. Porch does not follow any particular theory of aphasia. *See* Eisenson (1984);

Rosenbek et al (1989); Beech et al (1993).

Porch Index of Communicative Abilities in Children (PICAC) devised by Porch in 1971, it is a formal standardised assessment, for use with children with learning difficulties, either requiring special education or having a SPECIFIC DEVELOPMENTAL LANGUAGE DISORDER. It has two scales, one for children in the 2;0–6;0 age range while the other is for children in the 3;0–12;0 age range. As with PICA, Porch was concerned only with the child's communication, not necessarily with the linguistic or phonological aspects of the child's language. The principles for the 16-point scoring system are the same as for the PICA. *See* Porch (1971) in Appendix I; Beech et al (1993).

Portacom 40 a small communication aid with DIGITISED SPEECH which can be used by direct manual selection or by linear or row/column scanning with one or two switches. It has a keyboard of 40 keys. The keys can be grouped together to make larger keys. It has a system built into it which means the memory of the device will not be lost even if the batteries lose their charge completely or are removed.

Portage Early Education Programme devised in America in the late 1960s, it has been used in the UK since 1976. The Portage Early Education Programme is a major revision of the earlier Portage Checklist designed specifically for use in the UK. All Americanisms have been removed making the new materials more appropriate for users in the UK. It is a means of finding out the different abilities of children with the mental ages of 0–6 years. It is used mainly with those children who will require special education, severely physically handicapped children and those with a severe delay in acquiring various skills. It is designed for use in the home by parents under the supervision of a speech and language therapist, psychologist or district nurse. After analysing the results, the therapist can give the parents a programme to work on with the child. It assesses motor, cognitive, language and self-help skills and, for very young children, infant stimulation. The subtest on language skills was not appropriate for British children, so a new language subtest was devised – the Wessex Revised Portage Language Checklist. These changes have been incorporated into the revised programme. *See* Cameron and White; Shearer and Shearer (1974).

positron emission tomography (PET) radio-isotopes of oxygen or carbon dioxide are prepared in a cyclotron and injected into the bodies. The radio-isotope emits positively charged electron-like particles called positrons. These destroy the negative electrons which they find in the body and produce gamma rays. It is the gamma rays which are recorded. All the information is fed into a computer which produces a colour PET scan, showing the localisation of the radio-isotopes in the body. PET scans provide evidence of function in various parts of the body rather than of structures. Such scans provide information concerning blood flow in the BRAIN and HEART, the effects of CEREBROVASCULAR ACCIDENTS or heart attacks, cancerous growths, the chemical changes in SCHIZOPHRENIA, EPILEPSY, OBSESSIVE–COMPULSIVE DISORDERS and SENILE DEMENTIA. *See* Kolb and Whishaw (1990); Tortora and Grabowski (1993).

Possum there are several devices produced by Possum to help those who have communication disorders:

1. Porta-scan communicator: this device has a built-in plate switch. Six pictures can be placed on the communicator and the required picture indicated by illuminating a LED lamp at the top left-hand corner of the cell. It can be placed on a wheelchair.

2. Backlit communicator boards: the number following each name refers to the number of squares which can be lit up and hence the number of stimuli which can be placed on them. The communicators 4, 16 and 32 all have pictures or words which can be lit individually cell by cell. However, the communicator 100 has a 10×10 matrix, i.e. 100 cells. The patient indicates which cell is required by illuminating a LED lamp in the top left-hand corner of each cell. The light can be operated horizontally, vertically or diagonally. There are four overlays provided although therapists can make up their own. The memory can hold a message using 40 cells. It has an alarm cell to obtain attention when in difficulty. Any type of Possum input device can be used. A speech synthesiser or printer can be attached to it.

3. Typewriter systems:
   (a) overdeck typewriter conversion– this can be placed on the patient's own typewriter.
   (b) combination system– this system is supplied with a GCTW12 (an illuminating scanning board with characters), PEK (Possum Expanded Keyboard) for use with those patients who have gross uncontrollable movements and a minikeyboard for those patients with small controlled movements.

4. Text Processor Workstation: the most advanced communication aid designed by Possum. It comprises: (a) a tape library filing system; (b) an easy-read facility on TV screen (improves fluency and speed of reading and retrains visual scanning movements); (c) TV screen to precompose text before printing it or to store it in the memory of the microprocessor for future use; (d) a vocabulary of 800 words and phrases provided to increase the speed of composition; and (e) Tellink where two text processors can be connected to produce a telephone network. Possum also sup-

ply environmental control systems which control lights, televisions, radios and even curtains.

posterior pharyngeal wall the area at the back of the pharynx into which the superior, middle and inferior constrictor muscles (*see* PHARYNX) insert themselves. *See* Tortora and Grabowski (1993).

postlingual hearing loss a HEARING LOSS which occurs after language has been acquired.

postnatal the period of the baby's life following delivery.

postvocalic a description of a consonant following a vowel.

Power in Play devised by Gail van Tatenhove, it is a MINSPEAK APPLICATION PROGRAM for children with a mental age of 2;0–4;0 years. Power in Play is not a MAP which can be used for communicating needs but has been designed to stimulate language using games, story books, songs and role reversal. It comprises 7 eight-location overlays, 28 unique symbols, 3 symbols which are symbol reductions, 7 photographs and 292 messages. The messages are organised into themes (*see* TOUCH TALKER), each with a different two-symbol sequence. Each message within each theme can be accessed with either one or two key actuations. Changing between the themes is hidden under a coded symbol sequence which cannot be accidentally accessed by the child. To change theme, the 'tree' icon is depressed three times. It is not intended for the child to change between the themes but for the therapist or carer using Power in Play with the child. Some of the themes can be personalised for the child. *See* Van Tatenhove (1989).

PPA *see* PHONOLOGICAL PROCESS ANALYSIS.

PPVT *see* PEABODY PICTURE VOCABULARY TEST.

Prader-Willi syndrome diagnosed by Prader and his colleagues in 1956, children who have this syndrome will be obese and flaccid. They have almond-shaped facial appearance with strabismus. There will be varying degrees of LEARNING DISABILITY, an enormous appetite and breathing problems which could result in death. Parents should be advised of a suitable diet. The children will also have hypo-gonadism and, in some cases, diabetes mellitus. There is no specific treatment. The prevalence is about 1:10 000 and 1:25 000–30 000 births. The cause is uncertain but in the 1960s and 1970s researchers hypothesised about a localised effect in the hypothalamic region (*see* HYPOTHALAMUS). More recently, studies have tended to focus on an abnormality in chromosome 15 which affects about 50 per cent of those affected. Many researchers have proposed a delay in the child's speech and language with the major problems including multiple articulation errors, reduced intelligibility, language problems and voice problems (primarily hypernasality). DYSFLUENCY and flaccid dysarthria (*see* DYSARTHRIA) have also been found. Apraxia of speech has not been found. Therapy is aimed at improving the child's vocabulary, syntax and morphology. PRAGMATICS may also be a problem. It has been suggested that therapeutic programmes should be personalised for the child as the communicative profiles lack common features. There are differences in severity of articulation and language problems as well as in intelligibility, voice problems and fluency. *See* Hosking (1982); Smith (1985); Kleppe et al (1990).

pragmatics the analysis of language in use, e.g. by studying SPEECH ACTS, e.g. PERFORMATIVES, FELICITY CONDITIONS, etc. *See* van Dijk (1980); McTear (1985); Fromkin and Rodman (1993).

Pragmatics Profile of Early Communication Skills devised by Dewart and Summers in 1988 for children between 9 months and 5 years. Its aim

171

is to provide a descriptive and qualitative assessment of the pragmatic aspects of language or the way in which children use language. It is based on a structured interview in which the parent describes the child's typical behaviour in a wide range of communication settings. The profile gives qualitative information as a basis for treatment as well as for monitoring progress and efficacy of treatment. The profile takes into account three aspects of pragmatics plus the effect of different contexts on the child's communication:

1. The way the child uses messages to communicate.
2. The child's response to communication.
3. The child's participation in conversational activity.
4. The way the child modifies communication in relation to various contexts.

The questions in the profile are based on concrete and everyday events; thus the parents can use their own unique experiences and knowledge of the child's communication. *See* Dewart and Summers (1988) in Appendix I; Miller (1990); Beech et al (1993).

Pre-Verbal Communication Schedule devised by Kiernan and Reid in 1987 for children and adults with severe LEARNING DISABILITY who are either non-verbal or who have few words or symbols. It can provide comprehensive diagnostic information which can be used as the basis of a treatment programme. There is a 195-item checklist. It provides detailed diagnostic information about the person's pre-communicative, informal and formal communicative skills and receptive skills. Scores can be transferred to a special summary sheet which highlights strengths and weaknesses. It can be used with those who have a severe learning disability, non-speaking deaf children and those with a severe physical handicap, but it can also be used with non-handicapped infants. *See* Kiernan and Reid (1987) in Appendix I; Beech et al (1993).

Predictive Adaptive Lexicon (PAL) software designed by the team led by Professor Alan Newell at the Microcomputer Centre, Dundee University. It was designed for people who have a communication disorder and has been extended for use with children and older people with learning difficulties. PAL has a large dictionary of 5000 words. When the user types a letter, the five most frequently used words starting with that letter appear in a window on the screen. To access the word, the user actuates any of the first five function keys. In this way, the number of key actuations can be significantly reduced. The user continues typing in letters until the desired word is found. The team also developed a word processor called Palstar for use with PAL, although PAL can operate using any word processor. PAL can be operated on an IBM-compatible computer. *See* Swiffin et al (1987).

prelingual hearing loss The HEARING LOSS occurs before the acquisition of language, i.e. up to 18 months of age.

prenatal a stage occurring during pregnancy. At this time, the fetus can be affected by infections from the mother, e.g. TORCH, radiation, nutritional deficiency or abnormalities of the placenta. *See* Illingworth (1987).

preoperational stage the second stage of Piaget's theory of cognitive development. It lasts from about 2;0–7;0 and assumes the child can think independently about what he perceives using his developed sense of symbolisation. However, he may still have difficulties within his cognitive skills. When posed with a problem, the child can only see it from his own perspective, not from anyone else's viewpoint. This is egocentricity, e.g. three mountains test in

Donaldson (1987). Piaget introduced this theory of egocentricity into his theory of language development. He claimed a child could not understand the position of a listener in a two-way conversation and so children used collective monologues with which to communicate, not conversations. He called this egocentric speech. During this stage, the child fails to make inferences about various problems he is set. If the child is told, 'A is greater than B, B is greater than C', and asked what the relationship is between A and C, he fails to respond correctly. However, Donaldson has found that children can make inferences in real situations. Failure to conserve volume, weight, number, etc. also occurs during this stage according to Piaget. However, Donaldson (1987) has shown it depends on how the conservation task is presented to the child for him to succeed. *See* Beard (1969); Donaldson (1987); Atkinson et al (1993); Boden (1994).

preparatory blocks *see* BLOCK MODIFICATION.

preposition a constituent (*see* CONSTITUENT ANALYSIS) which is used to precede a NOUN PHRASE, noun or pronouns. It can function as a marker for possession, destination, direction, etc., while syntactically it has a particular place in a sentence. *See* Lyons (1968); Fromkin and Rodman (1993).

prepositional phrase a phrase found in CONSTITUENT ANALYSIS which can be expanded into a preposition plus a noun phrase, e.g. the man went INTO THE SHOPS. *See* Huddleston (1976).

presbycusis a HEARING LOSS which results from the normal ageing process. PURE-TONE AUDIOMETRY shows a high-frequency SENSORINEURAL HEARING LOSS which may also have a conductive component due to changes in the middle ear. People lose speech discrimination although they can have a good understanding of speech if the speaker speaks slower

rather than louder. There may also be a general slowing down of processing ability. *See* Katz 1985.

Prestel launched in 1980 by British Telecom, Prestel was the first videotex system in the world. In a similar way to Teletext, Prestel produces pages of data concerning news, weather, sporting information, etc. It uses a phone link to a network computer system to obtain data. *See* Bishop (1985).

preterm the description of a baby born before the normal duration of the pregnancy, usually before 37–38 weeks into the pregnancy. Premature labour can be caused by a trauma, e.g. car accident, a multiple pregnancy, or cervical incompetence. As the baby's lungs are immature, breathing problems can occur. The child is kept in a incubator. Liver problems occur producing a high level of bilirubin in the brain which in turn produces kernicterus (a condition involving CEREBRAL PALSY and HEARING LOSS). The child also has immature bone marrow producing anaemia and a lack of protection from infections. *See* Illingworth (1987).

prime mover *see* AGONIST, ANTAGONIST.

printer an output device for producing data in the form of a printout. The information usually comes from a word processor. There are three types of printer: daisy-wheel printers, dot-matrix printers and laser printers. *See* Bishop (1985).

PRISM *see* PROFILE IN SEMANTICS.

Prodos an operating system designed for use with the Apple II series of microcomputers. *See* Katz (1986).

Profile in Semantics (PRISM) devised by Crystal in 1982 to analyse the child's use of semantics. It was the most experimental of the profiles as very little research has gone into the acquisition of semantics. The profile is based on the acquisition of semantics/grammar and semantics/lexicon. PRISM-G is a three-page chart which analyses the relationship between meaning and grammatical elements of a sentence. PRISM-L is a 16-page analysis because of the amount of vocabulary it has to cover. It is possible for one chart to be used without the other but if the two are used together, an in-depth analysis of the child's semantic system can be discovered. *See* Crystal (1992).

Profile of Phonology (PROPH) devised by Crystal in 1982, it is a means of analysing the child's sound system (*see* PHONOLOGY). There is a transcription page plus a separate three-page section on ways of summarising the data. The therapist takes a language sample of about 100 words but need only transcribe as much of the sample as is necessary to work out the child's phonological problem. This sample is transcribed and then analysed into the segments used by the child. Error realisations are detailed in terms of single consonants, single vowels and consonant clusters. The three types of segments are divided into errors of place and manner of articulation (*see* ARTICULATION). Limited information is given about PHONOLOGICAL PROCESSES. Altogether this profile gives an in-depth analysis of the child's sound system. *See* Crystal (1992).

Profile of Prosody (PROP) devised by Crystal in 1982 to analyse the suprasegmental (*see* SUPRASEGMENTAL PHONOLOGY) patterns in the child's speech. It comprises a one-page chart on which is put the pitch, loudness, rate and rhythm patterns of the patient's speech. It is supposed to complement PROPH. A large part of the profile is devoted to the child's use of intonation since most linguistic errors come from this variable. The intonation section is divided into tones and tone units. A summary section is also provided. *See* Crystal (1992).

prolabium the middle part of the top lip which tends to protrude down further than the rest of the lip.

prolonged speech a treatment technique for use with patients who stammer. It has five parts:

1. Prolongation: a slowing down of the rate of articulation. This process simplifies the movement from one sound to another which is usually difficult for someone who stammers.
2. Flow: running the words together, thus reducing the stopping and starting in a stammerer's speech.
3. Light/soft contacts are encouraged between the articulators to reduce the tension in the mouth when producing such sounds as /p,b,t,d,k,g/.
4. Pausing: a stammerer believes pausing exhibits DYSFLUENCY and so finds it difficult to understand it is a normal process in daily conversation. The patient will have to be shown how he can use normal pausing.
5. Slowing down is encouraged to help the stammerer produce what is required in (1)–(4).

All these are intended to encourage the feeling of using fluent speech which some stammerers have never experienced. *See* Dalton (1983).

Promoting Aphasics' Communicative Effectiveness (PACE) devised by Davis in 1980, this is a treatment technique used with aphasic patients (*see* APHASIA). It has been designed to produce meaningful interaction between the therapist and the patient. Treatment sessions should resemble everyday face-to-face conversation. PACE is based on four principles: (1) equal participation between therapist and patient; (2) new information being conveyed between the therapist and patient; (3) a free choice of communication between modalities; and (4) feedback from the therapist sounding more natural. When PACE is used effectively, patients enjoy therapy because it is they who are communicating some new information to the therapist or another member of the group. *See* Eisenson (1984); Rosenbek et al (1989); Pulvermüller and Roth (1991).

pronoun a set of words which can be used to replace nouns or noun phrases. There are several types of pronoun:

1. Personal pronoun, e.g. I, you, he, etc.
2. Reflexive pronoun, e.g. myself, yourself, himself, etc.
3. Possessive pronoun, e.g. mine, yours, his, etc.
4. Demonstrative pronoun, e.g. this, that
5. Indefinite pronoun, e.g. anyone, anybody, etc.
6. Relative pronouns, e.g. who, which, whom, etc.

These pronouns are usually discussed in other areas of linguistics and are discussed under other terms such as DEIXIS (demonstrative pronouns), EMBEDDING (relative pronouns), ANAPHORA (reflexive pronouns). *See* Lyons (1968); Fromkin and Rodman (1993).

PROP *see* PROFILE OF PROSODY.

PROPH *see* PROFILE OF PHONOLOGY.

proprioception the ability to orientate one's limbs or joints in space, e.g. to touch one's nose with eyes closed. Such skills are used in a person's daily life, e.g. eating, walking, speaking, etc. If speech is dysarthric (*see* DYSARTHRIA), it may be caused by loss of proprioception, e.g. difficulty in moving the mouth to make the correct sounds. This results in a treatment programme including neuromuscular facilitation. *See* Tortora and Grabowski (1993).

proprioceptive neuromuscular facilitation (PNF) a therapeutic technique used to stimulate and facilitate movement in paralysed muscles. It is most commonly used in conjunction with PHYSIOTHERAPY. The aim is to bombard the affected neurons with a variety of different stimuli. Icing (wiping ice over particular muscle groups) is used extensively. *See* Langley (1987).

prosody a general description of the phonological features of tempo (*see* RATE), rhythm, loudness and pitch. *See* Fromkin and Rodman (1993); Cruttenden (1994).

prosthesis the technical term for a 'brace' used to correct positioning, e.g. teeth in the dental arches. For those with cleft palate, there are devices to put in the mouth to help the baby to feed, and for older children the palatal lift which raises the soft palate (*see* MOUTH) and reduces nasalisation in the child's speech. It is also used to describe any aid for the patient. Communication aids are often described as being 'prostheses'.

pseudobulbar palsy *see* BULBAR PALSY.

PSI *see* PERCEPTIONS OF STUTTERING INVENTORY.

psychiatry a branch of medicine which provides treatment for those who have a mental illness such as AFFECTIVE DISORDERS, neuroses (*see* NEUROSIS), PSYCHOSES and SCHIZOPHRENIA. The psychiatrist can give treatment in the form PSYCHOTHERAPY and/or drug therapy. *See* Stafford-Clark and Smith (1983).

psychoanalysis a psychological theory evolved by Sigmund Freud in 1900. The basis of the theory hinges on the two basic motivators in life – sex and aggression. Freud also believed people had certain instincts which guided them through life – the life instinct and the death instinct. The former, he believed, was concerned with the libido and sexual drives, while the latter was concerned with people's destructive feelings leading either to suicide or aggression against others. Both drives are found in young children but are often suppressed by their parents. Thus, the drives become unconscious motives and produce anxiety in the child as he knows he will incur his parents' disapproval if he tries to express them. Within the framework of psychoanalysis, Freud produced a theory for the development of one's personality using the unconscious motives of the id, ego and superego (*see* PERSONALITY). The child's emotional development was described in terms of PSYCHOSEXUAL STAGES OF DEVELOPMENT. In PSYCHOTHERAPY, psychoanalysis also plays a role. It is based on the Freudian concepts of free association, abreaction, insight, interpretation, transference and working through. During abreaction, the patient can release emotions in a safe environment. Following this, there is a period of insight when the patient is encouraged to discover the root cause of the conflict and how to interpret these emotions. Having discovered the cause, the patient transfers his emotional feelings to the therapist. Thus, patients begin to see the therapist in the role of person(s) with whom they have or have had difficulty in forming a relationship. It may be parents or friends with whom they are having such problems. By discussing such a transference, the patient is often helped to work through his feelings. See Atkinson et al (1993); Davison and Neale (1994).

psychodrama a therapeutic technique used in social skills training devised by Moreno in 1946. It can be used to produce insight, MODELLING, SYSTEMATIC DESENSITISATION, SOCIAL SKILLS and ASSERTIVE TRAINING. It helps people to share their problems and to make clear their emotions in certain situations, i.e. those in which the people have difficulty in expressing themselves. It can also improve empathy within the group. *See* Trower et al (1978).

Psycholinguistic Assessments of Language Processing in Aphasia (PALPA) produced by Kay and her colleagues in 1992, PALPA is a comprehensive psycholinguistic assessment of language processing in adult acquired APHASIA. The areas of language processing assessed are orthography and PHONOLOGY, word and picture SEMANTICS, MORPHOLOGY and SYNTAX. Responses are obtained from the client such as lexical decision, repetition and picture naming. Thus, the various tests assess spoken and written input and output. *See* Kay et al (1992) in Appendix I; Beech et al (1993).

psycholinguistics a subdivision of linguistics in which THEORETICAL LINGUISTICS come together with psychological theories to show the behaviour of children during the acquisition of language, how people are going to decide on what they are going to say, how they will produce it and how the listener understands it. *See* Clark and Clark (1977); Garnham (1985); Stackhouse and Wells (1993) (psycholinguistic assessment of developmental speech disorders).

psychology a science which studies behaviour and mental functioning in animals and man. The psychologist uses PSYCHOTHERAPY to treat people who produce abnormal behaviour, EMOTIONAL DISORDERS and CONDUCT DISORDERS, LEARNING DISABILITY and a lack of SOCIAL SKILLS. There are different branches of psychology to deal with such problems. The two main branches are clinical and educational psychology. However, psychologists also take part in industry, with firms and companies having their own psychologist, sometimes dealing with time and motion studies and with industrial disputes and personal problems affecting inter-staff relationships. *See* Atkinson et al (1993); Davison and Neale (1994).

psychoses psychotic disorders are those which cause the person to lose contact with reality. Such disorders include major AFFECTIVE DISORDERS, e.g. psychotic DEPRESSION, paranoia and SCHIZOPHRENIA. Such people may also have hallucinations and delusions. *See* Davison and Neale (1994).

psychosexual stages of development Freud proposed five distinct stages in the development of the child's personality. He believed children were more aware of different parts of their body at different ages and their manipulation satisfied the id (*see* PERSONALITY):

1. Oral stage: children are most conscious of their mouths. The pleasures which are satisfied by such manipulation are those of feeding and sucking.
2. Anal stage: satisfaction comes from the act of defaecation. Toilet-training usually occurs at this time.
3. Phallic stage: satisfaction comes from manipulation of the genitalia. The Oedipus complex begins to affect the child at this time.
4. Latency stage: not strictly a psychosexual stage of development as the child does not show sexual behaviour. The child turns away from the Oedipal conflict and begins to have an interest in outside friends, school, etc.
5. Genital stage: heterosexual relationships begin to develop.

Many critics believe these stages to be too simple to explain the development of personality. Erikson describes this development in terms of ATTACHMENT. *See* Atkinson et al (1993).

psychosomatic a description of disorders which produce changes in the body due to emotional reactions. *See* Stafford-Clark and Smith (1983); Atkinson et al (1993).

psychosurgery a treatment technique in which certain parts of the BRAIN are removed by cutting nerve fibres, usually between the frontal lobe and the limbic system or particular areas in the HYPOTHALAMUS. It is controversial therapy in the USA, as although the person is often happier and more relaxed, the brain has been so damaged that the person cannot function normally. New techniques have improved the situation, reducing the amount of intellectual impairment significantly. The procedure helps those with depression or who have suicidal feelings. *See* Kolb and Whishaw (1990); Atkinson et al (1993); Davison and Neale (1994).

psychotherapy different types of therapy used by psychologists and psychiatrists with the aim of modifying the person's behaviour, thoughts and emotions. Thus, it is hoped to improve their coping with stress and other behavioural problems. It includes BEHAVIOUR THERAPY, PSYCHOANALYSIS, PSYCHODRAMA, humanistic therapy and GROUP THERAPY. *See* Atkinson et al (1993); Davison and Neale (1994).

psychotic depression *see* DEPRESSION.

PTA *see* PURE-TONE AUDIOMETRY.

pterygoid plate *see* MUSCLES OF MASTICATION.

pull-out *see* BLOCK MODIFICATION.

punch-drunk syndrome a medical condition which can lead to DEMENTIA. It is caused by a subdural haematoma which can develop to affect the rest of the brain and produce dementia, tremor and seizures. *See* Stafford-Clark and Smith (1983).

pure agraphia a type of PURE APHASIA identified by the Boston school. Patients present with problems of writing and spelling. *See* Goodglass and Kaplan (1983).

pure alexia a type of PURE APHASIA identified by the Boston School. Patients present with problems of reading, although objects presented to the patient may still be recognised without difficulty. *See* Goodglass and Kaplan (1983).

pure aphasia a type of APHASIA identified by the BOSTON SCHOOL. Only one language modality is affected while all other allied modalities remain intact. *See* Goodglass and Kaplan (1983).

pure-tone audiometry (PTA) pure-tone testing involves the presentation of seven frequencies (125, 250, 500, 1000, 2000, 4000, 8000 Hz) at decreasing and increasing intensities in the range of −10 to 120 dB HL until the person identifies the tone as being present 50 per cent of the time or two-thirds of the time. The tones are given using two pathways of hearing:

1. Air conduction (AC): the sound waves enter the external auditory canal and are transmitted via the tympanic membrane to the ossicles in the middle ear, to the oval window from where they enter the inner ear. This action stimulates the hair cells on the basilar membrane. AC involves the whole hearing system, so any damage to any part of it will result in depressed thresholds for air conduction.

2. Bone conduction (BC): a vibrating unit is placed on the mastoid process although it has been suggested that placement provides more reliable results if the vibrator is placed on the frontal bone. Some researchers have proposed greater test–retest reliability and less inter-subject variability because of the kind of bone tissue making up the frontal bone and, by placing the vibrator on the frontal bone, there is less likelihood of interference from the middle ear and any disorders which may affect it at the time of testing. However, the sensitivity of testing bone conduction at this site is reduced. Bone conduction is intended to test the functioning of the inner ear. Depressed thresholds will only occur in bone conduction if there is a lesion or damage to the inner ear.

A CONDUCTIVE HEARING LOSS will have depressed AC thresholds but normal BC thresholds while a SENSORINEURAL HEARING LOSS shows depressed thresholds in both pathways. The machine which is used to carry out these tests is an audiometer. It produces the frequencies by means of an electronic oscillator. Pure tones are not used in everyday speech but their use in testing gives a good idea of how the person will cope with complex speech signals as they are made of pure tones. When testing for AC thresholds all seven frequencies are used while in BC only five are used (125 Hz and 8000 Hz are not tested). At 125 Hz, the intensity required to make the tone audible is so high that it would be approaching the person's threshold of pain, while at 8000 Hz so much energy would be required present audiometers would not be able to cope. There are not the same problems with AC. The results of pure-tone audiometry are displayed graphically on an audiogram. This gives frequencies along the horizontal axis and intensities down the vertical axis. The audiologist uses symbols to show which pathway has been tested and in which ear (*see* box below). When analysing the results on the audiogram, the tester should look for the presence of the air–bone gap, i.e. the difference between the AC and BC curves. This will reveal a conductive hearing loss. The degree of hearing loss is determined by the pure-tone average. The AC thresholds for 500, 1000 and 2000 Hz are added and divided by three. This gives only a reasonable prediction of the degree of hearing loss. The slope of the curves on the audiogram is also important:

1. Low frequency loss – usually conductive.
2. Flat loss across all frequencies – usually conductive or sensorineural.
3. Ski slope/high-frequency/sloping loss – usually sensorineural.

Audiograms can also show particular features of a person's hearing such as CARHART'S NOTCH, acoustic trauma, NOISE-INDUCED HEARING LOSS and PRESBYCUSIS. There are several classifications to show the degree of hearing loss such as that of D.S.Green (1978). *See* Katz (1985).

		Unmasked AC	BC	Masked AC	BC
Right ear (red)	R	O	<	Δ	[
Left ear (blue)	L	X	>	□	]

pure-tone average see PURE-TONE AUDIOMETRY.

pure vowels vowels that are not diphthongs. Most of the vowels in Scottish-English are pure vowels, e.g. /put/, /mek/, etc. The Scottish-English vowels system is:

i	ɪ	u
e	ʌ	o
ɛ	a	ɔ

ai	ʌu
ʌi	
ɔi	

See Cruttenden (1994).

pure word deafness a type of PURE APHASIA identified by the BOSTON SCHOOL. The patient's auditory comprehension fails although his expressive language remains unimpaired, as do his reading and writing. *See* Goodglass and Kaplan (1983).

pyramidal system/tract the fibres of the upper neuron (*see* NEURON) make up this system. As they come out of the BRAIN into the SPINAL CORD, they become known as the corticospinal tracts. They are responsible for voluntary movements. *See* Barr (1979); Kolb and Whishaw (1990); Tortora and Grabowski (1993).

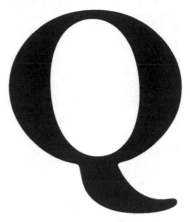

quadriparesis *see* QUADRIPLEGIA.

quadriplegia a physical paralysis which affects all four limbs. Often found in types of CEREBRAL PALSY. If paralysis is not complete and some movements persist, it is called quadriparesis. *See* Hosking (1982).

quality when used in AUDITORY PHONETICS, quality refers to the timbre or resonance of a sound constituted by its different frequencies. Quality can also be used to describe vowels and consonants, e.g. the difference between [i] and [e] can be said to be qualitative. When used in this way, quality is opposed to quantity (*see* LENGTH) or LENGTH. *See* Ladefoged (1993).

quantity *see* LENGTH.

Quinkey keyboard an input device for the BBC Microcomputer for those who cannot use a conventional QWERTY KEY-BOARD. It is a one-handed keyboard which bypasses the QWERTY keyboard. The operator produces combinations of keys to produce different characters. The Quinkey keyboard plugs into the analog port at the back of the computer. When the software which comes with Quinkey is loaded, the keyboard becomes operational. There is a Quinkey unit which can have four keyboards all interfaced into the computers for multi-users.

QWERTY keyboard the usual keyboard layout found on typewriters, computer keyboards and other high-tech communication aids manufactured in the UK. The name comes from the first six letters of the top alphabetic row of the keyboard. Similarly, on the Continent some keyboards are known as AZERTY keyboards. The positioning of letters on such keyboards depends on the frequency with which letters are used. It is opposed to keyboards which are set out alphabetically from A to Z.

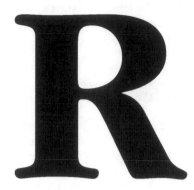

radical behaviourism *see* OPERANT CONDITIONING.

radiogram *see* RADIOGRAPHY.

radiography the process of observing structures within the body by X-rays. The film plates on which the images are printed are known as radiograms while those who carry out the X-rays are radiologists. A variety of specialised X-ray examinations are available, e.g. swallowing barium allows the examination of the act of swallowing. The swallowing may then be followed around the bowel. *See* Pracy et al (1974); Tortora and Grabowski (1993).

radiologist *see* RADIOGRAPHY.

radiotherapy a therapeutic technique used to treat malignant tumours without the patient undergoing surgery. Radiotherapy sometimes follows surgery as it is this combination which can be most effective for removing a tumour completely. *See* Pracy et al (1974).

raised intracranial pressure *see* INTRACRANIAL PRESSURE.

RAM *see* RANDOM ACCESS MEMORY.

Ramsay Hunt syndrome a syndrome which results from infection with herpes zoster (chickenpox virus). There may be facial paresis, hyperacusis, loss of taste which is unilateral, decreased salivation, pain in the ear and vesicles in the external canal and/or the eardrum. *See* Gilroy and Holliday (1982).

ramus of mandible *see* ZYGOMATIC ARCH.

random access memory (RAM) an area of the computer which is reserved for holding data in memory. Memory is held in either RAM or ROM chips. There are two types of RAM memory:

1. Static RAM holds information while the power is switched on.
2. Dynamic RAM will only retain information in memory if it is periodically 'refreshed' by the computer circuits.

All RAM memory loses the information it contains when the power is switched off. It is opposed to ROM (read-only memory). *See* Bishop (1985); Brookshear (1991).

randomisation *see* INDEPENDENT GROUP DESIGN.

range a measure of dispersion to show the spread of results received from an experiment. Range is calculated by subtracting the highest score from the lowest. However, there are times when this is not useful since one of the two groups of scores could have a highest score which is atypical and thus produce an inaccurate range. The statistician would use the interquartile range in such circumstances. *See* Miller (1975).

Rapid Screening Test (RST) this test forms part of the assessment used in the DERBYSHIRE LANGUAGE SCHEME. It is a quick way to find out the child's level of comprehension. After analysing the results, if it is found that the child requires further assessment for comprehension, the therapist will admininster the DETAILED TEST OF COMPREHENSION. *See* Masidlover and Knowles (1987) in Appendix I.

rate the speed at which people speak. It may also be described as tempo. An analysis of rate is made under SUPRASEGMENTAL PHONOLOGY. Rate is often tested in DYSARTHRIA assessments such as the ROBERTSON DYSARTHRIA PROFILE. It is often found that those who use a particularly fast rate have a DYSFLUENCY or DYSPHONIA. Thus, if they are made to slow down their rate of speech using techniques such as PROLONGATION or slowed speech, their dysfluency or dysphonia reduces significantly. *See* Robertson and Thomson (1986); Cruttenden (1994).

rational-emotive therapy (RET) a COGNITIVE BEHAVIOUR THERAPY developed by Ellis in the early 1960s. It is aimed at analysing the individual's distorted perception of life events, not the events themselves. Ellis listed twelve assumptions of distorted cognition which include such beliefs as: "'It is easier to avoid than to face life's difficulties and self-responsibilities", and "One has no control over one's emotions and one cannot help feeling certain things"' (Ellis, 1970, quoted in Rachman and Wilson, 1980, p.196). The therapy is aimed mainly at the neurotic population who do not always rehearse their distorted cognitions deliberately but appear suddenly and are pervasive in their influence. The onus is put on the individual to identify irrational thoughts and replace them with positive thoughts. The treatment procedure includes discussing the philosophical aims of RET; identifying the irrational thoughts by the client through discussion with the therapist; the therapist points out the irra-

tional thoughts and models a rational method of dealing with them; repetition of the rational thoughts aims at replacing the irrational thoughts; and, finally, the client is given behavioural tasks to reinforce the new rational thought processes. *See* Rachman and Wilson (1980); Davison and Neale (1994).

Raven's progressive matrices devised by Raven between 1938 and 1977 to assess a person's non-verbal comprehension. The black and white version was published in 1938 for use with adults. The coloured version was published in 1949 for use with young children and adults with varying degrees of LEARNING DISABILITY or other impairments. The advanced version was published in 1962 for use with those of above-average ability between the age of 11;0 and adulthood. The person is presented with a progression of abstract patterns from which a piece has been removed and hidden in an array of distracting pieces. The person has then to choose the correct piece to fit the pattern. Although designed for use by psychologists, it can be used with those who have APHASIA with associated comprehension deficits as a result of trauma to the brain, e.g. CVA, HEAD INJURY, TUMOUR IN THE CENTRAL NERVOUS SYSTEM, etc. It may be used as an alternative to the Token Test. *See* Aiken (1985).

raw score the score which a child or adult receives after an assessment has been carried out. This score can be turned into a STANDARD SCORE, AGE-EQUIVALENT SCORE or a PERCENTILE SCORE. *See* Atkinson et al (1993).

RDLS *see* REYNELL DEVELOPMENTAL LANGUAGE SCALES.

read when information is stored on a disk, the disk drive can be commanded by the computer to produce the information. This is done by a head in the drive reading the information from the disk and putting it in the computer's memory. It is a similar process to that of a stylus in a record player picking up what is said or sung from the grooves on the record. *See* Bishop (1985).

read-only memory (ROM) a chip in the computer which forms, with the RAM chip, the memory in a computer. It is not possible to write to this memory, the information can only be read from it. Thus, software which comes with ROM, e.g. the Microvoice, cannot accept information; it can only produce the information stored on the chip. It is opposed to RAM (*see* RANDOM ACCESS MEMORY). ROM retains its contents when the power is switched off. *See* Bishop (1985); Brookshear (1991).

Reading Comprehension Battery for Aphasia devised by LaPointe and Horner, this battery of tests is designed to provide the systematic evaluation of the type and severity of reading impairment in those with APHASIA. The intention was to produce a test, the results of which would lead the therapist to decide on appropriate therapy. The battery comprises 10 sub-tests:

I	Single word comprehension (visual)
II	Single word comprehension (auditory)
III	Single word comprehension (semantic)
IV	Functional reading
V	Synonyms
VI	Sentence comprehension (picture)
VII	Short paragraph comprehension
VIII & IX	Paragraphs: factual and inferential
X.	Morphosyntactic

See LaPointe and Horner (1979) in Appendix I; Rosenbek et al (1989).

realisation in speech pathology, the realisation of a sound usually refers to the wrong sound or PHONOLOGICAL PROCESS produced by a child. In articulation delay/disorder or phonological delay/disorder, it describes the differ-ence between the sound the child uses when producing certain words and the target sound, i.e. the correct sound. It is this difference which is analysed by the speech and language therapist. The aim of treatment is to match the realisa-tion to the target so that the differences disappear. *See* Grunwell (1987).

reality orientation therapy a therapeutic technique used with the confused elderly patient. The confusion is usually caused by trauma to the brain such as CVA, trauma, excess medication, etc. A regular daily routine is maintained while in the hospital with the patient's name, dates, schedule for meals and the patient's timetable. There is usually a reality orientation board in the ward to remind them of essential information. *See* Wertz (1981).

Rebus devised by Woodcock in 1969 in the form of *The Rebus Reading Series* for use with children with a mild LEARNING DISABILITY. A rebus is any pictorial representation which acts as a symbol to represent either individual words, phrases or sentences. It has been developed to help those children with language delay or language disorder who may or may not have learning disability. A computer program of rebus symbols has been designed for BBC microcomputers (*see* ACORN COMPUTERS). *See* Kiernan et al (1982); Beukelman and Mirenda (1992).

received pronunciation (RP) a non-regional accent of British English. It is an accent used to refer to other accents.

receptive aphasia the description of a comprehension (how language is 'received') deficit which someone with APHASIA might have. Its characteristics are similar to Wernicke's aphasia (*see* APHASIA (2)) and is opposed to EXPRESSIVE APHASIA. The degree of receptive aphasia can be determined by administering the TOKEN TEST, the TEST FOR RECEPTION OF GRAMMAR as well as comprehension subtests of formal aphasia assessments such as the BOSTON DIAGNOSTIC APHASIA EXAMINATION, the WESTERN APHASIA BATTERY or the MINNESOTA TEST FOR THE DIFFERENTIAL DIAGNOSIS OF APHASIA. *See* Eisenson (1984); Rosenbek et al (1989).

Receptive-Expressive Emergent Language Scale (REEL) devised by Bzoch and League in 1970, it is an observational checklist of language development undertaken jointly by the therapist and caregiver. It is suitable for use with children from birth to 3;0 years. Detailed questions about receptive and expressive ability can be asked corresponding to 1 month old, 2 months old and 3 months old; first year of life, second year and third year in normal child development. *See* Bzoch and League (1971) in Appendix I; Beech et al (1993).

recessive condition *see* CHROMOSOMES.

reciprocal assimilation *see* ASSIMILATION (2).

recruitment an accompanying problem to sensory hearing loss. It occurs when the intensity level of the sound is given a small increase but to the person it can become almost unbearable. For example, an increase of 20 dB may sound like an increase of 60 dB. Tests used to detect recruitment include direct tests for recruitment such as ALTERNATE BINAURAL LOUDNESS BALANCE TEST and the stapedius reflex threshold (*see* IMPEDANCE BATTERY), and indirect tests for recruitment such as finding out the DIFFERENCE LIMEN, the short increment sensitivity index and BÉKÉSY AUDIOMETRY. *See* Katz (1985).

recurrent laryngeal nerve palsy *see* LARYNGEAL NERVE PALSIES (5, 6); TRACHEA.

recurrent utterances also known as speech automatisms, these are stereotyped and repetitive productions made by those with a severe form of APHASIA. *See* Blanken (1991).

reduplication *see* PHONOLOGICAL PROCESSES (3).

REEL *see* RECEPTIVE-EXPRESSIVE EMERGENT LANGUAGE SCALE.

referent a process found in philosophical linguistics. A referent describes what a linguistic unit refers to in the outside world. For example, the word 'book' refers to the object 'book'. However, not all linguistic units have such obvious referents, e.g. the, a, and, is, etc. *See* Lyons (1981); Fromkin and Rodman (1993).

register the way in which people use their VOCAL FOLDS to change the type of voice they can produce. In speaking, there are different types of register such as breathy, creaky and hoarse voice while in singing there are the different voices such as tenor, soprano, falsetto, etc. These voice changes are caused by changes in the thickness, length and tightness in the vocal folds. *See* Catford (1977); Fromkin and Rodman (1993).

regressive assimilation *see* ASSIMILATION (2).

reliability if an assessment is to be worthwhile, it must be reliable, have validity and be discriminating. For an assessment to be reliable, each of the subtests must measure the same variable. For example, in assessments of language, all the subtests must be a measure of various aspects of language, e.g. word finding, reading aloud, comprehension, etc. Thus, there would not be subtests concerning social skills or other non-language functions. It must also be consistent over time, so that if children are tested with a particular test, they should have the same score when tested six months later if no improvement has taken place. This is known as test–retest reliability. *See* Purser (1982); Atkinson et al (1993).

remote-switch Intro Talker a high-tech communication aid which operates like the ordinary INTRO TALKER. Its main difference is the eight single switch sockets on the side of the device. When the device is used in 8-locations each of the individual locations can be operated by a switch. For example, if the device is used with children for group work, each child can have a switch and access a line of a song, poem or story. It is not a scanning device for which a POINT AND SCAN INTRO TALKER is required.

Renfrew Language Attainment Scales devised by Catherine Renfrew in the late 1960s, revised in the 1970s, 1980s and 1990s, to assess various modalities of the child's communication. There are five tests:

1. Bus Story: assesses continuous language.
2. Action Picture Test: assesses expressive language.
3. Word-finding Vocabulary Scale: assesses the use of words.
4. Auditory Discrimination Screening Test: assesses auditory comprehension.
5. Articulation Attainment Test: assesses use of English consonants.

See Clarke and Clarke (1974); Berry (1976).

repeated measures design a design used for carrying out an experiment the result of which will be analysed statistically. There are two groups but each group is made up of the same subjects. Each subject performs under all the conditions of the experiment. Thus, it is possible to find out how the two conditions affect the same subject. The subjects have to be counterbalanced, i.e. the groups are split in two and each half carries out both conditions separately. The most common parametric test used in this design is the related t-test (see T-TESTS) while the most common non-parametric test is the WILCOXON TEST. See Miller (1975).

repertory grids an assessment technique used in PERSONAL CONSTRUCT THEORY. If this theory is to be used effectively, the therapist has to find out how the person views the world and so the person's constructs have to be elicited. The person is provided with role constructs, e.g. someone you look up to, someone you dislike, someone who is successful, someone who is not successful, etc., and gives the names or initials of the people they think about. The person, however, should include himself/herself in the role constructs, e.g. me as I am now, me as I would like to be. Once the people have been identified, three are chosen and the person is asked the following question: 'Can you tell me in what important way two of these people are alike and thereby different from the third.' Thus, the person produces constructs. These can be divided into subordinate constructs, e.g. helpful/unhelpful, and superordinate constructs which the therapist finds out using the technique of laddering. In laddering, the therapist takes one of the bipolar constructs, e.g. helpful/unhelpful, and asks the person questions to obtain a more in-depth analysis of the person's personality. The therapist would stop the interview when it was thought a superordinate level had been reached. Both types of constructs (both subordinate and superordinate) are placed on a grid by the person using a rating system of 1–9. Correlations between the ratings of the constructs are worked out by a computer program. See Dalton (1983, 1994).

Reporter's Test devised by De Renzi and Ferrari in 1978, it is a formal assessment derived from the TOKEN TEST. Its full name is 'The Reporter's Test: A Sensitive Test to Detect Expressive Disturbances in Aphasics'. The same stimuli are used to test the person's expressive abilities as in the Token Test. So that the person becomes accustomed to the material, the 36-item Short Token Test (see TOKEN TEST) is given first. Following this, the 20 tokens are laid out in the prescribed manner. The person is told to pretend there is someone else next to him with a board placed between them. The therapist indicates by pointing to a token, which the person has to tell the 'other' person to point to. The scoring is based on whether the report would or would not allow a correct reproduction by the 'other' person. One point is scored if the response is correct after the first presentation and half a point after the second presentation. The correct names and adjectives must be used. If the score is 18–35 or less, there could be evidence of an EXPRESSIVE APHASIA. The weighting score scale measures the person's verbal output. If the score is 54 or less, there may be evidence for the person having APHASIA. See Eisenson (1984).

reserve volume in breathing, the full capacity of the lungs is not used all the time. Most people keep within the level of the TIDAL VOLUME. The rest of the air which could be used is the reserve volume of which there are two types:

1. Inspiratory reserve volume: the volume of air which can be used during varying degrees of deep inspiration.
2. Expiratory reserve volume: the volume of air which can be used for varying degrees of breath expiration.

See J.H. Green (1978); Tortora and Grabowski (1993).

residual air air remaining in the lungs as residual volume.

residual volume air which is always left in the lungs after total expiration. This amounts to about 1200ml. See J.H. Green (1978); Tortora and Grabowski (1993).

resonance a phenomenon found in ACOUSTIC PHONETICS to describe the setting in vibration of one structure at the frequency of the other structure which starts off the vibration. This occurs in the supraglottal part of the VOCAL TRACT. It occurs, in particular, when the air particles begin to vibrate in the nasal cavities. These cavities can change

shape, and increase loudness and frequency at the source of the sound. In disorders of nasality, the degrees of resonance will either be increased (hypernasality) or decreased (hyponasality). See Catford (1989).

respiration the process of breathing. There are two elements to respiration: inspiration (breathing in) and expiration (breathing out). The normal type of breathing in the male is ABDOMINAL-DIAPHRAGMATIC RESPIRATION while thoracic respiration (see CLAVICULAR) is more common in the female. See J.H. Green (1978); Tortora and Grabowski (1993).

respiratory capacity another name for vital capacity.

reticular system this system in the BRAIN receives almost all sensory input from the whole CENTRAL NERVOUS SYSTEM. It has a role in such functions of the brain as sleep-arousal cycle. Its neurons are connected to the motor areas of the brain and SPINAL CORD. See Barr (1979); Kolb and Whishaw (1990).

retract the action of the tongue to produce sounds in particular parts of the mouth, e.g. at the back by bunching the tongue at the back to produce velar sounds [k,g] and at the front of the mouth by raising the tongue to the post-alveolar area to produce sounds. See Catford (1977).

retrocochlear hearing loss a hearing loss which is caused by damage or a lesion behind the cochlea (see EAR), just below the BRAIN-STEM. It produces a neural hearing loss. See Katz (1985).

return key this key should always be actuated when the operator wants to communicate to the computer that a command has to be carried out when writing a program, carrying out an arithmetic function or when sending data or information to other peripheral units. On some computer keyboards, it is called the 'enter' key. Its function is derived from returning the carriage on a manual typewriter to the beginning of another line when typing a document. *See* Chandor et al (1985).

reversal a phenomenon used in PSYCHOLINGUISTICS. Traditionally, such problems are referred to as spoonerisms or metathesis. A very famous example is one of the many by William Spooner himself: 'You have hissed all my mystery lessons' for 'You have missed all my history lessons.' The phonemes [m] and [h] have been reversed in the mistaken utterance. *See* Clark and Clark (1977).

Revised Token Test *see* TOKEN TEST.

rewrite rules *see* CONSTITUENT ANALYSIS.

Reynell Developmental Language Scales (RDLS) devised by Reynell in 1969 (revised 1977, 2nd revision 1985), it is a formal, standardised assessment to assess the child's development of EXPRESSIVE LANGUAGE and COMPREHENSION. Although it can be used with children between 1;0 and 7;0, it is most sensitive for assessing children between 1;0 and 5;0. It can also be used with physically and visually handicapped children as well as those who have a HEARING LOSS. The RAW SCORE on the comprehension and expressive language tests can be converted to a STANDARD SCORE from which an AGE-EQUIVALENT SCORE can be derived. It was standardised originally on over 1300 UK children between the ages of 1;6 and 7;0. *See* Berry (1976); Reynell (1985) in Appendix I; Beech et al (1993).

RGB the first letters of the three primary colours used in a cathode ray display to make up pictures in colour – red, green, blue.

RGB monitor a monitor or VDU which uses the three primary colours to produce a clear display in colour by use of a cathode ray tube.

rhinitis a disorder found in the nose, affecting its mucous membrane which produces an excess of runny mucus. *See* Pracy et al (1974).

rhythm suprasegmental feature (*see* SUPRASEGMENTAL PHONOLOGY) of speech production in which the listener picks up a regular pattern of units in speech. Commonly, this pattern refers to the use of stressed and unstressed syllables, the use of short and long syllables or using high or low pitch in producing the sentence. In relation to a communication disorder, impaired rhythm is a characteristic of verbal dyspraxia (*see* DEVELOPMENTAL VERBAL DYSPRAXIA). In relation to movement, lack of rhythm is observed in the CLUMSY CHILD SYNDROME. *See* Gordon and McKinley (1980); Ladefoged (1993).

Robertson Dysarthria Profile devised by Robertson in 1982, it is a FORMAL ASSESSMENT to assess the severity of DYSARTHRIA. It concentrates on testing ARTICULATION, RATE, PROSODY and other suprsasegmental phenomena (*see* SUPRASEGMENTAL PHONOLOGY). There are seven subtests:

1. voice;
2. respiration;
3. facial musculature;
4. DIADOCHOKINESIS;
5. reflexes (e.g. swallow, cough);
6. articulation;
7. rate, prosody, intelligibility.

Unlike the FRENCHAY DYSARTHRIA ASSESSMENT, the profile does not produce an aetiology but, instead, will give an in-depth analysis of the dysarthric characteristics of the person's speech. *See* Robertson et al (1986).

robotics the capability of giving a machine commands via a computer. In education and speech and language therapy, the machine is often referred to as a TURTLE which the child can move by giving commands to it by the use of a computer keyboard or other input device. *See* Bishop (1985).

Rochester Method *see* EDUCATION OF HEARING-IMPAIRED CHILDREN.

Rogers *see* PHENOMENOLOGICAL APPROACH.

role reversal a therapeutic technique used commonly in training SOCIAL SKILLS. The person adopts the role of the assertive person and the supervisor takes the non-assertive role. If there is a role conflict, this type of therapy is often difficult to implement. It is part of ASSERTIVE TRAINING. *See* Trower et al (1978).

ROM *see* READ-ONLY MEMORY.

Royal College of Speech and Language Therapists the professional body concerned with the education of speech and language therapists and with standards of service throughout the United Kingdom. The College sets out a code of ethics which every therapist has to follow. It organises working parties to study all forms of communication disorders for which therapists provide treatment. The working parties can be approached at any time for advice on treatment programmes for a specific disorder. Membership of the College is open to all qualified speech and language therapists as well as to students studying speech therapy. College is financed by a yearly membership subscription for which therapists receive the *European Journal of Disorders of Communication* quarterly, the *Bulletin* (a magazine for therapists produced by therapists), a Directory of College members and a twice-monthly list of vacancies in Health Boards/Trusts in the UK and abroad. Information leaflets about different communication disorders are also available. College produces Position Papers concerning various aspects of speech and language therapy, e.g. dysphagia, dysphasia, use of AAC, etc. *See* Jennings (1984); Morris (1994).

RP *see* RECEIVED PRONUNCIATION.

RST *see* RAPID SCREENING TEST.

rubella also known as German measles. It forms part of the TORCH classification of infectious diseases which can adversely affect a fetus. If the fetus becomes infected, it may die or miscarry. If the fetus survives, there may be congenital heart disease, the brain may be underdeveloped producing CEREBRAL PALSY, AUTISM and LEARNING DISABILITY. The eyes may have cataracts and there may be a HEARING LOSS. The disease can be prevented by the mother undergoing immunisation before child-bearing years. This is usually carried out in the UK in the early senior school. *See* Hosking (1982).

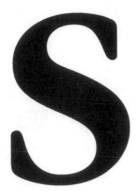

S-24 a shortened form of Erikson's (1969) S-scale, it is an assessment designed to find out the attitudes of a person to various communication situations. It is used commonly with stammerers. The individual is asked to give a true/false response to 24 statements, e.g. I often ask questions in groups. The statements cover how stammerers view their speaking ability, how they cope with anxiety-provoking situations, e.g. speaking in groups or to someone in authority, and what situations they try to avoid. *See* Dalton (1983).

S-indicator a device to help produce the correct [s] sound. An indicator panel with a needle plus a lamp give visual feedback as to the quality of the [s] produced. It can be used with the poorest of speakers. It can also be used to teach other voiceless fricatives. Tests in Sweden have shown that it can be used effectively with children of 6 years of age.

salivary glands there are three pairs of large salivary glands. The ducts from these glands open into the mouth. The glands are:

1. Parotid gland: wedge-shaped structure lying behind the MANDIBLE and below the EAR and in front of the mastoid process. It grows at the same rate as the person. Cranial nerve VII (*see* CRANIAL NERVES) runs through the gland. The duct runs over the buccinator and masseter muscle (*see* MUSCLES OF FACIAL EXPRESSION) and exits at the second molar. The secretion of the gland is to keep the mouth moist, lubricate the passage of food and initiate digestion by the presence of ptyalin which breaks down starch.

2. Submandibular gland: it opens through a duct in the floor of the mouth and runs posteriorly under the mandible. The gland measures 2–3 cm deep, wide and high. The duct opening is at the side of the lingual frenulum (*see* MOUTH). It is a mixed serous/mucus producing gland.

3. Sublingual salivary gland: it is situated under the floor of the mouth and is both the shape and size of an almond. It opens into the mouth by several ducts. It is a mixed serous/mucus producing gland.

These glands are controlled by secretory motor nerves. The parotid gland is supplied by the parasympathetic fibres from the glossopharyngeal nerve (*see* CRANIAL NERVES) while the other two salivary glands are supplied by the facial nerve (*see* CRANIAL NERVES). The salivary glands are compound racemose glands because they branch into several parts: lobes–lobules–branching ducts–dilated alveoli. These three glands together produce 1–1.5

litres of saliva per day. *See* Tortora and Grabowski (1993).

salpingopharyngeus muscle   *see* PHARYNX.

sample

1. A sample of language is often taken by a speech therapist for analysis as the person's language in a free situation is often more natural than in an assessment situation. It is an INFORMAL ASSESSMENT and can be analysed by any of the linguistic profiles devised by Crystal or just by the therapist's intuition and experience. *See* Crystal (1993).
2. *See* POPULATION.

Sandwell Bilingual Screening Assessment (SBSA) devised by Duncan et al for children of 6;0–9;0 years whose first language is Panjabi. It is a picture-based screening test for children who have problems acquiring English as a second language. By analysing the results of the SBSA, the therapist can decide if the problems are in the child's poor language skills or as a result of some pathological cause which will require therapeutic intervention from a speech therapist. The child is presented with 44 line drawings with questions being asked both in Panjabi and English. Two grammatical profiles are produced for each language. The scores in either language are compared with the norm tables in the manual to establish if problems exist in one or both languages. The norms have been obtained from 300 Panjabi and English children. *See* Duncan et al (1987) in Appendix I.

sarcoma a malignant tumour which arises from CONNECTIVE TISSUE. Thus, a fibro-sarcoma arises from fibrous tissue, an osteosarcoma arises from BONE while a chondrosarcoma arises from CARTILAGE. *See* Tortora and Grabowski (1993).

Saussure Ferdinand de Saussure (1857-1913) is the founding father of modern linguistics. The lingistic theories he proposed were set out in the '*Cours de Linguistique Générale*' in 1913. Saussure did not write this book himself. It was published posthumously from the notes of his students who had attended three series of lectures he gave before his death. When all the notes were collected, it was found there was repetition and some inconsistencies. However, all the information was gathered by Bally and Sechehaye and, to overcome the problems already mentioned, they concentrated their work on the third series of lectures as well as taking information from the other two series of lectures and Saussure's personal notes. Later, Rudolf Engler published Saussure's students' notes in 1967. There was much linguistic discussion before Saussure that was confined to the historical study of language. He proposed that it should be possible to stop at a particular time either past or present and describe the language processes which occur. This is the study of synchronic linguistics and is an important part of the historical description of linguistics. However, one of the main standpoints for his linguistics theory is 'language is a system of signs'. These signs are arbitrary by nature in that the 'signifier' for 'television' is a sequence of sounds which could be equally well respresented by other sound sequences such as 'bimp', 'gapo' or 'glick', etc. However, this arbitrariness is lessened with some processes such as onomatopeia, e.g. 'splash', 'miaow', etc. These words are not arbitrary as they are imitative of the action described. There are also sound sequences which are combined to produce new signs e.g. typewriter, as this sign is associated with the object it names. Saussure proposed a more complex explanation for the arbitrariness of the signifier and the signified. He tried to show they were arbitrary over time. For example, the word 'gay' in the nineteenth century and early part of the twentieth century meant 'happy', 'lively', etc. while in the last 20–30 years it has come to refer to someone's sexuality. Thus, the signifier and the signified are themselves arbitrary. 'La langue' describes the groups of forms which are used to make up a particular language while 'la parole' is the actual physical manifestation of language, i.e. the speech acts and how meaning is communicated. *See* Saussure (1916); Lepschy (1982); Culler (1986).

Scanning Director a stand-alone Environmental Control Unit which operates in a similar way to the DIRECTOR. By hitting a switch, users can scan through a list of appliances; when the appliance is selected, the device will scan through a list of functions, which have been previously 'learned' by the Scanning Director, to operate the appliance. When the function is selected, the appliance should operate as if operated by the usual infra-red remote control. The Scanning Director is also capable of being used with the X-10 system, which is capable of running a full domestic Environmental Control arrangement. *See* Appendix IV.

schema, schemata *see* ASSIMILATION (2).

schizophrenia a syndrome or group of mental illnesses characterised by specific psychological symptoms which interfere with an individual's thinking, emoting and behaviour and with each of these in a characteristic way. The person can have THOUGHT DISORDERS, FLATTENING OF AFFECT and disorders of speech and language. There are three main types of schizophrenia:

1. Hebephrenic schizophrenia: disorganised features of movements, ideas and moods.
2. Catatonic schizophrenia: odd movements caused by motor disturbances.
3. Paranoic schizophrenia: characterised by delusions which are often grandiose in nature.

As already mentioned, some people who have schizophrenia have associated problems in communication. These include: (1) PERSEVERATION in syntax; (2) repetition of words and syllables; (3) disruption of semantic memory; (4) clang associations; (5) ECHOLALIA and palilalia; (6) echopraxia; (7) mutism; (8) poverty of thought and speech; (9) concreteness; (10) PHONATION problems; and (11) FLATTENING OF AFFECT. A therapist will have to take a language sample for analysis and plan a treatment programme accordingly. Medical treatment can be treated by the PHENOTHIAZINE family of drugs. *See* Davison and Neale (1994).

Schuell in 1964, Schuell and her colleagues put forward a classification of aphasia comprising five major categories and two minor syndromes:

1. Simple aphasia: a breakdown in the symbolic use of language, resulting in a reduction in language, WORD-FINDING DIFFICULTIES with syntactic problems plus phonemic or jargon errors depending on the severity of the aphasia and comprehension errors depending on the length and complexity of what is said.
2. Aphasia with visual involvement.
3. Aphasia with persistent dysfluency.
4. Aphasia with scattered findings: the individual has some functional language, is not severely handicapped but may have dysarthria.
5. Aphasia with sensory motor involvement: mild aphasia with persistent dysarthria.

The two minor syndromes are:

1. Aphasia with intermittent auditory imperception.
2. Irreversible aphasia syndrome: a sudden loss in all modalities and loss of all functional language.

Schuell believed that aphasia was not modality-specific but affected all language modalities. Following this theory, she devised the MINNESOTA TEST FOR DIFFERENTIAL DIAGNOSIS OF APHSAIA (MTDDA). *See* Eisenson (1984); Rosenbek et al (1989).

schwa perhaps the most common vowel found in English. It is used to transcribe the last sound in 'after' [æftə], and when a stressed vowel becomes unstressed and is the pronounced sound in words such as 'a', 'an', 'the', etc. *See* Ladefoged (1993).

Schwann cell a cell which covers the myelin sheath covering the nerve's axon. It is divided into the sections of the nerve between the nodes of Ranvier. The myelin is formed by the membrane of the Schwann cell. When Wallerian degeneration takes place, it is the Schwann cells which are affected. *See* Barr (1979).

ScreenDoors an on-screen keyboard for Apple Mac computers, Screen-Doors produces a movable and resizeable window. It has good graphics and fonts on the keyboard. It offers word prediction and context specific dictionaries that can be created for different subjects. Selections are made through a puff switch. ScreenDoors runs in the MultiFinder environment on System 6.3 or higher. It requires a hard drive and at least two megabytes of RAM memory. *See* Appendix IV.

screening audiometry audiometric tests which are carried out quickly with individuals (usually children or in a pre-school clinic). The frequencies are tested at a constant intensity level. This is also known as sweep testing. *See* Katz (1985).

screening tests tests which can be carried out quickly to discover the severity of any disorder, e.g. APHASIA, DYSARTHRIA, etc. Such tests include the WHURR APHASIA SCREENING TEST and the FRENCHAY APHASIA SCREENING TEST (FAST). They are designed to provide an indication as to the type of in-depth assessment which should follow. *See* Byers Brown (1981).

192

scroll the continuous movement of characters forming lines of text which begins at the bottom of the screen and makes the other lines move up the screen. This occurs when a computer program is listed, text is produced by a wordprocessor and in some games which use text. Graphics often scroll across the screen in many arcade games.

SDLD *see* SPECIFIC DEVELOPMENTAL LANGUAGE DISORDER.

secondary articulation an articulation which occurs with little or no narrowing of the articulators while producing the secondary articulation. For example, a palatalised fricative where the friction is the primary articulation and the palatalisation is the secondary articulation. *See* Ladefoged (1993).

Secretary a high-tech communication aid which combines the message writing characteristics of the memowriter and the speech quality of the PARROT. It has a QWERTY KEYBOARD which produces messages on the display screen which can be printed on the internal printer. The recorded speech messages can call for attention or answer routine queries.

secretory motor nerves *see* SALIVARY GLANDS.

segmental phonology a study of the phonemes (*see* PHONOLOGY) in any given language. Phonemes are regarded as the segments under study. It is opposed to SUPRASEGMENTAL PHONOLOGY. *See* Hyman (1975).

seizure a descriptive term for fits or convulsions (compare EPILEPSY).

self-actualization *see* PHENOMENOLOGICAL APPROACH.

self-characterization an assessment used in PERSONAL CONSTRUCT THEORY. It is part of the 'credulous' approach. People are asked to describe themselves in a non-threatening way as if their best friend were making the description. The request is presented thus: 'I want you to write a character sketch of (person's name), just as if he were the principal character in a play. Write it as it might be written by a friend who knew him very intimately and very sympathetically, perhaps better than anyone ever really could know him. Be sure to write it in the third person. For example, start out by writing, "(person's name) is a..." *See* Dalton (1983, 1994).

self-instructional training (SIT) developed by Meichenbaum in 1977, SIT is a COGNITIVE BEHAVIOUR THERAPY. It is based in part on Ellis's RATIONAL-EMOTIVE THERAPY as well as on the developmental sequence which children use to develop internal speech and verbal-symbolic control over their behaviour. The therapist using SIT takes the client through the following stages:

1. The client is trained to identify maladaptive behaviour or thoughts (self-statements).
2. The therapist models appropriate behaviour while talking the client through effective action strategies using self-statements which are positive and stress the client's adequacy and reduce feelings of failure.
3. The client performs the target behaviour and rehearses the appropriate self-instructions aloud followed by rehearsing them internally. The therapist provides positive feedback to ensure constructive problem-solving self-talk which replaces anxiety-produced cognitions associated with the behaviour. *See* Rachman and Wilson (1980); Davison and Neale (1994).

self-theory *see* PHENOMENOLOGICAL APPROACH.

semantic field a conceptually identified group of lexical items, e.g. kinship relations, colour terms, constitutes a semantic field. The meanings of the lexical items that make up the field are in part determined by the sense relations they contract with one another within the field.

semantic relations one approach to the early utterance of children has tried to account for them in terms of semantic relations they express, rather than in terms of grammatical patterns. Such relations were proposed by Brown (1973):

agent + action	man put
action + object	kick ball
agent + object	mummy shoe
action + locative	go home
entity + locative	book table
possessor + possessed	daddy car
entity + attributive	cup blue
demonstrative + entity	that book

See Lyons (1981).

semantic-pragmatic disorder a rare disorder in which there is gross impairment of syntax and severely restricted pragmatic use of language Comprehension is also limited. Phonology may be normal or near normal.

semantics the study of meaning. Within modern linguistics, the most important areas have been lexical (structural) semantics which has concerned itself with structural relations in the vocabulary, e.g. autonymy, synonymy, hyponymy and truth-conditional semantics. This is an approach to sentence meaning which holds that (at least part of) sentence meaning is characterised in terms of the conditions (in the real or possible world) under which a sentence can be held to express a statement that is true. *See* Lyons (1981); Fromkin and Rodman (1993).

semi-vowels the sounds subsumed under this term are sometimes known as approximants (*see* ARTICULATION). They are classified as consonants but have a vowel-like quality in that they are produced without closure or friction. The sounds which follow this pattern in English are [j,w]. *See* Fromkin and Rodman (1993). Ladefoged (1993).

senile dementia *see* ALZHEIMER'S DISEASE.

sensation level (SL) a measure of the loudness of a sound above the person's hearing threshold. It is measured in decibels (dB). For example, if the hearing threshold is 60 dB HL and a sound is presented at 90 dB HL, the sensation level will be 30 dB SL (sensation level). *See* Katz (1985).

sensitivity training a therapeutic technique used commonly in SOCIAL SKILLS training. It takes the form of the participants learning from their own immediate and direct experiences within the group. It is not so much a procedure for learning social skills but a way of learning sensitivity to others, improving interpersonal relationships and improving the person's self-confidence. There are two types of techniques used for this end – ENCOUNTER GROUPS and T-GROUPS. *See* Trower et al (1978); Davison and Neale (1994).

sensorimotor stage the first of Piaget's four stages of cognitive development in children. The stage lasts from birth to 2 years of age and concerns the child's ability to perceive objects but not to think about them. In other words, the child can only act upon an object when it is within his vision but not if it is hidden. This is Piaget's theory of OBJECT PERMANENCE. The development of imitation and play are important in the child's ability to symbolise objects. Towards the end of this stage, the child may use deferred imitation, i.e. the ability to act out events which the child has stored in memory, and play with objects using them to symbolise other objects. This idea of symbolisation is the mainstay of Piaget's theory of language development. He believed a child could not develop language until the child had acquired symbolisation. More concisely, Piaget believed language did not appear until the cognitive events underlying symbolisation have been achieved and thus language develops out of cognition. *See* Beard (1969), Atkinson et al (1993); Boden (1994).

sensorineural hearing loss this is caused by a lesion or damage to the inner ear, to the auditory nerve, to the BRAIN-STEM or to the auditory cortex. It can only be improved by wearing a HEARING AID. Those with this type of hearing loss often talk too loudly because they cannot hear their own voice and sometimes they have vertigo and often TINNITUS. They have difficulty picking up speech especially if they are in a noisy environment or having a conversation in a group. There is no air–bone gap (*see* PURE-TONE AUDIOMETRY) whilst the loss varies from mild to severe. *See* Katz (1985); Atkinson et al (1993).

sensory aphasia acoustic agnosic APHASIA identified by Luria in 1966. The main difficulty lies in discriminating speech sounds and this leads to impaired understanding of word meaning. Because of the inability to analyse words into their sound components cueing-in through the initial sound of the word does not help. *See* Lesser (1989).

sentence the largest unit in grammar within which distributional patterns can be recognised. Lyons has referred to it as 'the largest unit of grammatical description' (Lyons 1968, p.172). Note, however, that it can be defined, either in traditional terms as a list of patterns defined in terms of some set of elements, e.g. SVO, SVA, SVC, etc., or more recently as the product of a set of defining rules. 'Sentence' is a theoretical term of linguistic description. *See* Lyons (1968); Fromkin and Rodman (1993).

Sentence Comprehension Test devised by Wheldall, Hobsbaum and Mittler in 1977 (revised 1987), it is a FORMAL ASSESSMENT to test the child's understanding of grammatical constructions. It can only be used with children of 3;0–5;6 years. It comprises 15 subtests, each of which have a different grammatical structure. Each subtest has four items from which the child has to choose the correct one. A subtest is passed if the child scores three or more in each subtest which produces a profile score out of 60 items from which the therapist decides whether or not therapy is required. Five subtests have been left out as well as several items (there are only ten subtests) and the pictures have been redrawn. There is also a Panjabi version. *See* Wheldall (1987) in Appendix I; Beech et al (1993).

separation anxiety a possible cause of EMOTIONAL DISORDER which children may have. Feelings of fear and anxiety are quite common and are normal reactions in children to certain circumstances but when these feelings begin to interfere with everyday life, they become abnormal. During children's early life, they are very sensitive and vulnerable to traumatic events and separation is one such event. The mother, often regarded by the child as being someone special (since she is usually the parent with whom bonding first takes place), may have to leave home suddenly, for example, to have another child or for other medical reasons. If the child has been adequately prepared for this separation, there will be less of a problem accepting the situation than if the mother disappears suddenly and no preparation has taken place. In the latter case, the child becomes 'lost' and has severe anxiety. PSYCHOTHERAPY of all kinds has been used successfully with such children. FAMILY THERAPY and/or parental counselling is also useful. *See* Rutter (1975); Davison and Neale (1994).

serial interface an interface where there is a serial exchange of information between the central processor and peripheral units. It is opposed to parallel interface. *See* Bishop (1985).

serial speech the type of language which is automatic to most people, e.g. days of the week, months of the year, alphabet, counting, etc. With some of those

with APHASIA, it may be the only language which is intact. Thus, in many aphasia assessments, subtests for serial speech are included. *See* Eisenson (1984).

serous cells these produce a water-like substance. *See* SALIVARY GLANDS.

serous otitis media *see* OTITIS MEDIA (3).

servo system in speech, a cybernetic theory proposed by Fairbanks in 1954 to explain speech production. He describes an effector unit, a feedback loop and a comparator device whereby output may be compared with intention, error detected and necessary connections made.

sex chromosomes *see* CHROMOSOMES.

Sheffield Screening Test for Acquired Language Disorders devised by Syder and colleagues in 1994, this screening test can be used to assess the presence of high level language disorders as a result of trauma to the brain. It is in three sections; the first allows some assessment of the person's functional communication while the second and third allow an assessment of receptive and expressive language problems. It takes 10 minutes to administer. The test has been standardized on 112 people aged 30–91 years. *See* Syder et al (1994) in Appendix I.

Short Token Test *see* TOKEN TEST.

shunt a device fitted into the BRAIN to drain the fluid causing pressure in the FOURTH VENTRICLE in people with hydrocephalus. There are two types of shunt treatment – Spitz-Holter shunt and the Pudenz shunt. *See* Hosking (1982).

shwa *see* SCHWA.

sibilant a subtype of fricative (*see* ARTICULATION). The fricatives in English are [f, v, θ, ð, s, z, ʃ,ʒ]. Some fricatives are produced with greater acoustic energy and hence a higher pitch. This produces a loud hissing noise. These fricatives, i.e. [s,z,ʃ,ʒ] are sibilants and thus opposed to the non-sibilants. ie, [f,v,θ, ð]. *See* Ladefoged (1993).

sibling rivalry it is common knowledge that there is almost always some degree of rivalry between or among siblings. This may take the form of play-fighting or trying to do better at school, etc. It is usually caused by just wanting to do better than the other sibling to obtain more praise from parents. However, if parents go out of their way overtly to show preference to one sibling rather than to another, the one to whom preference is not given may produce feelings of aggression either to the other sibling or to parents or both. These feelings can produce either CONDUCT DISORDERS or EMOTIONAL DISORDERS such as ELECTIVE MUTISM. For example, if children wish to be vindictive towards the parents, they may decide not to speak at school and so make life as difficult as possible. See Rutter (1975).

sigh/yawn technique see YAWN/SIGH APPROACH.

sign languages a type of ALTERNATIVE AUGMENTATIVE COMMUNICATION system taught to those who have difficulty in using EXPRESSIVE LANGUAGE. A sign language has its own grammar and has similar characteristics to any oral language, i.e. historical change, puns, humour, arbitrariness, etc. Such languages include BRITISH SIGN LANGUAGE (BSL) and American Sign Language (ASL) for use with those who have a hearing loss. See Kiernan et al (1982); Beukelman and Mirenda (1992).

sign systems a type of ALTERNATIVE AUGMENTATIVE COMMUNICATION system taught to those who have difficulty in using expressive language or whose speech is significantly unintelligble. A sign system is not a language in itself although it has signs which represent words and, in some cases, morphological endings. It does not have its own grammar but follows the order in spoken English as it has a sign for each keyword in the sentence. Such examples are the PAGET-GORMAN SIGN SYSTEM and MAKATON Vocabulary. See Kiernan et al (1982); Beukelman and Mirenda (1992)

signed English this SIGN SYSTEM is designed to represent oral English. The hand signs are used with speech which makes the message to be communicated very clear. It can be used with children who have a HEARING LOSS. Each sign has a semantic relationship with each English word. There are about 2500 sign words and 14 sign markers for morphological endings. See Bornstein and Hamilton (1978); Beukelman and Mirenda (1992).

signifier, signified, sign see SAUSSURE.

simple aphasia proposed by Schuell in the 1960s, it refers to a reduction in the ability to use all language modalities without accompanying DYSPRAXIA or DYSARTHRIA. See Eisenson (1984).

simple depression see DEPRESSION.

singer's nodes/nodules see VOCAL NODULES.

single case study in studies of the efficacy of certain treatment techniques, it has been found to be insufficient to use test designs such as the INDEPENDENT GROUP, MATCHED PAIRS and REPEATED MEASURES. Thus, statisticians proposed the single case study. In this type of study, the subjects have to act as their own CONTROL GROUP. The aim is to test the subject during periods of treatment and non-treatment. The best design for such studies is the ABA design. This means that during 'A' (no treatment) the person is tested, during 'B' treatment is given followed by 'A' when the person is retested using similar stimuli as were used during the treatment sessions. For example, if the person has naming problems and therapy is given to improve his naming skills, the therapist might take 50 pictures, test the person, take half the cards and give treatment to help him to name these pictures and then retest using all 50 pictures. See Coltheart (1983).

SIT *see* SELF-INSTRUCTIONAL TRAINING.

skew *see* CENTRAL TENDENCY.

ski slope hearing loss *see* PURE-TONE AUDIOMETRY.

Skinner's boxes *see* OPERANT CONDITIONING.

skull a structure formed by the bones of the cranium and MANDIBLE. The bones all fit together strongly except for the mandible which swings quite freely so that the mouth can open and close. The function of the skull is to protect the BRAIN. Other areas of the skull are the orbits which are filled by the eyes and their respective nerves and muscles, the nasal cavities (*see* NOSE) and the MOUTH. *See* Tortora and Grabowski (1993).

SL *see* SENSATION LEVEL.

slit a particular configuration of the TONGUE for producing fricatives (*see* ARTICULATION). The tongue is flat for the fricatives [f,v,ʃ,ʒ] while it is grooved for the fricatives [s,z]. *See* Catford (1977).

sloping hearing loss *see* PURE-TONE AUDIOMETRY.

smooth muscle produces slow contraction over long distances. It is supplied by the AUTONOMIC NERVOUS SYSTEM (ANS). Its fibres are spindle-like and have thin ends while the central part is thicker containing the nucleus of the muscle. Smooth muscle is involuntary muscle tissue and innervated by involuntary nerves and certain hormones. It is found in the gut, respiratory passages, urinogenital system, iris of eye and blood vessel walls. *See* Leeson et al (1985) ; Tortora and Grabowski (1993).

social skills a phenomenon in which a person produces socially acceptable behaviour and the behaviour produces the desired effect on others. Any child or adult who does not possess such skills has to be given a treatment programme to teach him/her how to cope in various situations through experience. Such treatment takes the form of ASSERTIVE TRAINING,

SENSITIVITY THERAPY and PSYCHODRAMA. *See* Trower et al (1978); Davison and Neale (1994).

Social Use of Language Programme devised by Rinaldi in 1992, this programme is designed to improve the social communication skills of children and adolescents with mild to moderate learning disabilities, speech impairment or hearing difficulties. It is possible to assess a person's different social communication skills, both verbal and non-verbal, as well as implement an effective educational therapy programme. It uses group activities such as games, role-playing exercises and problem solving for assessment and remediation. *See* Rinaldi (1992) in Appendix I.

socialised conduct disorder *see* CONDUCT DISORDER.

sociolinguistics the study of accents and dialects used in different regions of a country. It also studies the different varieties of language used in social contexts and the role of linguistic minorities in a multiracial society. *See* Trudgill (1974).

sodium valproate a drug treament for EPILEPSY.

soft copy information which is produced from the keyboard and appears on the monitor only. It is opposed to hard copy.

soft palate *see* MOUTH.

software the computer programs which can be stored on disk. It can also refer to published programs which the operator may require to assemble his program in machine code, to debug his programs or to copy one file to another using utility programs and so on. It is also possible to obtain software for particular purposes such as making up wages or annual accounts for which the operator can use a spreadsheet. *See* Bishop (1985).

sonorant a MAJOR CLASS FEATURE proposed by Chomsky and Halle to distinguish sounds produced without any blocking of the VOCAL TRACT [+SONORANT], i.e. liquids, nasals and laterals, from those which are produced with an obstruction [−SONORANT]. *See* Fromkin and Rodman (1993); Ladefoged (1993).

sonority a phenomenon in auditory phonetics which examines loudness relative to pitch, stress and duration. *See* Ladefoged (1993).

sound pressure level measured at a given point along the propagation of the sound wave. It decreases as distance from source increases. It is measured in dynes/cm² or pascals (Pa). *See* Denes and Pinson (1973).

sound system *see* PHONOLOGY.

source features a classification in Chomsky and Halle's DISTINCTIVE FEATURES. The others are MAJOR CLASS FEATURES, cavity features, manner of articulation features and prosodic features. The features describe the modification which happens to the airstream producing voice and strident sounds. *See* Hyman (1975).

spastic cerebral palsy *see* CEREBRAL PALSY.

spastic dysarthria *see* DYSARTHRIA.

spastic dysphonia a type of DYSPHONIA in which the voice becomes strained and staccato owing to intermittent spasm of the vocal folds. It occurs equally frequently in men and women. The cause is not understood as there appears to be no obvious pathology. *See* Greene and Mathieson (1989).

spasticity a condition produced by a lesion to the upper motor neurons (*see* NEURONS) causing hypertonia of the muscles. The person's speech is characterised by spastic DYSARTHRIA. *See* Tortora and Grabowski (1993).

speak more fluently a technique of remediation for those who stammer. Little attention is paid to any underlying psychological causes. It concentrates on removing the stammer completely and making the person totally fluent. Therapists using this theory aim for total fluency – an ACCEPTABLE STAMMER is regarded as failure. The MONTEREY FLUENCY PROGRAMME is based on this theory, as

is PROLONGED SPEECH. *See* Dalton (1983).

SpeakEasy a basic message system which can hold twelve single messages totalling 4 minutes and 20 seconds while six keys allow for 10-second messages, four keys allow for 20-second messages and two keys allow 60-second messages. Each of these can be accessed by a switch although there is no scanning. The device can be attached by a cable to toys which can be operated with auditory reinforcement. It can be carried by a shoulder strap. *See* Appendix IV.

speaker's nodes/nodules *see* VOCAL NODULES.

special education a description of the education received by children who have varying degrees of LEARNING DISABILITY. The classes are often small, and outside agencies such as SPEECH AND LANGUAGE THERAPY, PHYSIOTHERAPY and PSYCHOLOGY are involved in the education of these children. However, it is becoming more usual for these children to be integrated into mainstream education with their own support teacher who works with them on a one-to-one basis, although there are subjects in which they participate with the rest of the class.

Special Needs Assessment Software devised by Douglas in 1990, it aims to establish the educational needs of young children with severe physical difficulties and/or LEARNING DISABILITY. There are two separate tests:

1. Cognitive development test: assesses the child's cognitive skills in such tests as visual discrimination matching, observational memory, visual sequencing, etc. Results can be interpreted using a criterion-referenced scoring system, or by comparison with norms for able bodied children aged 2;6 to 6;0 years.

2. Verbal comprehension test: a test of the child's language comprehension in such areas as the use of preposi-

tions, verb tenses, adjective comprehension and use of number concepts. Interpretation of results is similar to that of the cognitive development test.

Responses for both tests can be made using any input device suitable for the child. The software can run on a BBC B or Master microcomputer with a single 40-track disk drive. A hard copy of the results can be obtained from a printer although the results also appear on the screen. *See* Douglas (1990) in Appendix I.

specific developmental language disorder (SDLD) a communication disorder affecting children. The causes are not the same as those which produce LANGUAGE DELAY. The child will have one of the following:

1. A phonological delay during the child's early years.
2. A grammatical problem with expressive language.
3. A high non-verbal IQ and a low verbal IQ.
4. Disorder of prosody.
5. Limited symbolic play.
6. Visual sequential memory superior to auditory sequential memory.
7. Degree of frustration from producing a language performance below the child's intellectual level.

If a child is to be diagnosed as having SDLD, he may or may not present with some of the following causes:

1. Developmental articulatory, verbal or constructional apraxia.
2. Minor neurological problems.
3. Comprehension problems.
4. LANDAU-KLEFFNER SYNDROME.
5. DYSLEXIA or DYSGRAPHIA.

This DIFFERENTIAL DIAGNOSIS from language delay, which has a different set of causes, can only be carried out by a speech and language therapist. SDLD must be differentiated from language delay, if treatment is to be successful.

See Wyke (1978).

specific language impairment (SLI) *see* SPECIFIC DEVELOPMENTAL LANGUAGE DISORDER.

spectrography the acoustic measurements of sounds. The spectrograph was invented in the late 1940s. Every sound consists of frequencies with each of these frequencies shown on the spectrograph. The spectrogram has a time scale along the horizontal axis while the frequency is measured down the vertical axis. The frequencies show up as light or dark marks depending on their intensity. In a typical spectrogram, there are dark bands known as formants, i.e. groups of harmonics whose intensity is greater than those of the surrounding harmonics. Each formant is numbered from the bottom of the spectrogram. The lowest formant is F1, while the next formant is F2, etc. *See* Ladefoged (1993).

speech acts speech acts describe the presumed intention of the speaker when expressing an utterance in relation to the hearer. Speakers may, for instance, be directive, commanding or requesting a hearer to do something. Or they may be expressive, in using utterances to convey their own feelings or attitudes, e.g. apologising, welcoming. Various other categories have been proposed. Searle has stated, 'speech acts are the basic or minimal units of linguistic communication' (Searle, 1969, p.16) *See* Searle (1969); Clark and Clark (1977); Fromkin and Rodman (1993).

speech and language therapist a term used in the UK to describe the person who assesses, diagnoses and treats people with communication disorders.

speech and language therapy the profession responsible for the assessing, diagnosing and treatment of all types of communication disorders as well as DYSPHAGIA, DYSPHONIA and LARYNGECTOMY affecting both children and adults. In

199

1990, it was decided by a ballot of all members of the ROYAL COLLEGE OF SPEECH AND LANGUAGE THERAPY to change the name of the profession in the UK from speech therapy to speech and language therapy. *See* Crystal (1984).

speech audiometry an audiometric test to give the audiologist a better measurement of the person's hearing as real speech is used instead of pure tones (*see* PURE-TONE AUDIOMETRY) which are not used in everyday speech. Those with a RETROCOCHLEAR HEARING LOSS and a CENTRAL HEARING LOSS may do reasonably well with pure tones but still have poor speech discrimination. This type of audiometry also allows the tester to assess the person's social disability, find a lesion in the auditory pathway, predict the outcome of surgery, assess the value of LIPREADING or auditory training, etc., and assess the efficiency of HEARING AIDS. Any speech from monosyllabic words to sentences and discourse is used. However, monosyllabic and bisyllabic words are used most often. Whatever linguistic material is used, it must be within the person's abilities to understand it. The stimuli are usually presented by the tester in one room while the person sits in the other and hears the stimuli through earphones or out of loudspeakers. There can be variability between testers but stimuli should be presented as a suitable speech for each person. A tape recording could also be used. A free-field presentation is used with children. Two types of test are carried out:

1. SPEECH RECEPTION THRESHOLD.
2. SPEECH DISCRIMINATION TEST.

See Hood (1981); Martin (1996).

speech chain the means by which a speaker transmits information to a listener. The speaker forms an utterance by selecting the words and making-up the correct order in the BRAIN. This is the performance part of the speech chain. These words are sent by nerve impulses along the VOCAL TRACT, uttered by the articulators, whereupon they are transferred into sound waves. These waves are acoustic energy which are sent across the gap between speaker and listener. The latter receives them through his/her EAR where they undergo a physiological change in the form of nerve impulses to the brain where they are decoded so that the listener can understand the utterance. Thus, one human can communicate through the medium of speech to another human – a feature of Man's existence which raises him above other animal life. In speech and language therapy, the therapist has often to find out which part of this chain is broken, e.g. the route taken by the nerve impulses to activate the facial nerve (*see* CRANIAL NERVE VII) and muscles of the tongue is interrupted as in DYSARTHRIA. It could also be that the person has difficulty in formulating an utterance either by not finding the required word to use or not being able to put the words in the correct order, as in APHASIA, or it may be the feedback system which does not function, as with a HEARING LOSS. When this broken link is found by ASSESSMENT, a TREATMENT PROGRAMME can begin to repair it. *See* Denes and Pinson (1973).

speech discrimination test a test used in SPEECH AUDIOMETRY for assessing the person's ability to understand speech at levels above the threshold of hearing. Usually lists of ten words are presented to the person. The words have been phonetically balanced. One list is presented at ±30 dB above SPEECH RECEPTION THRESHOLD. Correct repetitions are scored as percentages. The next list is presented at 10 dB higher followed by another list at 10 dB higher than the previous list. The curve of discrimination scores is shown on a graph. *See* Hood (1981).

speech pathology

(1) The title used for speech and language therapy in the US and Canada.
(2) The study of disordered communication.

speech reception threshold (SRT) the level in dB, at which 50 per cent of bisyllabic words are repeated accurately. Three words are presented at a level of ±25 dB above PTA. The person repeats the words and then the test level descends in 5 dB steps until the person fails to repeat one or more words. This is followed by six words at each level. The SRT is the level at which three or four words out of six are repeated correctly. *See* Hood (1981).

speech synthesis the production of speech by use of a microprocessor to simulate the human voice. It is also called voice synthesis. The quality of the speech output depends on the cost of the synthesiser used. During 1989 and 1990, researchers at the Microcomputer Centre at Dundee University were trying to develop a speech synthesiser to produce emotion in speech. Thus, if the operator produces the statement on the computer 'I am happy', the speech output will sound happy and a similar outcome will happen for other emotions such as 'sadness', 'doubting', etc. The software which allows this to happen is known as HAMLET (Helpful Automatic Machine for Language and Emotional Talk). At the present time, DECTALK is regarded as being the best speech synthesis available and is being used with many voice output communication aids. *See* Bishop (1985); Edwards (1990); Keller (1994).

SpeechPAC a high-tech communication aid with a QWERTY keyboard, a small internal printer, a mini cassette drive, LCD display screen and an internal speech synthesiser. It can be programmed to store hundreds of messages which can be transferred for speech output by depressing the 'talk' key. The SpeechPac uses a specialised programming language 'Lolec'. Using this software, the user can program and retrieve complete sentences up to 250 characters long. It operates on the hypothesis that each programmed sentence will be a logical thought which will be programmed by a logical letter code. For example, if the users wish to give the message 'I want a cup of tea', they will program the keys 'C' (cup), and 'T' (tea) to 'speak' the given sentence. When 'CT' is followed by actuating the 'talk' key, the voice output will give the complete sentence. The memory can hold 17 000 characters. It is operated with rechargeable batteries and can be accessed by various input systems as well as with an expanded membrane board and it can be mounted on wheelchairs.

spina bifida a congenital abnormality of the SPINAL CORD. The most common condition is spina bifida occulta. It occurs between the lumbar vertebrae and the sacral vertebrae. There is a failure in the fusion of the vertebral arch and an abnormality in the overlying skin. Twenty per cent of children with a closed lesion have normal intelligence and no physical handicaps. HYDROCEPHALUS commonly develops in children with spina bifida. According to recent research, children with spina bifida form the largest subgroup of the hydrocephalic population. In the USA, research was undertaken to find out if there were language problems in this group. It had been thought, that these children had an inability to produce utterances that met basic semantic-pragmatic requirements. This problem had been found to take several forms:

1. Production of numerous utterances of the topic or task in hand.
2. Utterances are often over-personalised.

201

3. Production of automatic social phrases such as 'thank you' and 'how are you' at an abnormally high rate and inappropriately.
4. Often imitate words and phrases of others rather than answer questions or otherwise contribute to the discussion.
5. Utterances are often semantically anomalous or bizarre. There were also thought to be problems in comprehension as well as expressive language.

Syntax was at the age-appropriate level although there were semantic-pragmatic problems. The conclusions of the study showed that, although children with spina bifida hydrocephalus may have some language difficulties, those who are intellectually normal do not have such problems – at least in the semantic-pragmatic domain. The authors propose it may be the degree of associated LEARNING DISABILITY that will account for linguistic difficulties. *See* Hosking (1982); Byrne et al (1990).

spinal cord a cylinder-like structure which is situated in the canal of the vertebral column. It is about 45 cm long and about 1 cm wide. It extends up the magnum foramen to the MEDULLA OBLONGATA. At the end of the spinal cord is the causa equina (a collection of lumbosacral roots); in the middle of these roots is the filum terminale which attaches to the coccyx. There are two enlargements which enervate the limbs:

1. Cervical enlargement supplies the upper limbs.
2. Lumbosacral enlargement supplies the lower limbs.

It is composed of grey and white matter. *See* Barr (1979); Tortora and Grabowski (1993).

Splink an early high-tech communication aid, comprising a small electronic word board which has 950 basic words, letters, numerals, common phrases and various prefixes/suffixes plus instructions. It can fit onto the person's knee and transmits a signal by infra-red to a microprocessor box which is plugged into the aerial socket of an ordinary TV set. Thus, the words appear on the screen. There are no wires but the person must keep within 12–15 feet of the TV set. Two or more word boards can be used with a single microprocessor so that Splink can be used with groups. Splink is an acronym for 'Speech Link'. *See* Code and Müller (1989).

split screen the process by which information can be output on screen from two separate computer programs but which can appear together on the same screen.

spontaneous recovery spontaneous recovery occurs without the intervention of professional skills. It can occur during the first 2–6 months following the onset of a disorder such as APHASIA, but some people may not go through spontaneous recovery. *See* Eisenson (1984).

spontaneous speech a description of language which a person produces every day. It is opposed to elicited language (*see* ELICITATION) or speech where the therapist is trying to get the person to say particular words or phrases. A language assessment, whether it is formal or informal, should always include a subtest from which an analysis could be made of the person's spontaneous speech.

spread an aspect of lip movement when producing vowels such as [i,e,ɛ,a] found in the primary CARDINAL VOWEL SYSTEM. It is opposed to lip rounding. *See* Ladefoged (1993).

spreadsheet a piece of software which can be used for a particular purpose, e.g. producing annual accounts, keeping running totals for budgets. It can SCROLL both horizontally and vertically if there is not enough space on the screen to take the full spreadsheet. The computer carries out calculations when certain formulae are used. These formulae may vary according to the particular spreadsheet being used. *See* Bishop (1985).

SRT *see* SPEECH RECEPTION THRESHOLD.

stammer a disorder of fluency which appears to have a multifactorial aetiology. Consequently there are many theories of intervention. Chief among putative causes are: (1) organic factors such as minimal brain damage; a forced change in CEREBRAL DOMINANCE; heredity or IQ level; (2) neurotic causes in the form of emotional predisposition; a compulsive neurosis; CONVERSION REACTION or learnt behaviour. This last proposition makes use of CLASSICAL CONDITIONING and OPERANT CONDITIONING. Avoidance reaction is another psychological cause which has been proposed. However, nowadays it is argued that stammering could be caused by a combination of some of these factors. Treatment techniques fall into two main theories – SPEAK MORE FLUENTLY and STAMMER MORE FLUENTLY. *See* Dalton (1983).

stammer more fluently a treatment approach used with those who have a STAMMER. It takes into account the underlying psychological symptoms which may affect the stammerer. One of the major therapeutic techniques used is van Riper's BLOCK MODIFICATION. This approach is also known as stutter more fluently. *See* Dalton (1983).

standard deviation a process in DESCRIPTIVE STATISTICS used for finding out how far from the mean (*see* CENTRAL TENDENCY) in a NORMAL DISTRIBUTION a person's score is. The standard deviation is worked out as the square root of the variance of the dispersion of scores. *See* Miller (1975).

standard score a score obtained in various assessments from the RAW SCORE. It

is based on the STANDARD DEVIATION. *See* Atkinson et al (1993).

Standard Theory an early form of TRANSFORMATIONAL GRAMMAR (TG) proposed by Chomsky (1965) (*see* CHOMSKYAN LINGUISTICS). In it he proposed a deep structure from which, by a series of transformations, a surface structure would appear. It is the surface structure which is spoken or written. *See* Chomsky (1965); Huddleston (1976).

standardisation *see* STANDARDISED TESTS.

standardised tests to standardise a test it must be given to a large number of the population covering the age range for which it is intended to be used. In this way, the tester can discover the most frequent or normal responses of the different age groups, and thence be enabled to compare the scores obtained from those with a particular disorder with those of the norm for the age groups. In some tests, the mental age and resulting IQ can also be calculated.

Stanford-Binet Intelligence Scales assessments to test children's intelligence levels. Binet published his first test in 1905 with the help of Theodore Simon (1873–1961), a French psychologist. These tests became known thoroughout the world and translations into English followed. The scale, which became widely used, had been translated and adapted by Lewis Terman of Stanford University. Terman introduced the INTELLIGENCE QUOTIENT to the scales, while Stern, a German psychologist, proposed the IQ scale. There have been three editions subsequently since 1916. The latest edition (4th edition) was published in 1985. Its age range is similar to that of the other editions – 2 years to adulthood. It tests four areas:

1. Cognitive ability.

2. Verbal reasoning.

3. Quantitative reasoning.

4. Abstract/visual reasoning and short-term memory.

The scale comprises fifteen subtests: vocabulary, comprehension, verbal relations, pattern analysis, matrices, paper folding and cutting, copying, quantities, number series, equation building, memory for digits, sentences, objects and beads. *See* Aiken (1985).

stapedectomy the removal of the stapes (*see* EAR) by surgery. *See* Pracy et al (1974).

stapedius reflex *see* IMPEDANCE BATTERY.

stapes *see* EAR.

Starset software which allows the operator to produce or adapt computer programs for use with the concept keyboard.

statementing following the 1981 Education Act, Education Authorities have a statutory obligation to see that SPECIAL EDUCATION is provided for all those children in need. To this end a multidisciplinary asssessment is carried out and a written statement of advice is given. This formal statement is reviewed annually. Children with language impairment are included in this process.

static impedance *see* IMPEDANCE BATTERY.

static memory *see* RANDOM ACCESS MEMORY.

statistics a study which makes theories into realities. Psychology is often said to be common sense, but the use of science makes it into a science. There are two main types of statistics – INFERENTIAL STATISTICS and DESCRIPTIVE STATISTICS. In the former, measures of CENTRAL TENDENCY and dispersion are used, while in the latter parametric and non-parametric tests (*see* PARAMETRIC TESTS) are used to analyse the score obtained from experiments. *See* Miller (1975).

status epilepticus *see* EPILEPSY.

sternocleidomastoid muscle a muscle in the neck which runs from behind

the EAR to the clavicle. *See* Tortora and Grabowski (1993).

sternohyoid muscle *see* LARYNX.

stirrup *see* EAR.

stoma a hole left in the neck after LARYNGECTOMY or TRACHEOTOMY. It is used for breathing. If a person collapses who has this operation, mouth-to-mouth resucitation will not help, he will have to be given mouth-to-stoma resuscitation. People who have undergone this operation can produce OESOPHAGEAL VOICE by occluding the stoma. *See* Edels (1983).

stop a description of a sound which is produced by a complete blocking of the air in the mouth. Thus, stops can be used to classify plosives (*see* ARTICULATION). *See* Ladefoged (1993).

stress

(1) *See* SUPRASEGMENTAL PHONOLOGY.

(2) *See* HYSTERIA.

striated muscle this type of muscle is also known as skeletal muscle. It is innervated by the somatic nervous system. *See* Leeson et al (1985); Tortora and Grabowski (1993).

strident a DISTINCTIVE FEATURE proposed by Chomsky and Halle to distinguish sounds produced with high frequency and intensity (*see* ACOUSTIC PHONETICS) as in [f,s,ʃ,ʒ] [+STRIDENT] from those produced with low frequency and intensity [−STRIDENT]. It is opposed to non-strident. *See* Hyman (1975).

string a set of characters or digits used in a computer program. *See* Bishop (1985).

stroke the layman's term for CEREBROVASCULAR ACCIDENT (CVA).

structural brain disease a possible cause of EPILEPSY. Almost any disease of the BRAIN which produces a focus for discharging neurons will cause epileptic convulsions. The disease could be due to a TUMOUR OF THE CENTRAL NERVOUS SYSTEM, a BRAIN ABSCESS or degenerative disorders causing degeneration of neurons, etc. *See* Draper (1980).

structured programming a method of designing a program which breaks the task down into functional units or modules and builds the program from these modules. This is also called top-down programming.

Sturge-Weber syndrome its main characteristics are a port-wine naevus on the scalp, and other vascular abnormalities both intracranially and elsewhere in the body. These may produce LEARNING DISABILITY (about 30 per cent), HEMIPLEGIA (about 30–40 per cent) and EPILEPSY (about 90 per cent). *See* Salmon (1978).

stutter *see* STAMMER.

Stuttering Prediction Instrument for Young Children devised by Riley, the instrument is designed to let clinicians determine the severity and potential chronicity of childhood dysfluency and can be used with children between 3 and 11 years of age. There are five sections including the history of the child; the child's, parents' and others' reactions to the child stammer; part-word repetitions; prolongations and the frequency of the stammer. *See* Beech et al (1993).

Stuttering Severity Instrument for Children and Adults devised by Riley, the instrument is a STANDARDISED assessment of the quantity and quality of the dysfluency and can be used with either children or adults. It measures three parameters:

1. frequency of repetition, prolongation of sounds and syllables;
2. estimated duration of the longest blocks;
3. observable physical concomitants.

The scores from these categories give a RAW SCORE, and the total is converted into a PERCENTILE SCORE and severity rating. The tape records speech samples

for analysis and the therapist notes any EXTRANEOUS MOVEMENTS rating them from 0 (none) to 5 (severe and painful). *See* Beech et al (1993).

stuttering stages a description, proposed by van Riper, of the sequences found in stammerers as their dysfluency progresses:

1. Primary stuttering stage: easy repetitions of words, syllables of a sentence without emotion or stress.
2. Secondary stuttering stage: the person becomes more conscious of his DYSFLUENCY and begins to anticipate the situation in which the person will stammer.
3. Transitional stuttering stage: occurs between the primary and secondary stages in which emotions accompany the easy repetitions of the primary stuttering stage.

See Dalton and Hardcastle (1989).

Stycar Hearing Test devised by Sheridan to be used with children between the ages of 6 months and 7 years. It uses very simple and familiar objects, words and pictures. Its aim is to test the child's ability to hear meaningful speech with different frequency and intensity components. The test contains several different subtests for different age groups. These subtests take the form of toy tests, cube tests, doll vocabulary, picture vocabulary, word lists and sentences. Thus, the tester can identify sounds which are producing difficulties for the child. *See* Sheridan (1973) in Appendix I.

Stycar Language Test devised by Sheridan to assess the normal development of children concerning comprehension, expression and use of language forms such as mime, models, picture and especially spoken-verbal language. It can be used with 'normal' children (1–7 years) and older children with developmental delay. It uses real objects, toys and pictures and the child's performance is recorded descriptively. The clinician makes a detailed observation of the child's ability to use 'language codes' such as verbal, gestural and two-dimensional as well as other symbolic activity such as play and other aspects of development such as physical manipulation. There are three tests: Common Objects Test, Miniature Toy Test and Picture Book Test. *See* Sheridan (1976) in Appendix I; Beech et al (1993).

Stycar Tests devised by Sheridan in 1973, this is a series of assessments plotting normal development from birth to 5;0 years. Four parameters of development are examined: motor, vision, hearing and speech, and social and play development.

styloglossus muscle *see* EXTRINSIC MUSCLES OF THE TONGUE.

stylohyoid muscle *see* MUSCLES FOR SWALLOWING.

styloid process a projection found in the skull which extends down and forward from the temporal bone and measures 2 cm long and 3 mm wide. It is the attachment point for muscles and ligaments which are marked by using stylo- as a prefix to their complete name. *See* Tortora and Grabowski (1993).

stylopharyngeus muscle *see* MUSCLES FOR SWALLOWING.

subarachnoid space this is the space which contains the CEREBROSPINAL FLUID and is enclosed by the arachnoid membrane. Berry aneurysms (*see* CEREBROVASCULAR ACCIDENT) cause bleeding into the subarachnoid space. *See* Barr (1979).

subglottic a description of the position of all structures or lesions below the GLOTTIS. It is opposed to supraglottic.

sublingual salivary gland *see* SALIVARY GLANDS.

submandibular salivary gland *see* SALIVARY GLANDS.

submucous cleft palate *see* CLEFT PALATE.

subroutine part of a computer program in which specific functions take place which do not occur in the main program. It is a subsection or submodule of the whole program. *See* White (1985); Bishop (1985).

suction a DISTINCTIVE FEATURE proposed by Chomsky and Halle to describe sounds made in a specific way by the GLOTTIS and velum such as implosives and clicks (*see* VELARIC AIRSTREAM) [+SUCTION]. *See* Hyman (1975).

suffix MORPHOLOGY identifies separate units which are used in the formation of words. Those that occur at the ends of words are referred to as suffixes, e.g. '-ness' in 'happiness', '-er' in 'robber', '-s' in 'hats', etc. *See* Matthews (1974).

sulcus in the BRAIN, a sulcus appears as a groove surrounded by elevated areas called gyri (*see* GYRUS). *See* Barr (1979).

sulcus terminalis *see* TONGUE.

superego *see* PERSONALITY.

superior constrictor muscle *see* PHARYNX.

supplementary movements a classification for DISTINCTIVE FEATURES proposed by Chomsky and Halle. They are used to distinguish manner of articulation (*see* ARTICULATION). The two distinctive features subsumed by this term are SUCTION and PRESSURE which describe such sounds as EJECTIVES, IMPLOSIVES and clicks. *See* Hyman (1975).

suppurative otitis media *see* OTITIS MEDIA.

supraglottic a description of the position of the structures or lesions found above the GLOTTIS. It is opposed to subglottic.

suprasegmental phonology the study of stress and intonation. Stress often marks the difference between verbs and nouns, e.g. re'cord/'record; (') is the diacritic used to mark stress. A speaker's intonation contours are usually described in terms of pitch direction, e.g. fall–rise. The pitch range could be higher or lower than the average range or widened or narrowed until it becomes a monotone. A tone group is the part of the sentence which contains changes in pitch. In the tone group, there is normally one single syllable which receives a major pitch change – the tonic syllable or nuclear syllable. The direction change of the tonic syllable, also known as the nucleus, is most important in understanding speech since it usually gives information concerning attitudes of the speaker:

`yes (falling)	–	the answer is 'yes'
´yes (high-rise)	–	did you say 'yes'
‚yes (low-rise)	–	please go on I'm listening
ˇyes (fall-rise)	–	I'm doubtful
^yes (rise-fall)	–	I'm certain
		(based on Ladefoged).

Thus, a person can show by changing their way of producing the tonic syllable the meaning of what they say. Some people who have DYSARTHRIA have lost the distinctions used in stress and intonation patterns and so cannot make changes to meaning as exemplified above. *See* Fromkin and Rodman (1993); Ladefoged (1993).

surface structure *see* TRANSFORMATIONAL GRAMMAR.

swallowing the transfer of the food bolus from the MOUTH to the stomach avoiding the airway, i.e. the TRACHEA. It is also known as the process of deglutition. The bolus goes through stages before it reaches the stomach after it is prepared by the saliva from the SALIVARY GLANDS:

1. Oral stage: the food is chewed in the mouth and prepared into a bolus. It is transferred to the back of the mouth by the tip of the tongue being raised towards the alveolar ridge. As the tongue contracts, the bolus is moved near the PHARYNX. This is a wholly voluntary process.

2. Pharyngeal stage: the bolus leaves the mouth and enters the oropharynx (*see* PHARYNX), the muscles of which are stimulated from the MEDULLA OBLONGATA via the glossopharyngeal nerve (*see* CRANIAL NERVES). The bolus could leave this area by four potential routes - the mouth, nasoph-arynx (*see* PHARYNX), LARYNX/TRACHEA or OESOPHA-GUS but muscle contraction closes off all the exits except the one to the oesophagus.

3. Oesophageal stage: the bolus reaches the top of the oesophagus. As it is a flat tube, the bolus has to wait for the muscle at the top to relax and produce a contraction to push the bolus into it. The bolus is propelled down the oesophagus by a series of peristaltic waves. When the bolus reaches the lower end of the oesophagus, there is a sphincter into the stomach which the last peristaltic contraction opens to allow the bolus to enter into the stomach.

See Tortora and Grabowski (1993).

sweep testing *see* SCREENING AUDIOMETRY.

switches most high-tech communication aids and specially designed computer software can be operated by various kinds of switches for those who cannot operate the communication aid or computer by the keyboard. Particular companies which produce communication aids often produce switches designed for their own aids. However, nearly all the switches produced are similar in their function. The most common switches used are:

1. Plate switch: by touching a rocking plate the aid can be operated. In some models, it may be a double switch so that the person can operate the device in two ways.

2. Foot switch: for gross foot movement.
3. Joystick: allows for scanning up/down, side to side and diagonally, or any combination of these. There are 4-way and 8-way joysticks.
4. Wobblesticks: can be hit in any direction to operate the scanning. Used with those who have gross uncontrollable movements.
5. Head-operated: either microswitches can be placed on a neck halter so that the person can operate them with the chin, or a switch can be attached to the back of the chair and can be operated by head movement.
6. Flexitube switch: operated by the person sucking or blowing down the tube.

It is important that the therapist carries out a good motor assessment, so that the appropriate switch can be chosen to help the person use the communication aid or computer. *See* Enderby (1987); Beukelman and Mirenda (1992).

syllable a unit of a word. Each unit can be pronounced as a single unit as in 'picture'. A syllable has been described in different ways. One way of describing it is as an increase in the pressure in the speaker's lungs and as being more sonorous than other parts of the word. In PHONOLOGY, the syllable is described in terms of PHONOTACTICS. *See* Fromkin and Rodman (1993); Ladefoged (1993).

Symbolic Play Test devised by Lowe and Costello in 1976 (revised 2nd edition 1988), it is an observational assessment for very young children and provides information about symbolic and conceptual development. It takes the form of a collection of small toys with which the child plays. The level of play is assessed against a checklist. There is practically no verbal requirement on the part of either the assessor or the child. *See* Lowe and Costello (1988) in Appendix I; Lewis et al (1992); Beech et al (1993).

symbolisation *see* SENSORIMOTOR STAGE.

sympathetic nervous system becomes highly active when the person becomes very excited. Thus, it is often known as the 'fight, fright, flight' system. The chemical transmitted to the muscle is noradrenaline. As part of the AUTONOMIC NERVOUS SYSTEM (ANS), it innervates SMOOTH MUSCLE. *See* J.H.Green (1978); Tortora and Grabowski (1993).

symphysis menti *see* MANDIBLE.

synapse a junction between two nerves where there is a transfer of nerve impulses by the emission of chemicals from one to another. *See* J.H.Green (1978).

synchronic linguistics *see* SAUSSURE.

syndrome a grouping of several characteristic clinical features common to a particular disease or condition. *See* Tortora and Grabowski (1993).

syntactic-pragmatic syndrome a rare disorder in which there is gross impairment of syntax and severely restricted pragmatic use of language. Comprehension is also limited. Phonology may be normal or near normal.

syntagmatic relations the linear description of sentences. Rules define the order in which elements occur. *See* Lyons (1968).

syntax grammar is sometimes subdivided into MORPHOLOGY, the study of the formation of words, and syntax, the study of the formation of sentences. Within this very general definition, there are a variety of approaches in the modern era to the characterisation of the structure of sentences. *See also* GENERATIVE GRAMMAR and CASE GRAMMAR. *See* Lyons (1968); Stockwell (1977); Fromkin and Rodman (1993).

systematic desensitisation a BEHAVIOUR THERAPY based on CLASSICAL CONDITIONING. It has as its aim the gradual reduction of a learned anxiety. The client tells the therapist what is causing the anxiety. He is relaxed and asked to rate his fear on a fear thermometer. Thus, the therapist can construct an anxiety hierarchy. As the client continues to relax he is asked to imagine the least feared stimulus and after it has been overcome due to the relaxation, the next most feared stimulus is treated similarly and so on. However, it is uncertain for how long fears can be extinguished using this procedure. *See* Atkinson et al (1993).

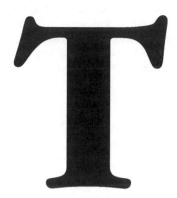

t-groups a therapeutic technique used in the sensitivity training approach to social skill training. In these groups, the clients make their own decisions as the therapist takes a backseat. They have to make up their minds who is going to be a group leader and what their feelings for each other are, while some may fail to participate completely. If necessary, the therapist will show them how to express such feelings for each other and their reactions to each other, and will encourage openness. The clients themselves may provide a model. *See* Trower et al (1978).

t-tests there are two types of *t*-tests depending on whether a parametric or a non-parametric test (*see* PARAMETRIC TESTS) is used. If the former is being used with an INDEPENDENT GROUP DESIGN, the independent *t*-test will be used, while if the latter is being used with a REPEATED MEASURE DESIGN, the related *t*-test is used. As with other tests, degrees of freedom are used so the experimenter can find out how many scores can vary; this is usually $n-1$ with n being the mean. *See* Miller (1975).

tabulation the movement of a typewriter carriage or cursor on a word-processor to predetermined positions. This is often abbreviated to tab, which marks the key on a keyboard which is used for this operation.

TACL *see* TEST FOR AUDITORY COMPREHENSION OF LANGUAGE.

tactile a description of the action of touching an object. *See* Tortora and Grabowski (1993).

tag question a structure with interrogative form which is placed at the end of an utterance and has a particular discourse function:

1. It's raining, isn't it?
2. She isn't coming, is she?

Generally, the tag question in English (other languges, e.g. French, with an unchanging structure, *n'est-ce pas*, provide a simpler form) is a subject pronoun which matches the number and gender of the subject noun phrase of the sentence to which it is attached. It also generally repeats the auxiliary verb of the main sentence but has reverse polarity to the main sentence (though there are exceptions to both these statements). The tag has a conversational function in seeking or encouraging a response by one's conversational partner. The type of response depends on the intonation of the tag. *See* Brown and Miller (1991).

talking brooch a very early high-tech communication aid designed by Alan Newell at Southampton University in 1974. It comprised a display contained in a lapel brooch, a keyboard and a control box. The message was typed out on the keyboard and appeared on the display. The message ran from right to left across the display. *See* Enderby (1987).

Talking Lifestyles devised by Whitton and Zloch, a vocabulary package for the ORAC communication aid. It is designed to give users a vocabulary to suit their needs. The overlay is divided into three areas for grammatical parts of speech, the symbols where the majority of the vocabulary is stored and alternate keys which produce opposites etc. There are over 20 000 pre-stored words, phrases and messages on a 128-overlay. *See* Whitton and Zloch (1995).

Talking Notebook a high-tech communication aid with a QWERTY keyboard and facility for speech synthesis. It can store information in a memory for over 3 weeks, even if the batteries fail or the machine is switched off. It is a complete word processor contained in a lightweight portable computer with an eight-line, 40-character display. It also has a facility for quickly recalling frequently used phrases. To obtain hardcopy, a printer can be attached.

Talking Scratchpad the talking notebook becomes a communication aid as the machine 'speaks' each word as it is typed and will repeat the whole phrase or sentence on command.

Talking Screen a DYNAMIC DISPLAY application with symbols. It is possible to create pages from 1 symbol up to 128 symbols. It can be used with IBM PC computers using DOS or WINDOWS. It uses Mayer-Johnson symbols as well as scanned-in photographs and images from CD-ROMs. It uses the DECtalk speech synthesis system as well as allowing for recorded speech and sound and an environmental control. It also can cope with Multimedia. *See* Appendix IV.

tamber *see* TIMBRE.

target a description of the correct production of a sound. It is opposed to REALISATION.

taste the tongue is the organ in the body which is responsible for the sense of taste. For this purpose, it is divided into the following parts:

1. The anterior two-thirds of the tongue detects a bitter taste and is innervated by cranial nerve VII (*see* CRANIAL NERVES).
2. The posterior one-third of the tongue detects a salt/sweet taste and is innervated by cranial nerve IX (*see* CRANIAL NERVES).
3. The anterior two-thirds of the tongue (except the taste buds) are supplied by the chorda tympani nerve, a branch of cranial nerve VII (*see* CRANIAL NERVES).

See J.H.Green (1978); Atkinson et al (1993); Tortora and Grabowski (1993).

taste buds these produce the sensation of taste and are found in the papillae which cover the anterior two-thirds of the tongue. There are three types of papillae:

1. Circumvallate papillae: mushroom-shaped and surrounded by a ditch or moat in which are found rows of taste buds (8–12 in a row) in front of the sulcus terminalis.
2. Fungiform papillae: little puff-like balls with a moat around them in which are found more taste buds.
3. Filiform papillae: small, conical-shaped lumps which contain no taste buds.

The taste buds are supplied by cranial nerve IX (*see* CRANIAL NERVES). *See* Tortora and Grabowski (1993).

teacher's nodes/nodules *see* VOCAL NODULES.

Teaching Talking devised by Locke and Beech in 1992, Teaching Talking allows for structured screening and intervention programmes to help teachers in mainstream nursery, infant and junior schools. It is suitable to be used with children between the ages of 3 and 11 years. *See* Locke and Beech (1992) in Appendix I.

teeth bone-like excrescences developing out of the jaw. Their function is to chew food and grind it down into smaller pieces for digestion. Each person has 32 teeth, 8 incisors, 4 canines, 8 premolars and 12 molars. *See* Tortora and Grabowski (1993).

Teflon injection a method whereby Teflon is injected in a paralysed vocal fold to provide an increase in mass and thus facilitate approximation with the normally functioning vocal fold. It is used in the treatment of LARYNGEAL NERVE PALSIES. *See* Fawcus (1991).

Teletext in the UK, there are two teletext systems in use – Ceefax (BBC) and Teletext (ITV and Channel 4). Television produces picture images on lines but some lines are not used for producing such images. It is these spare lines which the television uses to produce the text when switched to teletext mode. These systems can also be used with a computer if a suitable converter is purchased. It is possible to store teletext information on disk or print it out by this means. *See* Bishop (1985).

tempo *see* RATE.

temporal lobe *see* CEREBRAL HEMISPHERES.

temporalis muscle *see* MUSCLES OF MASTICATION.

temporary tracheostomy *see* TRACHEOTOMY.

temporomandibular joint a joint between the temporal and mandibular bones. It allows the jaw to open and close.

temporomandibular joint syndrome the failure of the joint to allow the jaw to open and close which leads to difficulty in chewing (*see* MUSCLES OF MASTICATION). There may be other characteristics to the syndrome affecting the person's hearing as well as causing discomfort in the muscles and a clicking of the joint. *See* Tortora and Grabowski (1993).

tensor veli palatini muscle the muscle which operates the soft palate (*see* MOUTH) and is shaped like a triangle as it starts from the skull and runs along the eustachian tube (*see* EAR). It has its apex at the pterygoid hamulus. Its nerve supply comes from cranial nerve Viii (*see* CRANIAL NERVES). Its functions are to open the auditory tube and, on contraction, to tense the soft palate (*see* MOUTH). *See* Edwards and Watson (1980).

terminal data can be fed to or taken from these machines. Thus, a monitor is often thought of as a terminal, as is a computer which is connected to a host computer. *See* Bishop (1985).

Test for Auditory Comprehension of Language (TACL) devised by Carrow-Woolfolk in 1976 (revised, 1985), it is an assessment which has been standardised to test the child's auditory verbal understanding of semantic, syntactic and morphological structures. It takes the form of line drawings and involves the selection of one out of four in response to an auditory stimulus. It covers an age range of 3;0–10;0 years. Raw scores can be converted into STANDARD SCORES, AGE-EQUIVALENT SCORES or PERCENTILES. It is standardised on a North American population. A Spanish version is also available. *See* Carrow-Woolfolk (1985) in Appendix I; Beech et al (1993).

Test for Reception of Grammar (TROG) devised by Bishop in 1984, it is a formal, standardised assessment to test children's auditory verbal comprehension. However, it can be used to gain a more in-depth analysis of an aphasic person's auditory verbal comprehension, although it has not been standardised for this population. The material consists of 80 line drawings which are divided into four blocks of 20, each containing four test sentences of increasing syntactic complexity. All four items in each section must be correct before proceeding to the next level. Scoring is either according to AGE-EQUIVALENT SCORES or PERCENTILES when used with children. *See* Bishop (1984); Beech et al (1993).

Test of Word Finding devised by German in 1986, it assesses children aged 6;0–12;0 years who have a lexical retrieval deficit. It comprises four different types of naming task. Results are based on accuracy and speed of response. Scores are computed as STANDARD SCORES and PERCENTILES. It is standardised on a North American population. *See* German (1986); Beech et al (1993).

TG *see* TRANSFORMATIONAL GRAMMAR.

thalamus a large part of the DIENCEPHALON which measures about 3 cm. It comprises two oval shaped pieces of grey matter and it forms the side of the THIRD VENTRICLE. Each piece can be found deep in the CEREBRAL HEMISPHERES above the MIDBRAIN. Various nuclei can be found within it, e.g. those for hearing, vision and general sensation plus taste. Some of the other nuclei act as synapses controlling voluntary motor actions and arousal. It acts also on information from the senses such as temperature, touch and pressure. *See* Barr (1979); Tortora and Grabowski (1993).

theoretical linguistics a term used to contrast particularly with applied linguistics. Some linguists would disavow the possibility of a distinction. *See* Lyons (1968).

thermal paper special paper which can be used with dot-matrix printers. The paper has a special coating which is removed by the electric current from the styluses on the printing head to produce the required characters.

third ventricle it is divided by the THALAMUS and between the lateral ventricles which are linked to the third ventricle by the interventricular foramen. The CEREBROSPINAL FLUID flows into the third ventricle from its initial starting point in the lateral ventricles and before it enters the FOURTH VENTRICLE from where it passes around the rest of the BRAIN. *See* Barr (1979); Tortora and Grabowski (1993).

thoracic respiration *see* CLAVICULAR.

thought disorder a symptom of SCHIZOPHRENIA. There are two different kinds of thought disorder – form and content. The former consists of:

1. Incoherence in conversation.
2. Neologisms.
3. Loose associations: while the person communicates successfully with the listener, he has difficulty sticking to the one topic.
4. Clang association: the words used are put in a certain order because of their rhyme rather than their syntax.
5. Poverty of speech: either the amount of discourse is increased or it conveys little information.
6. Perseveration.
7. Blocking.

The latter consists of:

1. Delusions.
2. Delusional percept: a normal perception which has a special meaning for the person and an often delusional system develops quickly.
3. Somatic passivity: inability to rouse the person by outside forces operating on his body.
4. Thought insertion: thoughts, different from those of the person, are placed in the person's mind from an outside agent.
5. Thought withdrawal: the person believes their thoughts are being removed from their mind without warning.
6. Thought broadcast: the person believes their thoughts are being transmitted to others.
7. 'Made' feeling.
8. 'Made' volitional acts.
9. 'Made' impulses.

See Davison and Neale (1994).

thyrohyoid muscle *see* LARYNX.

thyroid cartilage *see* LARYNX.

thyroid gland *see* TRACHEA.

TIAs *see* TRANSIENT ISCHAEMIC ATTACKS.

tic repeated jerky movements usually of the face or neck. GILLES DE LA TOURETTE

SYNDROME is a grouping together of symptoms, one of which is meaningless grunting. *See* Stafford-Clark and Smith (1983); Tortora and Grabowski (1993).

tidal volume the amount of air taken into the LUNGS when breathing normally. *See* RESERVE VOLUME. *See* Tortora and Grabowski (1993).

timbre the ability on the part of the listener to distinguish different characteristics of sound even if the loudness, pitch and length (*see* AUDITORY PHONETICS) are the same. It is often referred to as QUALITY or tamber. *See* Abercrombie (1967).

timing the process of moving the articulators into the correct sequences for producing sounds and making them into words. This can produce important features in rhythm (*see* PROSODY) and other prosodic features. *See* Clark and Clark (1977).

tinnitus a condition which is found in any type of HEARING LOSS and in normal hearing. The person will often complain of rushing, roaring, ringing noises in the ear. It is a very annoying condition and there is no real treatment for it although it is possible to help the person with a tinnitus masker, HEARING AIDS as well as COUNSELLING. The tinnitus masker is placed behind the ear to control the amount of tinnitus experienced by the patient. In many cases, the sound can only be heard by the person, but with certain types of tinnitus, other people can hear it. *See* Katz (1985).

tinnitus masker *see* TINNITUS.

toggle function key a key which can switch between one of two functions.

token economy a behaviour therapy technique based on OPERANT CONDITIONING. Basically, people will receive a reward if they overcome the anxiety-provoking situation. The tokens which are given are intended to act as sufficient reinforcers to reduce the aberrant behaviour and promote the behaviour of the norm. *See* Kazdin (1981).

Token Test devised by DeRenzi and

Vignolo in 1962, it is a formal assessment to test the auditory comprehension of those with APHASIA. The test material comprises 20 tokens which differ in size, shape and colour. The original token test was divided into five parts; the first four used auditory commands of increasing length while the fifth contained commands of increasing grammatical complexity. DeRenzi and Faglioni reported their use of a shortened form of the Token Test where 36 graded commands are presented in six sections. The Revised Token Test devised by McNeil and Prescott in 1978 gives more control over the syntactic variables, and performance can be plotted graphically to reveal variance in performance patterns across subtests. The Short Token Test was devised by Spellacy and Spreen in 1969. *See* DeRenzi and Vignolo (1962) in Appendix I; DeRenzi and Faglioni (1978) in Appendix I; McNeil and Prescott (1978) in Appendix I; Johns (1981); Rosenbek et al (1989).

Token Test for Children devised by DiSimoni, it is a test of children's comprehension and is based on the TOKEN TEST. It can be used with children between the ages of 3;0 and 12;6 years of age. Various objects (usually shapes of different colours), are placed in a standardised manner. Spoken commands are given to the child to manipulate the objects. The commands become progressively longer and more complex. It is a rapid screening test which may indicate further testing of the lexicon and syntax is required. *See* DiSimoni (1978) in Appendix I; Beech et al (1993).

tone *see* SUPRASEGMENTAL PHONOLOGY.

tone decay there are two main types of tone decay depending at what point it is measured:

1. Threshold tone decay is measured at or near threshold. It is a decrease in threshold sensitivity resulting from the presence of a barely audible sound.

2. Suprathreshold tone decay is measured well above threshold. It is a loss of audibility as a result of a stimulating tone which is present at a high presentation level.

A differential diagnosis can be made between retrocochlear and other lesions depending on whether a significant tone decay is present or absent. Both BÉKÉSY AUDIOMETRY and PURE-TONE AUDIOMETRY have been used to test for tone decay. However, pure-tone audiometry is usually used to detect tone decay. The quantity of tone decay, measured in dB, is the difference between the initial threshold and the threshold at which the test is ended. There are several different procedures which have been proposed which makes classification and comparing test results between people difficult. *See* Katz (1985).

tone group *see* SUPRASEGMENTAL PHONOLOGY.

tongue the floor of the mouth is formed by the tongue, which when lifted is held down by the MUCOUS MEMBRANE – the lingual frenulum. On either side of the frenulum are two papillae or bumps on top of which is the opening of the sub-mandibular SALIVARY GLANDS, while below the tongue there are two swellings which are called sublingual salivary glands (*see* SALIVARY GLANDS). The tongue can be divided into two parts and the line where the division occurs is the sulcus terminalis, i.e. the inverted 'v' shape. The foramen caecum is at the apex of the 'v' or small depression. The surface is covered by stratified squamous epithelium partly keratinised. The anterior two-thirds are covered by papillae while the underside is smooth mucous membrane similar to the rest of the surface. In these papillae, the taste buds can be found. The posterior one-third is covered by the lingual tonsil. Immediately behind the tonsil are two depressions or val-leys called vallecula while behind the ridge is the EPIGLOTTIS. The tongue is moved by six muscles – three INTRINSIC MUSCLES OF THE TONGUE and three EXTRINSIC MUSCLES OF THE TONGUE. The tongue is an active articulator used in speech and is also used in the processes of swallowing and chewing. *See* Tortora and Grabowski (1993).

tongue thrust the involuntary forward movement of the tongue, often found in children who have CEREBRAL PALSY. It can produce ARTICULATION DELAY or ARTICULATION DISORDER, and can affect the eating process as the food can be pushed out by the tongue. Treatment for both problems can be given by speech and language therapy.

tongue-tie the layman's term for ANKYLOGLOSSUS.

tonic a stage in which all the muscles contract during a fit in grand-mal EPILEPSY. It can also be a minor fit producing muscle contractions, keeping the muscles tight. *See* Gilroy and Holliday (1982).

tonic syllable *see* SUPRASEGMENTAL PHONOLOGY.

tonicity *see* SUPRASEGMENTAL PHONOLOGY.

tonsil there are three tonsils at the back of the mouth - the pharyngeal, palatine and lingual tonsils. *See* Tortora and Grabowski (1993).

tonsillectomy the operation which removes infected and enlarged tonsils. The palatine tonsil or true tonsil is removed. It may produce hypernasality which can be treated by speech and language therapy. *See* Pracy et al (1974).

TORCH an acronym for the four conditions which can affect a fetus:

1. TOXOPLASMOSIS.
2. RUBELLA.
3. CYTOMEGALOVIRUS.
4. HERPES SIMPLEX.

total communication *see* EDUCATION OF HEARING-IMPAIRED CHILDREN.

Toucan communicator a high-tech communication aid which is operated by two switches. The display comprises two circles of coloured LED lamps. The outer circle contains the most frequently used characters such as letters, numbers and some punctuation marks. The inner circle is used less frequently. There are two displays, one facing the user and one facing the 'listener'. Each display can hold 870 characters. The memory can be accessed to provide urgently required phrases or to plan future conversations. All messages can be prepared in advance and stored in the device's memory. The speed at which the characters are chosen can be varied. An alarm button can be used to call for attention. It can be connected to many types of computer, printer and the Toucan portable speech synthesiser. It has rechargeable batteries.

touch-sensitive screen an input device which allows a computer program to be operated without the use of a keyboard. The operator touches the screen surface to make selections.

Touch Talker a high-tech communication aid with synthetic speech output (DECTALK). It uses MINSPEAK to organise vocabulary to store into the device. It has a memory of about 40K. It can only be accessed by direct manual selection. The device can be set into 8, 32 or 128 locations and if the Touch Talker uses the ENHANCED MINSPEAK OPERATING SYSTEM (EMOS) it can also be set into the 'alternative' overlay. There are various MINSPEAK APPLICATION PROGRAMS (MAPs) which can be transferred into the device. The memory can be backed up on a computer. It can also be used for computer emulation and can be linked to the DIRECTOR, an environmental control. *See* Appendix IV.

toxoplasmosis an infection which can cause brain damage if transferred *in utero* through the placenta to the fetus. It is caused by ingestion of food which has come into contact with protozoal organisms found in cat faeces. It forms part of the TORCH classification of infection which can affect a fetus. Many adults have serological evidence of previous infection which has not been identified by a clinical illness. *See* Gilroy and Holliday (1982).

ToyPac a high-tech means for physically handicapped children to operate radio-controlled toys. It can be used to increase the child's eye-hand coordination, switch control, scanning, etc. In single switch operation the scanning speed of light on the control panel is set. When the light reaches the switch the child wishes, he presses it. The toy will go either forward or back, left or right, or open or close. A double switch can be used for children who have difficulty with scanning. A second switch or a double switch is attached to the control box which stops the light scanning. Pressing one switch selects the desired action for the toy and the second switch makes the toy carry out the action. A directional switch or a joystick can also be used.

trace conditioning *see* CLASSICAL CONDITIONING.

trachea the trachea is commonly referred to as the windpipe. It is about 10 cm long and 2 cm wide, extending from the sixth cervical vertebra down to the fifth thoracic vertebra. At this point, it divides into the left and right bronchi. In outline, it is more or less circular but it is actually flattened at the back because running down its whole length is the OESOPHAGUS. It is surrounded by three important structures in the neck – carotid artery, jugular vein, vagus nerve (*see* CRANIAL NERVES). The nerve behind the trachea is the recurrent laryngeal nerve which supplies nearly all the muscles of the LARYNX. It can be easily picked out on X-ray as it has twenty tracheal rings made of hyaline while the rest of the wall comprises CONNECTIVE TISSUE and SMOOTH MUSCLE. It is lined by ciliated columnar EPITHELIUM with mucus cells. At the front, opposite the third tracheal ring is the thyroid gland. On inspiration, the trachea lengthens and changes shape as its walls are elastic. Its main function is to provide air during inspiration. *See* Tortora and Grabowski (1993).

tracheostomy *see* TRACHEOTOMY.

tracheotomy an operation to open into the TRACHEA when a person has severe problems in breathing. A tube is inserted into a hole in the neck to aid breathing. *See* Pracy et al (1974); Tortora and Grabowski (1993).

trackball an input device which can be used instead of the QWERTY keyboard to operate a computer program. It consists of a ball which can be rolled by the palm of the hand to move the cursor or draw lines to produce graphics.

traditional grammar *see* SYNTAX.

trait approach an approach to psychology which has as its aim finding out the characteristics which make the person act the way he does. Traits are descriptions of behaviour characteristics such as aggressiveness, emotional stability, agreeableness, etc. In fact, a trait is any characteristic which differs significantly from person to person. It does not explain the person's behaviour. A method for measuring traits is factor analysis. The method allows the therapist to reduce a large number of measures to a small number of independent dimensions. Cattell developed a 16 personality factor questionnaire. The client is asked over 100 questions to which he need only reply 'yes/no', and from his replies Cattell could work out the person's personality profile. For the trait approach to be effective, each person's profile should be compared in different situations to find out in which situation the person's traits are most affected. *See* Atkinson et al (1993).

transcortical motor aphasia a major form of APHASIA described by the BOSTON SCHOOL. It produces non-fluency, but repetition and comprehension remain relatively intact while naming, reading aloud and writing are impaired. The lesion occurs in the perisylvian areas of the BRAIN. *See* Goodglass and Kaplan (1983); Rosenbek et al (1989).

transcortical sensory aphasia a major form of APHASIA described by the BOSTON SCHOOL. It produces fluent language full of neologisms (*see* JARGON APHASIA (4)) and PARAPHASIAS, impaired comprehension, naming, reading comprehension and writing, while reading aloud is affected to varying degrees and repetition remains unaffected. *See* Goodglass and Kaplan (1983); Rosenbek et al (1989).

transcription systems ways in which a person's speech can be represented usually by the symbols on the IPA chart (*see* Appendix III). When it is carried out by a speech and language therapist, it shows which sounds have changed and to what they have changed. There are three types of transcription:

1. Phonemic transcription, also known as broad transcription. Each symbol represents all allophonic (*see* PHONOLOGY) variations.

2. Allophonic transcription, also known as narrow transcription. A more technical transcription as it requires the representation of all allophonic variations of each phoneme (*see* PHONOLOGY). DIACRITICS are also used to make the transcription as accurate as possible.

3. Impressionistic transcription is carried out without regard to the phonemic or allophonic interpretation of the sounds.

In speech and language therapy, (1) and (2) are the most commonly used to transcribe the speech of children with ARTICULATION DELAY or ARTICULATION DISORDER, or PHONOLOGICAL DELAY or PHONOLOGICAL DISORDER. *See* Abercrombie (1967); Grunwell (1987).

217

transformational grammar (TG) a theory of SYNTAX proposed by Chomsky (*see* CHOMSKYAN LINGUISTICS) in 1957 after he had set aside the other two theories of finite state GRAMMAR and PHRASE STRUCTURE GRAMMAR. His initial description of such grammar was : 'a grammatical transformation T operates on a given string..with a given constituent structure and converts it into a new string with a new derived constituent structure' (Chomsky, 1957, p.44). In 1965, he put forward the STANDARD THEORY of TG. The transformations which he proposed to operate between the deep and surface structures were designed to delete, substitute, insert, move and raise strings so that the person could arrive at the spoken or written utterance. Chomsky believed the most important study for linguists was the syntactic component of language, and to arrive at the correct syntactical structures it was not necessary to deal with the semantic component. Both surface and deep structures represent the phonetic and semantic components interpreted in language. Chomsky went so far as to claim syntax was 'autonomous' and had little to do with semantics. Chomsky found he had to revise the standard theory and so he proposed the Extended Standard Theory (EST). In this theory, Chomsky began to accept the role of semantics in the surface structure. This apparent change was caused by the failure of the Standard Theory to account for the use of stress. In such sentences, the meaning change depends on which word is stressed. Chomsky's problem was: do such sentences all have the same deep structure or different deep structures?

1. Is Bill coming on TUESDAY?
2. Is BILL coming on Tuesday?
3. IS Bill coming on Tuesday?

In the Standard Theory, Chomsky would have had to give all these sentences the same deep structure because transformational rules could not change the meaning of the deep sentence between the deep and surface structures. To overcome this problem, he proposed transformational rules which allowed for markers to be placed in the deep and surface structures so that both structures would affect the semantics of the sentence. This is sometimes called Interpretive Semantics Grammar. In 1973, Chomsky revised EST to the Revised Extended Standard Theory (REST). This theory removed the relationship of the deep structure to the semantic component as in EST, so that all semantic information could be read off from the surface structure. To accomplish this, he introduced the Trace Theory. A trace 't' is an empty node left behind after a NOUN PHRASE has been removed. Thus, the passive transfromation becomes as shown in the box below: (1') shows the trace from where the NP 'John' has been removed to the beginning of the sentence. Thus, traces are like chains in that when linked together, the NP can be traced to its original position. The latest development of Chomsky's theory is referred to as 'Government and Binding'. *See* Chomsky (1982); Steinberg (1982); Salkie (1990); Lyons (1991); Fromkin and Rodman (1993).

transient ischaemic attacks (TIAs) episodes of temporary ischaemia of the BRAIN or BRAIN-STEM. It is a transient loss of cerebral function presumed due to a vascular event which resolves within 24 hours. The attacks begin

deep structure	(1)	Mary kissed John
surface structure	(1')	John was kissed t (by Mary)
		i i

suddenly and symptoms and signs are present for a few minutes before disappearing. The common symptoms and signs are weakness of a limb or face, loss of sensation or transient blindness in one eye (amaurosis fugax). Some people may have just a single attack while others have several at different time intervals. There are many possible causes for TIAs and it is likely that no cause will be found. It is believed the vast majority of attacks are due to small emboli formed from blood platelets with some fibrin thrombus. These emboli originate chiefly in the first centimetre of the internal carotid artery (*see* CAROTID ARTERY) which has become ulcerated due to the formation of atheroma (*see* above). In addition, they may originate on the aortic valves, the damaged wall of the left ventricle (after a heart attack) or in the mitral valve or left atrium (*see* HEART) in people with rheumatic heart disease. Other suggested causes are abnormalities of the blood constituents such as hypercoagulability or reduced cerebral perfusion such as diminished effective cardiac output, steal syndromes, kinking and compression of extracranial vessels. *See* Gilroy and Holliday (1982); Kaye (1991); Tortora and Grabowski (1993).

transverse muscle *see* INTRINSIC MUSCLES OF THE TONGUE.

trauma any injury which occurs to parts or structures in the body or severe feelings of stress caused by the external environment. *See* Kaye (1991).

Treacher Collins syndrome a syndrome described by Treacher Collins in 1900, although the first reported case was made by Thomson in 1846. In the 1940s, the condition was also known as mandibulofacial dysostosis. About 40 per cent of those with this condition have a CLEFT PALATE. The characteristic facial appearance is downward slanting eyes with an underdeveloped mandible and maxilla. There are also abnormalities of the

EAR such as lack of a pinna causing HEARING LOSS. The hearing loss may produce learning difficulties but the syndrome is not associated with learning disability. *See* Edwards and Watson (1980); Smith (1985).

treatment programme the plan of therapy produced by a therapist for each individual client based on the assessments which have been carried out. This may include some published therapeutic techniques, e.g. PROMOTING APHASICS' COMMUNICATIVE EFFECTIVENESS, MELODIC INTONTATION THERAPY, NUFFIELD DYSPRAXIA PROGRAMME, etc., various forms of ALTERNATIVE AUGMENTATIVE COMMUNICATION or therapy devised by the therapist based on experience of what has worked best in the past with those with similar disorders. However, there must be flexibility built into a treatment programme if the person does not respond appropriately.

tree diagram a hierarchical structure which is used to analyse constituents (*see* CONSTITUENT ANALYSIS). The constituents are all linked by branches and the points where the branches meet are nodes:

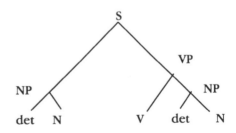

The 'S' sentence is said to dominate the NP and VP which are said to dominate their respective lower constituents. Trees are known as phrase markers. *See* Huddleston (1976); Fromkin and Rodman (1993) (phrase structured trees).

tremor a rhythmic, involuntary and purposeless contraction of muscle groups. There are three main types of tremor:

1. Essential tremor: a benign tremor which is usually bilateral, beginning in the fingers and hands. It may be inherited as an autosomal dominant trait (see CHROMOSOMES). It is caused by an imbalance of neurotransmitter substances in the BASAL GANGLIA. It can appear in either young children or the elderly. The tremor worsens if the person is emotionally upset. It is associated with mild cerebellar signs. The main drug treatment is a ß-receptor blocker such as propranolol and diazepam.

2. Intention tremor: it increases with movement and involves upper extremities, often occuring at the end of the movement. This may be found in those with cerebellar disease. The same drug treatment is used as for essential tremor.

3. Parkinsonian tremor (see PARKINSON'S DISEASE).

See Gilroy and Holliday (1982); Tortora and Grabowski (1993).

tricyclics see ANTIDEPRESSANT DRUGS.

trigeminal nerve see CRANIAL NERVES.

trill see ARTICULATION.

triplegia a physical handicap which affects three limbs – usually both legs and one arm – and is often found in those who have CEREBRAL PALSY.

trisomy-21 see DOWN'S SYNDROME.

TROG see TEST FOR RECEPTION OF GRAMMAR.

true tonsil see MOUTH.

tuberous sclerosis often thought to have been described first by von Recklinghausen over 100 years ago, Bournville is usually credited for its recognition in 1880. Hamartomatous lesions develop in many tissues, especially the skin and the brain. A condition which has three principal features:

1. EPILEPSY;
2. LEARNING DISABILITY;
3. skin disorder.

However, not every child has all three features. About 40 per cent have skin disorder while 60 per cent have a degree of learning disability and almost all have a form of epilepsy. See Hosking (1982); Smith (1985).

tumour the medical term for a cancerous (see CANCER) growth found in tissues in the body.

tumours of the central nervous system these are some of the commonest cancerous (see CANCER) growths in the glia of the BRAIN:

1. Oligodendrogliomas: these tumours, which may become malignant, produce a greyish-red area in the brain giving a honeycomb effect. It is most often found in the frontal lobe of the CEREBRAL HEMISPHERES. As they grow slowly, they produce a gradual headache and a generalised seizure. They appear in people between the ages of 30 and 40 years. They comprise 5 per cent of all gliomas. Treatment takes the form of surgical removal followed by RADIOTHERAPY with the post-operative life span likely to be about 5–7 years.

2. Meningiomas: these comprise 10 per cent of all intracranial tumours. They usually appear in the later years of life and are more common in women. Treatment takes the form of surgical removal. The prognosis is good as long as complete removal has taken place. Otherwise the tumour may reappear and necessitate a second operation a few years later.

3. Neurofibromas: this type of tumour can be inherited as an autosomal dominant trait (see CHROMOSOMES). These peripheral tumours may be associated with intracerebral gliomas. They may appear on the cranial or peripheral nerves of the brain and SPINAL CORD and produce raised pressure in the head, aphasic symptoms (see APHASIA), HEMIPLEGIA, problems in the visual fields as well as seizures. Headaches are not a common symptom. There may also be café-au-lait spots on the skin. The tumours are

usually multiple and some may become malignant.

4. Astrocytomas: these tumours are locally invasive. They appear most commonly in the frontal, temporal and parietal lobes (*see* CEREBRAL HEMI-SPHERES), basal ganglia and occipital lobes (*see* CEREBRAL HEMISPHERES) in decreasing order of frequency. Headaches are often felt on one side of the brain which become more generalised, and raised INTRACRANIAL PRESSURE develops. Treatment takes the form of surgical removal followed by radiotherapy.

5. Medulloblastomas: these grow very quickly and are very invasive from metastatic seeding. These tumours account for about 20 per cent of all intracranial tumours in childhood. They are common in children below the age of 10 years and rarer in older children. The posterior fossa is the site for these lesions. As they grow near the FOURTH VENTRICLE, HYDRO-CEPHALUS can often develop. Treatment takes the form of surgical removal followed by radiotherapy while the hydrocephalus can be treated with ventricular SHUNTS. The prognosis depends on how much of the tumour has been removed and the efficacy of the radiotherapy.

See Gilroy and Holliday (1982;) Kaye (1991).

turn a sociolinguistic phenomenon. Turn taking in conversation is crucial for a conversation to take place. *See* Clark and Clark (1977).

turn taking the pattern of reciprocal interchange which takes place in normal conversational situations. It is absent or deficient in some types of language disorder.

Turner's syndrome Turner described, in 1938, a condition which involved small stature, sexual infantilism, webbed neck and cubitus valgus in seven females. It is a sex chromosome (*see* CHROMOSOMES) where 45 chromosomes are present with one X but no Y chromosome. Thus, it is also known as an XO syndrome. It is not particularly associated with LEARNING DISABILITY. However, there can be associated disorders of the neck, kidneys, ovaries and heart. The child is likely to have educational difficulties such as reading problems. *See* Salmon (1978); Smith (1985).

turtle either a robotic machine which can be moved by a child giving it commands from the computer or a small triangle which can be moved about the screen. *See* LOGOTRON.

twinkle eye-controlled switch an input device which can be used for both the BBC and Apple microcomputers. Two sensors which produce electrical signals when the eyes move are placed on the person's temples close to the eyes. When the eyes move to the right, the left sensor is closed and vice versa. There is a connection to the analog port of the BBC and BBC Master and to the games port of the Apple II.

tympanic membrane *see* EAR.

tympanogram classification *see* IMPEDANCE AUDIOMETRY.

tympanometry *see* IMPEDANCE AUDIOMETRY.

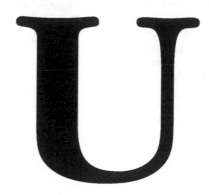

U

ultrasonography a non-invasive technique originally devised to assess the growth of the fetus. It can show how the fetus is placed in the placenta, the amount of fetal growth which has taken place and can identify any disorder of the spine, thus showing any possibility of the child having SPINA BIFIDA. It may also show if there are to be multiple births. It is now more widely used as an imaging technique for organ enlargement, tumours, blood flow, presence of gallstones, etc. It is a popular technique because it is totally safe, cheap and easily repeatable. *See* Tortora and Grabowski (1993).

unconditioned response *see* CLASSICAL CONDITIONING.

unconditioned stimulus *see* CLASSICAL CONDITIONING.

unconscious motives *see* PSYCHOANALYSIS.

underextension the opposite of OVEREXTENSION. During the stage of underextension, the child uses one word for a particular object. So, the child may use the word 'teddy' for his own teddy but not for the teddies belonging to his siblings or friends. However, at a later stage, he could call other teddies by their correct name and overextend its use to an object which may have similar characteristics to a teddy bear, but is another object. *See* Clark and Clark (1977).

understanding *see* COMPREHENSION.

undifferentiated jargon *see* JARGON APHASIA (1).

unilateral a lesion or disease which affects one side of the body or structure in the body. It is opposed to bilateral.

unilateral abductor paralysis *see* LARYNGEAL NERVE PALSIES.

unilateral adductor paralysis *see* LARYNGEAL NERVE PALSIES.

unintelligible speech the speech of a person who has a very severe communication problem. For children, this may be an articulation or phonological delay or disorder. For adults, this may be caused by an ACQUIRED DYSPRAXIA or severe DYSARTHRIA. It is often the case close relatives can make out what the person is saying but strangers fail. *See* Grunwell (1987).

unit any item in a syntactic, phonetic, semantic or morphological description. A unit in any of these areas of linguistics describes the focus for discussion. *See* Lyons (1968).

Unity/128 devised by Badman et al, it is a MINSPEAK APPLICATION PROGRAM designed using the WORDS STRATEGY paradigm and similar overlay. It is aimed at any age range and from mild learning disability to no learning disability. Unity can start at about 3 years of age and is suitable for childhood, adolescence and adulthood, so there will be no need to learn a new program when the child reaches the cut-off point with a program like IEP+. It uses symbols combining with grammatical labels for nouns, verbs and all their endings, adjectives, prepositions and adverbs as well as using categorisation for a larger set of vocabulary. There are four overlays, the main difference being the gradual increase of grammatical labels until the third and fourth overlays when all the grammatical labels are on the overlay. On the third overlay these labels are represented with icons while on the fourth there is just the written label as with Words Strategy. *See* Badman et al (1995).

upper motor neuron *see* NEURON.

UR (unconditioned response) *see* CLASSICAL CONDITIONING.

US (unconditioned stimulus) *see* CLASSICAL CONDITIONING.

utterance as opposed to sentence, or some other theoretical term referring to an identifiable linguistic unit, i.e. defined within some theoretical approach, utterance is a pre-theoretical term referring to some stretch of speech prior to analysis. *See* Lyons (1968).

uvula a piece of tissue hanging down from the back of the soft palate and between the isthmus of fauces (*see* MOUTH). The uvular muscle runs along the middle of the soft palate (*see* MOUTH) and moves the uvula. Although this may not have been thought to be of much use, research now suggests that the muscle contracts and leads to a VELOPHARYNGEAL closure. *See* Edwards and Watson (1980); Tortora and Grabowski (1993).

uvular *see* ARTICULATION.

uvular muscle *see* UVULA.

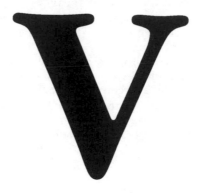

vagus nerve *see* CRANIAL NERVES.

vallecula *see* TONGUE.

vascular a description of structures or problems in the blood supply to the body.

VDU *see* VISUAL DISPLAY UNIT.

velar *see* ARTICULATION.

velaric airstream an airstream used to produce clicks which are also described as velaric ingressive stops. Clicks which can be produced are bilabial click [.], tongue tip [!], lateral click [11] (as in the 'gee-up' sound for horses), retroflex click [‡]. In English, clicks are only used to express the speaker's feelings and not linguistically as in such languages as Hottentot in which all four types of clicks are used to produce linguistic meaning. *See* Ladefoged (1993).

velopharyngeal a description of structures or disorders between the soft palate (*see* MOUTH) and the back wall of the nasopharynx (*see* PHARYNX). When the structures in this area close, it is known as velopharyngeal closure. This closure takes place during speech and swallowing so that the oropharynx (*see* PHARYNX) is separated from the nasopharynx by the raising of the soft palate and the moving inward of the walls of the pharynx. A failure of this closure is known as velopharyngeal incompetence. If the soft palate or velum fails to reach the back wall of the pharynx because of damage or because it is too short to reach the wall, it is known as velopharyngeal insufficiency. *See* Edwards and Watson (1980).

velopharyngeal closure *see* VELOPHARYNGEAL.

velopharyngeal incompetence *see* VELOPHARYNGEAL.

velopharyngeal insufficiency *see* VELOPHARYNGEAL.

ventricles *see* THIRD VENTRICLE; FOURTH VENTRICLE.

verb particle a term used in some grammatical approaches to refer to the unit in phrasal verb sequences in English which are preposition-like but do not always function as prepositions, e.g. 'up', 'off', 'away' as in (1)–(3).

(1) We ran a bill up.
(2) She took her hat off.
(3) He threw the rubbish away.

See Crystal et al (1976).

verb phrase *see* CONSTITUENT ANALYSIS; Fromkin and Rodman (1993).

verbal auditory agnosia a very severe form of AGNOSIA. Superficially the child may appear deaf and there may be some HEARING LOSS but this is not sufficient to account for complete lack of AUDITORY COMPREHENSION. Consequently EXPRESSIVE LANGUAGE is also severely affected. Also known as congenital auditory imperception.

verbal dyspraxia *see* DEVELOPMENTAL VERBAL DYSPRAXIA.

verbal paraphasia *see* PARAPHASIA.

vertical muscle *see* INTRINSIC MUSCLES OF THE TONGUE.

vestibular system *see* EAR.

vestibulocochlear nerve also known as acoustic nerve. *See* CRANIAL NERVE VIII.

videofluoroscopy a radiographic technique to visualise the movement of contrast medium in the body, e.g. the pharyngeal stage of swallowing. The person is given barium mixed with small quantities of food or fluid. The swallowing process is recorded on video film for subsequent analysis which is carried out frame-by-frame so that the therapist can accurately assess the time taken for the person to trigger a swallow and examine closely what happens during different stages of the swallow. Since a lateral view and a head-on view are given of the person swallowing, the therapist can see all the structures in the head and neck which may be defective in the swallowing process. The findings may include aspiration of the bolus, pooling in the vallecula or the pyriform sinuses, the destination of pooled material, spillage of material into the PHARYNX before the swallow is triggered, and delay in the activation of the swallow reflex. *See* Langley (1987).

visible speech *see* FINGER SPELLING.

Visispeech a real-time analysis and display system. It can be used with the BBC microcomputer and Apple microcomputer. Visispeech shows many aspects of voice visually. It can help in the assessment of voice quality of people with DYSPHONIA or HEARING LOSS and those with DYSARTHRIA who have pitch problems. There are three displays:

1. pitch;
2. energy;
3. voicing.

Visispeech II has an easy key access as it operates with one actuation of each of the function keys on a BBC computer. There is also a histogram program which provides graphical representations of the frequency distribution. Histograms and the three energy displays can be saved on disk as well as being printed out so that an assessment can be kept and progress monitored accurately.

visual display unit a unit which displays text or graphics produced from the memory of the computer. It forms the display section of a terminal.

vital capacity the greatest TIDAL VOLUME, i.e. the biggest breath a person can take in and let out. *See* J.H. Green (1978); Tortora and Grabowski (1993).

Vocaid a high-tech communication aid with speech synthesis. It is a dedicated communcation aid in that there are prestored messages in the device and only those can be activated. Users cannot make up their own messages. It is supplied with a set of printed overlay cards with 32 squares providing 35 utterances and an on/off square. Each card covers specific topics, e.g. illness, leisure, etc. Each card has a special code that decides the program to be used. As one of the squares is actuated, the word or phrase is produced. The back of each overlay card has blank squares so that it can be adapted for a system of symbols, e.g. photographs, Blissymbols, Makaton symbols or rebus symbols. It is easily portable.

vocal abuse *see* VOCAL NODULES.

vocal cords *see* VOCAL FOLDS.

vocal folds found in the LARYNX, they vibrate while a person is speaking. It is the vibration which produces the voice quality in speech. The process of producing voice is known as PHONATION. They may also be called vocal cords. Any growths or structural damage to the folds can produce DYSPHONIA. *See* Catford (1977); Tortora and Grabowski (1993).

vocal misuse *see* VOCAL NODULES.

vocal nodules growths that appear on the posterior third of the vocal folds. They can occur in both children and adults through vocal abuse or misuse. This takes the form of excessive shouting, abnormal phonation patterns and excessive strain on the vocal folds. The nodules increase in size because of the persistent rubbing together of the strained folds, compare the appearance of corns on the feet after wearing ill-fitting shoes. The nodules prevent the folds from closing normally during phonation and harsh or hoarse voice can occur. Treatment takes the form of relaxation exercises and voice exercises which prevent the vocal folds from coming together harshly, e.g. YAWN/SIGH APPROACH. Voice rest, where the person has to use the voice as little as possible, may be necessary. This may require the person to take time off work and not live such an active social life for a period of time. Voice rest gives therapy the optimum conditions for improving the voice. See Fawcus (1991).

Vocal Profile Analysis devised by Laver in 1980, it is based on a phonetic analysis of voice quality. The interrelationship of different points in the vocal tract is considered together with different types of phonation. Analysis is based on visual and auditory information. Specialised courses are offered for training in the skills necessary to carry out the analysis. See Fawcus (1991); Beech et al (1993).

vocal tract the whole system through which sounds are produced. It begins with an expulsion of air from the LUNGS which moves up through the TRACHEA and LARYNX in which the VOCAL FOLDS are located. From this point,

the air reaches the MOUTH where it is modified by the muscles of the face and tongue to produce the required sound. See Catford (1977).

vocalic a MAJOR CLASS FEATURE set up in the DISTINCTIVE FEATURE theory of PHONOLOGY. It distinguishes sounds which are made with a free passage of air through the VOCAL TRACT. In a spectrogram (see SPECTROGRAPHY), there is a distinct formant structure [+VOCALIC]. See Hyman (1975).

vocalis muscle see LARYNX.

voice disorders see DYSPHONIA.

voice onset time (VOT) a phenomenon found in the production of any plosive (see ARTICULATION). There is a period of time between the articulators coming together and then releasing to make the sound. This delay occurs in all plosives except for fully voiced stops. Such a gap shows up on a spectrogram (see SPECTROGRAPHY). See Ladefoged (1993).

voice quality see REGISTER.

voice rest see VOCAL NODULES.

voice synthesis see SPEECH SYNTHESIS.

voicing see ARTICULATION.

volatile memory computer memory which loses its contents when power is switched off. See Brookshear (1991).

VOT see VOICE ONSET TIME.

vowel see CARDINAL VOWEL SYSTEM.

vowel system different languages have different vowel systems as have different accents of the same language. There are also a number of varieties of English which have different systems such as Scottish English, American English, Australian English, etc. See Fromkin and Rodman (1993); Ladefoged (1993).

VP (verb phrase) See CONSTITUENT ANALYSIS.

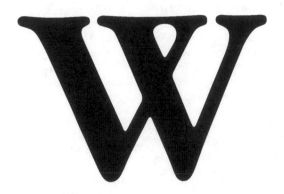

WAIS-R *see* WECHSLER ADULT INTELLIGENCE SCALE – REVISED.

Walker Talker a high-tech communication aid using digitised speech output. It uses MINSPEAK to organise vocabulary to store into the device. It has a memory of one minute standard speech and two minutes extended speech. There is an extra memory card which will increase the memory to four minutes standard speech and eight minutes in extended speech. It is worn on a waist strap on which is a pouch with a 16-location symbol pad. However, it is possible to have symbol sequences of up to three symbols in a sequence so the client will not be restricted to 16 messages. The larger part on the waist strap has the battery pack, the amplifier with in-built microphone and the control panel for storing messages into the device. Memory can be backed up on a computer disk. *See* Appendix IV.

warble tone a tone emitted from a machine which varies in intensity levels. It is part of the DISTRACTION TESTS used to test the hearing of young children. If the child hears the tone, he will turn his head to the side on which the tone has been presented. If he cannot hear the tone, he will continue to look at the person in front of him who is distracting him with toys.

Warnock Report a UK Government report published in 1978 entitled 'Children with Special Needs'. It recommended use of the term 'children with learning difficulties' to replace the former 'educationally subnormal'. They were then to be graded as being mild, moderate or severe with an additional 'specific' category where the difficulty related to one area. *See* Beech et al (1993).

Wechsler Adult Intelligence Scale – Revised (WAIS-R) the first version of WAIS was published in 1939 and revised in 1955. The latest edition was published in 1981. There are eleven subtests, five performance tests and six verbal tests. It can be used with adults in the age range of 16–74 years of age. The subtests have been designed from the easiest to the most difficult and administration is stopped after the person has failed a certain number of items. The RAW SCORE is converted into a STANDARD SCORE with a mean of 10 and a STANDARD DEVIATION of 3. When the six scaled scores of the verbal subtests and the five performance subtests are added together as well as the scaled scores on all the eleven subtests, the three sums are converted to IQ scores – verbal, performance and full-scale. The IQs have deviations with a mean of 100 and a standard deviation of 15. *See* Aiken (1985); Atkinson et al (1993); Beech et al (1993); Davison and Neale (1994).

Wechsler Intelligence Scale for Children–Revised (WISC-R) the original WISC was first developed in 1949. The revised version of WISC was published in 1974. It can be administered to children between the ages of 6;0 and 16;0. There are five verbal and five performance subtests with an additional two alternative subtests which are to be used with the child if one of the performance subtests is spoiled or proves difficult to administer. The test usually lasts one hour and the tester receives verbal, performance and full-scale IQ. *See* Aiken (1985); Atkinson et al (1993); Davison and Neale (1994).

Wechsler tests tests produced by David Wechsler in the 1930s and 1940s. He produced a test for children – WECHSLER INTELLIGENCE SCALES FOR CHILDREN – REVISED (WISC-R) – and for adults – WECHSLER ADULT INTELLIGENCE SCALES – REVISED (WAIS-R). *See* Kolb and Whishaw (1990).

Wernicke-Korsakoff syndrome a SYNDROME which can lead to DEMENTIA. It is produced by a vitamin deficiency of thiamine in the BRAIN. Such deficiency of thiamine occurs in alcoholism, starvation and malnutrition. It has two stages:

1. Wernicke's encephalopathy: the person becomes disoriented in time and place, becomes drowsy, develops abnormalities of the eyes and ataxia. This is caused by the person taking alcohol only, without having anything to eat. Such a condition could be fatal unless the person is given an injection of thiamine. If there is a delay in giving thiamine, the person may recover but will be left with Korsakoff's syndrome.
2. Korsakoff's syndrome: during this part of the syndrome, the person has problems with short-term memory. Proceeding from Wernicke's encephalopathy, the person cannot remember what he has been doing. He cannot find his way to places, and if he does, he cannot get back. People have difficulty forming new memories and they make up stories as they go along. The person should be put on adequate diet with vitamin supplementation and should abstain from alcohol.

See Stafford-Clark and Smith (1983); Kolb and Whishaw (1990).

Wernicke's aphasia a type of APHASIA first described by Wernicke in 1874 and one of the major types of aphasia identified by the BOSTON SCHOOL. It occurs in Wernicke's area (*see* CEREBRAL HEMISPHERES) and consequently the predominant feature is impairment in auditory verbal comprehension. *See also* APHASIA (2). *See* Goodglass and Kaplan (1983); Rosenbek et al (1989); Kolb and Whishaw (1990).

Western Aphasia Battery (WAB) devised by Kertesz, it is an assessment of APHASIA following the LOCATIONIST position whereby the aphasic person is classified into an exclusive category depending on the results, and it uses the modality approach whereby the different modalities of expression, auditory comprehension, reading and writing are tested. The subtests in the Western Aphasia Battery aim to assess content, fluency, auditory comprehension, repetition and naming as well as reading, writing and calculation. RAVEN'S PROGRESSIVE MATRICES are also included in the battery to assess non-verbal visual thinking and there are also subtests for assessing drawing, block design and praxis. After the test is completed, there are two scores–the Aphasia Quotient and a Cortical Quotient. *See* Kertesz (1982) in Appendix I; Rosenbek et al (1989); Beech et al (1993).

wh- questions question words which begin with 'wh-', i.e. why, what, who, when, which, where. 'How' is also included in this classification as it behaves in a similar way to other 'wh-' words. This type of question is opposed to YES/NO QUESTIONS. *See* Fromkin and Rodman (1993).

wh- words *see* WH- QUESTIONS.

Wilcoxon test a non-parametric test (*see* PARAMETRIC TESTS) used with the REPEATED MEASURES design for statistical analysis. It is the equivalent of the related *t*-test (*see* T-TESTS). The scores should be ranked in an interval ranking scale. *See* Miller (1975).

Window

1. Used in icon software (*see* ICON) to show the choices on a menu. It can also be used in graphics where text can be written in a window to explain features of the graphics or as a bit of text referring to the graphic.

2. Users of IBM PCs and compatibles can use Microsoft Windows which is an OPERATING SYSTEM, allowing the operator to use a MOUSE to carry out various functions on the computer without having to type in command words as when using the DOS operating system. Each window has a menu bar with a number of pull-down menus which allow the operator to save, open, edit a file or change the fonts and size of print or choose the type of graphic to draw etc.

3. Operators of Apple Macintosh computers use a Window in a similar way although this type of operating system first appeared on an Apple Macintosh. There is a common menu bar with pull-down menus which changes according to the application which is being used at the particular time.

WISC-R *See* WECHSLER INTELLIGENCE SCALE FOR CHILDREN-REVISED.

WiViK 2.0 an on-screen keyboard, WiViK produces a movable, resizeable window and offers a number of different keyboards. Keyboards can be customised to contain letters, numbers, short words and phrases and functions. Selections are made either through a puff switch or by holding the cursor on a character for an adjustable length of time. WiViK 2.0 can also be bundled with a writing rate enhancement package (WREP) to add word prediction and abbreviation expansion features. WiViK 2.0 runs best on an IBM or compatible 386 with two megabytes of RAM memory and a hard disk drive. It also requires the Windows 3.1 operating environment. See Appendix IV.

WiViK WREP a means of speeding up typing into WiViK, WiViK WREP (Writing Rate Enhancement Package) contains two methods of increasing speed of text entry: word prediction and abbreviation expansion. When the user types the first letter of a word, word prediction causes a group of words to be displayed. If the desired word appears, the user selects it and that word is immediately sent to the working application. If the desired word is not listed, typing an additional letter will refine the word list. Abbreviation expansion allows short sequences of letters such as N & A to stand for longer phrases such as 'Name and Address'. WiViK WREP will only work if WiViK 2.0 is already installed in the computer. See Appendix IV.

word a unit of grammar used in the construction of phrases and sentences. It is recognised intuitively (*see* INTUITION) by a native speaker but when examined more scientifically by linguists, 'what is a word?' becomes a more complex problem. For example, it is necessary to distinguish between individual word forms occurring in utterances such as 'scream', 'screams', 'screamed'. At a more abstract level, however, linguists would like to recognise all three as forms of a word 'scream'. The latter is sometimes referred to as a lexeme. *See* Lyons (1968); Fromkin and Rodman (1993).

word and paradigm (WP) *see* MORPHOLOGY.

word-final the description of a sound which occurs at the end of a word. For example, in the word /buk/ ('book'), the sound [k] is said to appear word-finally.

word-finding difficulty *See* LEXICAL SYN-TACTIC DEFICIT.

Word-Finding Vocabulary Scale devised by Renfrew in 1968 (2nd edition 1972, 3rd edition 1988). It includes 45 pictures each line-drawn on a separate card and arranged in order of frequency of recognition. A guide is given as to which picture testing should start, relative to the child's age and also guidance as to the number of failures made before discontinuing the test. It is useful for finding whether a child has difficulty retrieving words to which he would respond correctly when named. The test is standardised in the UK and norms are supplied for children of 3;6–8;0 years. *See* Renfrew (1988).

word-form dyslexia *see* ACQUIRED DYSLEXIA.

word-initial the description of a sound which occurs at the begining of a word. For example, in the word 'bin', the sound [b] is said to appear word-initially.

word-medial the description of a sound occuring in the middle of the word. For example, in the word /bʌtə/ 'butter', the sound [t] is said to appear word-medially.

word order the sequence of words used to construct phrases and sentences. In English the word order is fixed (*see* SYNTAGMATIC RELATIONS) while in German it is more variable with adverbial phrases and verbs floating around the sentence as long as the verb remains the second idea, not necessarily the second word, of the sentence. *See* Lyons (1968).

word processor a machine for typing any kind of document by the use of computer technology. It can also refer to the piece of software for use with a microcomputer. Some advantages in using a word processor instead of a manual or electronic typewriter include:

1. The text appears on the screen and can be edited before it is printed or saved on disk.

2. Corrections, which can be made quickly, can be carried out on text which is on disk and then resaved.

3. A letter format can be put on disk and used time after time.

See Bishop (1985).

Words Strategy devised by Bruce Baker in the late 1980s, it is a MINSPEAK APPLICATION PROGRAM (MAP) for use with the older child, adolescent or adult. Words Strategy has a large core vocabulary with over 2500 individual words and phrases. Almost all the vocabulary is coded by icons and grammatical labels. Some grammatical labels have only one form while others have many forms. The multiple forms are Words Strategy's greatest strengths. No selection requires more than three icon actuations, the majority only require two. In practical usage, Words Strategy has a 66–75 per cent reduction in actuation for spelling. The user does not require to know the grammatical concepts as a prerequisite to using the system. Many acquire vocabulary on an item-by-item basis and understand at a later date the grammatical categories. Words Strategy is not an end point. The preprogrammed vocabulary and grammatical functions can be deleted so that it can be customised for each client to reflect his personality and environment, etc. Grammatical labels on the overlay can be changed to graphic symbols or Minsymbols or even Blissymbols. *See* Baker (1989).

working through *see* PSYCHOANALYSIS.

WP (word and paradigm) *see* MORPHOLOGY.

write the opposite process from read. Data are transferred to a storage device such as a disk. Data can be read from a disk, if they have been previously written to the disk.

wug an imaginary bird-like creature used in an experiment to find out the order of acquisition of grammatical morphemes. In 1958, Berko proposed that if a child had learnt the correct morphological affixes for nouns and verbs, then he could put the correct endings on imaginary words. She drew pictures of imaginary creatures, of which the 'wug' was one. The picture was presented to the child, who was told what it was, and then another picture of the same creature was presented. To the first one, the child was told 'This is a wug, here is another, we have two....', and usually the child replied correctly: 'wugs'. *See* Clark and Clark (1977).

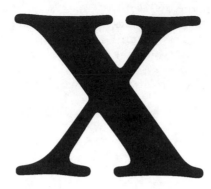

X chromosome *see* CHROMOSOMES.

X-ray *see* RADIOGRAPHY.

xeroradiography a type of X-ray imaging system which enhances contrast in soft tissue by producing a high kilovolt X-ray. It produces an image on a xerographic plate from the effects of X-rays on an electrically charged plate. This technique has been used to examine the VOCAL TRACT during PHONATION. Information about the functioning of the PHARYNX can be assessed along with laryngographic recordings. *See* Greene and Mathieson (1989); Fawcus (1991).

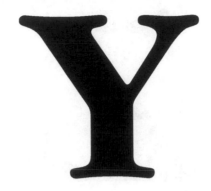

Y-cord hearing aid *see* HEARING AID.

yawn/sigh a technique advocated by Boone in 1977 for treating VOCAL NODULES, it is a means of producing voice without the hard glottal attack which produces vocal nodules. The person is advised to relax completely, take in a deep breath and let it out gradually as a yawn or a sigh and, during this stage, begin to phonate, thus preventing the VOCAL FOLDS from rubbing together harshly. *See* Fawcus (1991).

yes/no questions the type of question which will require the answer 'yes' or 'no'. In general, these questions are formed by inversion of the verb and subject or first noun phrase, i.e. NP1:
(1) He can play football.
(1') Can he play football?
Yes/no questions can be contrasted with WH-QUESTIONS. *See* Clark and Clark (1977).

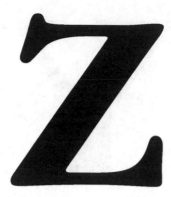

Z scores a score or rank which shows how many of the norm group are above the person's RAW SCORE. For example, if a person receives a Z score of 21 per cent, this means there are 79 per cent of the norm group above this score. It is part of DESCRIPTIVE STATISTICS. *See* Miller (1975).

zero hearing level sound pressure level required to make any frequency barely audible to a person with normal hearing. *See* Katz (1985).

zygomatic arch the arch of bones which form the cheeks. The bones which form the arch and the protruding part of the cheek are the zygomatic bones. *See* Tortora and Grabowski (1993).

Appendix 1:
Tests and assessments

The publishers given at the end of these references are either the publisher of the test or the UK supplier of the test.

Assessment References

Aarons, M., Gittens, T. (1992). *The Autistic Continuum: an assessment and intervention schedule.* Windsor: NFER-Nelson.

Anthony, A., Bogle, D., Ingram, T.T.S., McIsaac, M.W. (1971). *Edinburgh Articulation Test.* Edinburgh: Churchill Livingstone.

Berry, P., Mittler, P. (1981). *Language Imitation Test.* Manchester: Manchester University Press.

Bishop, D.V.M. (1984). *Test for Reception of Grammar.* Manchester.

Blomert, L., Kean, M.-L., Koster, Ch., Shokker, J. (1994). Amsterdam-Nijmegen Everyday Language Test: construction, reliability and validity. *Aphasiology,* **8;4,** 381-407.

Boehm, A.E. (1976). *Boehm Resource Guide for Basic Concept Teaching.* New York: The Psychological Corporation.

Boehm, A.E. (1986a). *Boehm Test of Basic Concepts: Preschool Version.* New York: The Psychological Corporation.

Boehm, A.E. (1986b). *Boehm Test of Basic Concepts: Revised.* New York: The Psychological Corporation.

Bolton, S.O., Dalshiell, S.E. (1984) *Interaction Checklist for Augmentative Communication.* California: Imaginative Communication Products.

Brimer, M.A., Dunn L.M. (1962). *English Picture Vocabulary Tests: Manual.* Awre, Glos.: Education Evaluation Enterprises.

Brimer, M.A., Dunn, L.M. (1973) *English Picture Vocabulary Tests: Administration Manual.* Awre, Glos: Education Evaluation Enterprises.

Bzoch, K., League, R. (1971). *Receptive-Expressive Emergent Language Scale.* Windsor: NFER-Nelson.

Carrow-Woolfolk, E. (1974). *Carrow Elicited Language Inventory.* Windsor: NFER-Nelson.

Carrow-Woolfolk, E. (985). *Test for Auditory Comprehension of Language,* revised edn. Windsor: NFER-Nelson.

Connery, V., Henry, C., Hammond, C., Williams, P., Riley J. (1985). *Nuffield Centre Dyspraxia Programme.* London: Nuffield Hearing and Speech Centre.

Dabul, B. (1979). *Apraxia Battery for Adults.* Tigard: C.C. Publications.

Dean, E., Howell, J., Hill, A., Waters, D. (1990). *Metaphon Resource Pack.* Windsor: NFER-Nelson.

De Renzi, E., Faglioni, P. (1978). Normative data and screening power of a shortened version of the Token test. *Cortex,* **14,** 41-49.

De Renzi, E., Ferrari, C. (1978). The Reporter's Test: a sensitive test to detect expressive disturbance in aphasics. *Cortex,* **14,** 279-293.

De Renzi, E., Vignolo, L.A. (1962). The Token Test: a sensitive test to detect receptive disturbances in aphasics. *Brain*, **85,** 665-678.

Dewart, H., Summers, S. (1988). *Pragmatics Profile of Early Communication.* Windsor: NFER-Nelson.

DiSimoni, F. (1978). *The Token Test for Children.* Windsor: NFER-Nelson.

Douglas, J. (1990). *Special Needs Assessment Software.* Windsor: NFER-Nelson.

Duncan, D., Gibbs, D., Singh Noor, N., Mohammed Whittaker, H. (1987). *Sandwell Bilingual Screening Assessment.* Windsor: NFER-Nelson.

Dunn, L.M. (1969). *Peabody Picture Vocabulary Test.* Circle Pines, MN.: American Guidance Service.

Dunn, L.M., Dunn, L.M., Whetton, C., Pintilie, D. (1982). *British Picture Vocabulary Scales.* Windsor: NFER-Nelson.

Elliott, C.D., Murray, D.J., Pearson, L.S. (1990 rev). *British Ability Scales.* Windsor: NFER-Nelson.

Enderby, P. (1988). *Frenchay Dysarthria Assessment and Computer Differential Analysis.* Windsor: NFER-Nelson.

Enderby, P., Wood, V., Wade, D. (1987). *Frenchay Aphasia Screening Test.* Windsor: NFER-Nelson.

German, D.J. (1986). *Test of Word Finding.* DLM Teaching Resources.

Goldman, R., Fristoe, M. (1972). *Goldman-Fristoe Test of Articulation.* Windsor: NFER-Nelson.

Goldman, R., Fristoe, M., Woodcock, R.W. (1976). *Goldman-Fristoe-Woodcock Auditory Skills Test Battery.* Circle Pines, Minn.:American Guidance Service.

Goodenough, F.L., Harris, D.B. (1963). *Goodenough-Harris Drawing Test.* New York: The Psychological Corporation.

Goodglass, H., Kaplan, E. (1983). *Boston Diagnostic Aphasia Examination.* Philadelphia: Lea and Febiger.

Grunwell, P. (1985a). *Phonological Assessment of Child Speech.* Windsor: NFER-Nelson.

Grunwell, P. (1985b). *PACS Pictures: Language Elicitation Materials.* Windsor: NFER-Nelson.

Grunwell, P. (1995). *PACS Toys Screening Test.* Windsor: NFER-Nelson.

Gutfreund, M. (1989). *Bristol Language Development Scales.* Windsor: NFER-Nelson.

Hitchings, A., Spence, R. (1991). *Personal Communication Plan.* Windsor: NFER-Nelson.

Holland, A.L. (1980). *Communicative Abilities in Daily Living.* Austin, Tex.: PRO-ED.

Jones, S. (1989). *INTECOM.* Windsor: NFER-Nelson.

Kaplan, E., Goodglass, H., Weintraub, S. (1983). *Boston Naming Test.* Philadelphia: Lea & Febiger.

Kay, J., Lesser, R., Coltheart, M. (1992). *Psycholinguistic Assessments of Language Processing in Aphasia.* Hove: Erlbaum.

Kertesz, A. (1982). *Western Aphasia Battery.* New York: The Psychological Corporation.

Kiernan, C., Reid, B. (1987). *Pre-verbal Communication Schedule.* Windsor: NFER-Nelson.

Kirk, S., McCarthy, J., Kirk, W. (1969). *Illinois Test of Psycholinguistic Abilities.* Windsor: NFER-Nelson.

LaPointe, L.L. (1977). Base-10 programmed stimulation: Task specification, scoring and plotting performance in aphasia therapy. *Journal of Speech and Hearing Disorders*, **42**, 90-105.

LaPointe, L.L., Horner, J. (1979). *Reading Comprehension Battery for Aphasia*. Austin, Tex.: PRO-ED.

Lee, L.L. (1969). *The Northwestern Syntax Screening Test*. Evanston, Ill.: Northwestern University Press.

Leiter, R. G. (1969). *The Leiter International Performance Scale*. Chicago: Stoeting & Co.

Locke, A. Beech, M. (1992). *Teaching Talking*. Windsor: NFER-Nelson.

Lowe, M., Costello, A. (1988). *Symbolic Play Test*, 2nd edn. Windsor: NFER-Nelson.

McKenna, P., Warrington, E. (1983). *Graded Naming Test*. Windsor: NFER-Nelson.

McNeil, M., Prescott, T. (1978). *Revised Token Test*. Baltimore: University Park Press.

Masidlover M., Knowles, W. (1987). *Derbyshire Language Scheme, revised edn*. Educational Psychology Service, Derbyshire County Council, Ripley.

Miles, T.R. (1982). *Bangor Dyslexia Test*. Wisbech, Cambs.: LDA.

Morgan-Barry, R. (1988). *Auditory Discrimination and Attention Test*. Windsor: NFER-Nelson.

Mulhall, D. (1989). *Functional Performance Record*. Windsor: NFER-Nelson.

Newton, M., Thomson, M. (1976). *Aston Index*. London: LDA.

Paraskevopoulus, J.N., Kirk, S.A. (1985). *The Development and Psychometric Characteristics of the Revised Illinois Test of Psycholinguistic Abilities*. Champaign: University of Illinois Press.

Porch, B. (1967). *The Porch Index of Communicative Ability*. Palo Alto: Consulting Psychologists Press.

Porch, B. (1971) *The Porch Index of Communicative Ability in Children*. Palo Alto: Consulting Psychologists Press.

Raven, J. (1977). *Raven's Progressive Matrices*. Windsor: NFER-Nelson.

Renfrew, C.E. (1989). *Renfrew Language Attainment Scales*. Oxford: Churchill Hospital.

Renfrew, C.E. (1988). *Word Finding Vocabulary*, 3rd edn. Oxford: the author.

Reynell, J. (1985). *Reynell Developmental Language Scales*, 2nd edn revised by M Huntley. Windsor: NFER-Nelson.

Rinaldi, W. (1992). *Social Use of Language Programme – enhancing the social communication of children and teenagers with special educational needs*. Windsor: NFER-Nelson.

Rustin, L. (1987). *Assessment and Therapy Programme for Dysfluent Children*. Windsor: NFER-Nelson.

Schuell, H. (1973). *Minnesota Test for the Differential Diagnosis of Aphasia*, revised edn. Windsor: NFER-Nelson.

Sheridan, M. (1973). *STYCAR Hearing Tests*. Windsor: NFER-Nelson.

Sheridan, M. (1976). *STYCAR Language Test*. Windsor: NFER-Nelson.

Shriberg L., Kwiatowski, J. (1980). *Natural Process Analysis*. New York: Wiley.

Skinner, C., Wiez, S., Thimpson, I. and Davidson, J. (1984). *Edinburgh Functional Communication Profile: An observation procedure of the evaluation of disorderd communication in elderly patients*. Winslow, Bucks: Winslow Press.

Spellacy, F.J., Spreen, O. (1969). A short form of the Token Test. *Cortex*, **5**, 390.

Stutsman, R. (1926-1931). *Merrill-Palmer Pre-School Performance Scale*. Steolting Co.

Syder, D., Body, R., Parker, M., Boddy, M. (1994). *Sheffield Screening Test for Acquired Language Disorders*. Windsor: NFER-Nelson.

Thorndike, R., Hagen, E., Sattler, J. (1985). *Stanford-Binet Intelligence Scale,* 4th edn.Windsor: NFER-Nelson.

Thorndike, R., Hagen, E., Sattler, J. (1986). *Stanford-Binet Intelligence Scale: Guide for Administering and Scoring the Fourth Edition.* Chicago: Riverside.

Wechsler, D. (1981). *Wechsler Adult Intelligence Scale–Revised.* New York: The Psychological Corporation.

Wechsler, D. (1991). *Wechsler Intelligence Scale for Children–Revised.* San Antonio: The Psychological Corporation.

Weiner, F.F. (1979). *Phonological Process Analysis.* Baltimore, Maryland: University Park Press.

Wheldall, K. (1987). *Sentence Comprehension Test.,* revised edn. Windsor: NFER-Nelson.

Whurr, R. (1974). *The Aphasia Screening Test.* London: Whurr.

Wiig, E.H. (1982a). *Let's Talk –Developing Prosocial Communication Skills.* New York: The Psychological Corporation.

Wiig, E.H. (1982b). *Let's Talk – Inventory for Adolescents (LTIA).* New York: The Psychological Corporation.

Wiig, E.H. (1983). *Let's Talk –For Children.(LTC).* New York: The Psychological Corporation.

Wiig, E.H. (1984). *Let's Talk - Intermediate Level (LTIL).* New York: The Psychological Corporation.

Wiig, E.H. (1987). *Let's Talk –Inventory for Children (LTIC).* New York: The Psychological Corporation.

Wiig, E.H. (1988a). *CELF-R Scoring Assistant.* New York: The Psychological Corporation.

Wiig, E.H. (1988b). *CELF-R Screening Test.* New York: The Psychological Corporation.

Wiig E.H. (1994). *Clinical Evaluation of Language Fundamentals - Revised Edition,* UK Adaptation (CELF-R^{UK}). New York: The Psychological Corporation.

Appendix II:
Speech and language development

Age	Description.
0;0–0;3	Cries and reflexive sounds.
0;3–1;0	Babbling begins; babbling and intonation sounds like human language, i.e. babbling drift.
1;3–2;6	Lexical overgeneralisation, i.e. protowords or vocables.
1;0–1;9	First word stage: later in this stage, intonation is used meaningfully.
1;9–2;3	Second word stage; the child begins to use semantic categories; his language begins to become more complex.

Acquisition of syntax.

Verb phrase – tense, aspect, mood

(a) Simple present
(b) Progressive
(c) Past tense (use of 'did')
(d) Future (use of 'going to')
(e) Passive (develops between 6;0-9;0)

Auxiliary

(a) Can't ⎫ used as
(b) Don't ⎭ negatives
(c) No/not – alternatives
(d) Did
(e) Will
(f) Can

Negation

(a) No/not (used at start of sentence)
(b) Can't ⎫ used as
(c) Don't ⎭ negatives
(d) No/not – used as alternatives
    e.g. I no eat meat
    e.g. I not eat meat

Noun phrase – demonstratives/articles, pronouns, adjectives

Order of appearance in:

1. Demonstratives/articles
   (a) this/that
   (b) indefinite article
   (c) definite article
2. Pronouns
   (a) (i) 1st person subject – I (me/mine)
       (ii) 3rd person inanimate – it (object)
   (b) (i) 1st person object – me, mine
       (ii) 3rd person inanimate – it (subject)
   (c) he, she, him, her
   (d) remainder includes second person and plurals
3. Adjectives
   (a) adjectives of size
   (b) adjectives of affection
   (c) adjectives of colour

Some adjectives appear at two-word stage

Adverbials

(a) Location – two word stage
(b) Time – 6 months after start of two-word stage
(c) Manner – end of first year of developing syntax
(d) Sentence adverbials – 4;0

Prepositions

(a) In, on, under
(b) Back, front, between (+featured object)
(c) Back, front (+unfeatured object)
(d) Left, right

Interrogative

(a) Yes/no questions   – marked by intonation and gesture
                       – auxiliaries added not necessarily correctly formed, e.g. does lions walk?
                       – auxiliary-subject inversion correctly used
(b) Wh- questions   – wh- words without auxiliary or inversion, e.g. where me sleep?
                       – wh- word with auxiliary but without inversion, e.g. where me do sleep?
                       – wh- word used correctly with both auxiliary and inversion, e.g. where do I sleep?

Acquisition of wh- words

(a) What
(b) Where – used for locatives in two-word stages
(c) Why   ⎫ large gap between the development
    What ⎬ of these three and first two seems
    Where ⎭ to reflect cognitive/social development

Conjunctions

(a)   And, but (early)
(b) So, if, because, when ⎫ developed by
(c) Before, after   ⎬ almost 4;0

Acquisition of morphology

Inflectional morphology

1. The form of morpheme occurs as a free variant with the root form:
   (a) third person simple present
             [s] after voiceless C
   {z} ⤵ [z] after voiced C
             [ɪz] after sibilants
   (b). past tense
             [t] after voiceless C
   {D} ⤵ [d] after voiced C
             [ɪd] after /t,d/

2. The morpheme occurs correctly and consistently but is not always used where it would be obligatory in adult language.

3. The morpheme occurs correctly and consistently although the actual phonological form may vary.

Note: The transition between (2) and (3) may take several months so it is difficult to say when the morpheme is used correctly; it is best to say it is present when it occurs on 90 per cent of occasions where it would occur in adult language. Using such a criterion the order of inflectional morphemes is as follows:

(a) Present progressive {be...ing}
(b) Plural
(c) Past
(d) Third person singular present

Note: these forms are only acquired in this order, not necessarily with meaning (*see also* MEAN LENGTH OF UTTERANCE).

Acquisition of lexis

Comprehension of words is very likely to be ahead of their production.

1. Production averages (words):
By 1;6	100–200
By 2;6	500
By 5;0	2000
By 6;0–7;0	4000

2. Words learnt in order:
   (a) names for classes of food
   (b) body parts
   (c) articles of clothing
   (d) small household/garden objects
   (e) animals
   (f) vehicles
   (g) toys
   (h) pictures in picture books

3. Word meaning:
   (a) reference – most words learnt this way; the object is present when named but could lead to mislearning.
   (b) linguistic induction – at 3;0–4;0. The children begin to guess the meaning of the new word by knowing the meaning of the words in the immediate environment of the new one.
   (c) learning by deduction – comes later, perhaps not until the child's early years at school.

Note: These have been found in research and are based on Cruttenden (1979). As there is variation in children's acquisition of speech and language, all ages given and the order of various items should be treated with caution.

Appendix III: The International Phonetic Alphabet (revised to 1989)

CONSONANTS

	Bilabial	Labiodental	Dental	Alveolar	Postalveolar	Retroflex	Palatal	Velar	Uvular	Pharyngeal	Glottal
Plosive	p b			t d		ʈ ɖ	c ɟ	k g	q ɢ		ʔ
Nasal	m	ɱ		n		ɳ	ɲ	ŋ	N		
Trill	ʙ			r					R		
Tap or Flap				ɾ		ɽ					
Fricative	ɸ β	f v	θ ð	s z	ʃ ʒ	ʂ ʐ	ç ʝ	x ɣ	χ ʁ	ħ ʕ	h ɦ
Lateral fricative				ɬ ɮ							
Approximant		ʋ		ɹ		ɻ	j	ɰ			
Lateral approximant				l		ɭ	ʎ	L			
Ejective stop	p'			t'		ʈ'	c'	k'	q'		
Implosive	ƥ ɓ			ƭ ɗ			ƈ ʄ	ƙ ɠ	ʠ ʛ		

Where symbols appear in pairs, the one to the right represents a voiced consonant. Shaded areas denote articulations judged impossible.

DIACRITICS

◌̥ Voiceless	n̥ d̥	◌̹ More rounded	ɔ̹	◌ʷ Labialised	tʷ dʷ	◌̃ Nasalised	ẽ
◌̌ Voiced	s̬ t̬	◌̜ Less rounded	ɔ̜	◌ʲ Palatalised	tʲ dʲ	◌ⁿ Nasal release	dⁿ
◌ʰ Aspirated	tʰ dʰ	◌̟ Advanced	u̟	◌ˠ Velarised	tˠ dˠ	◌ˡ Lateral release	dˡ
◌̈ Breathy voiced	b̤ a̤	◌̠ Retracted	i̠	◌ˤ Pharyngealised	tˤ dˤ	◌̚ No audible release	d̚
◌̰ Creaky voiced	b̰ a̰	◌̈ Centralised	ë	~ Veralised or pharyngealised	ɫ		
◌̼ Linguolabial	t̼ d̼	◌̽ Mid-centralised	ë̽	◌̝ Raised	e̝ (ɹ̝ = voiced alveolar fricative)		
◌̪ Dental	t̪ d̪	◌̩ Syllabic	ɹ̩	◌̞ Lowered	e̞ (β̞ = voiced bilabial approximant)		
◌̺ Apical	t̺ d̺	◌̯ Non-syllabic	e̯	◌̘ Advanced tongue root	e̘		
◌̻ Laminal	t̻ d̻	◌˞ Rhoticity	ə˞	◌̙ Retracted tongue root	e̙		

243

VOWELS

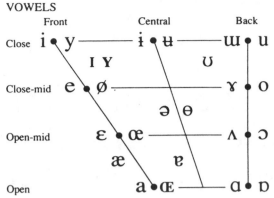

Where symbols appear in pairs, the one to the right
represents a rounded vowel.

OTHER SYMBOLS

ʍ	Voiceless labial–velar fricative	ʘ	Bilabial click
w	Voiced labial–velar approximant	ǀ	Dental click
ɥ	Voiced labial–palatal approximant	ǃ	(Post)alveolar click
ʜ	Voiceless epiglottal fricative	ǂ	Palatoalveolar click
ʢ	Voiced epiglottal fricative	ǁ	Alveolar lateral click
ʡ	Epiglottal plosive	ɺ	Alveolar lateral flap
ɕ ʑ	Alveolopalatal fricatives	ɧ	Simultaneous ʃ and x
ɝ	Additional mid-central vowel		

Affricates and double articulations can be represented
by two symbols joined by a tie bar if necessary. k͡p t͡s

SUPRASEGMENTALS

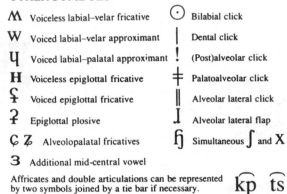

ˈ Primary stress ˌfoʊnəˈtɪʃən

ˌ Secondary stress

ː Long eː

ˑ Half-long eˑ

˘ Extra-short ĕ

. Syllable break ɹi.ækt

| Minor (foot) group

‖ Major (intonation) group

‿ Linking (absence of a break)

↗ Global rise

↘ Global fall

TONES and WORD ACCENTS

LEVEL

e̋ or ˥	Extra high	
é ˦	High	
ē ˧	Mid	
è ˨	Low	
ȅ ˩	Extra low	
↓	Downstep	
↑	Upstep	

CONTOUR

ě or ˩˥	Rising	
ê ˥˩	Falling	
e᷄ ˧˥	High rising	
e᷅ ˩˧	Low rising	
e᷈ ˧˩˧	Rising–falling etc.	

Appendix IV: acknowledgement of trademarks and UK suppliers of aac devices and software

Many high-tech communication aids and computer software have been described in the dictionary. The author would like to acknowledge the trademarks of these products where known to him. The names of the suppliers in the UK are also given.

AllTalk, EvalPAC, RealVoice, SpeechPAC, ToyPAC, DAC are all trademarks of Adaptive Communication Systems and are supplied in the UK by Rainbow Rehab, Unit 15, 7 Airfield Rd., Christchurch, Dorset, BH23 3TQ.

Alpha Talker, Blissymbol Minspeak Component Words Strategy (BMW), Communic-Ease, Delta Talker, Director, EMOS, HeadMaster, Interaction, Education and Play (IEP+), Intro Talker, Language, Learning and Living (LLL), Liberator, Light Talker, Minspeak Application Programs, Power in Play, Scanning Director, Stories and Strategies for Communication (SSC), Topics to Learn Communication (TLC), Touch Talker, Unity/128, Walker Talker, Words Strategy are all trademarks of Prentke Romich Company. These products are supplied in the UK by Liberator Ltd., Whitegates, Swinstead, Lincs, NG33 4PA and in Europe by Prentke Romich Europe at the same address.

BIGmack, Big Red switches, Jelly Bean switches, SpeakEasy, are all trademarks of AbleNet Ltd. and are supplied in the UK by Liberator Ltd., Whitegates, Swinstead, Lincs, NG33 4PA.

CAMELEON, CommPac, EZ Keys, FingerFoniks, MessageMate, System 2000/Versa, Talking Screen are all trademarks of Words + and are supplied in the UK by Cambridge Adaptive Communication, The Mount, Toft, Cambridge, CB3 7RL.

Canon Communicator is a trademark of Canon and is supplied in Scotland by BCF Technology Ltd., 8 Brewster Square, Brucefield Industrial Park, Livingston, West Lothian EH54 9BJ and in the rest of the UK by Easiaids.

DAVE, Fourtalk is supplied by Quest Enabling Designs.

DECtalk is a trademark of Digital Equipment Corporation.

DynaVox, DynaSyms, Dyna Write and DynaCard are registered trademarks of Sentient Systems Technology. DynaVox is supplied by Rainbow Rehab, Unit 15, 7 Airfield Rd., Christchurch, Dorset, BH23 3TQ.

Echo is a trademark of Street Electronics.

HeadMouse is a trademark of Origin Systems and is supplied in the UK by Don Johnstone Special Needs Ltd, c/o NW SEMERC, 1 Broadbent Rd., Watersheddings, Oldham, OL1 4HU.

Ke:nx is a registered trademark of Don Johnstone Development Equipment, Inc. In the

UK, contact Jamie Munro, Don Johnston Special Needs Ltd, 18 Clarenden Court, Calver Rd, Winwick Quay, Warrington WA2 8QP.

Lightwriter is manufactured and supplied by Toby Churchill Ltd, 20 Panton St., Cambridge, CB2 1HP.

Macaw and Parrot are trademarks of Zygo Industries. Zygo equipment is supplied in the UK by Toby Churchill Ltd, 20 Panton St., Cambridge, CB2 1HP.

Minspeak is a trademark of Semantic Compaction Systems.

Persona is supplied by Hugh Steeper Ltd.

ScreenDoors, Telepathic and Magic Cursor are trademarks of Madenta Communications Inc. and are supplied by Liberator Ltd and Don Johnstone Special Needs Ltd.

SmoothTalker is a trademark of First Byte.

Talking Lifestyles is a vocabulary set written for the Orac. Orac is manufactured and supplied by Mardis, Business Development Centre, Fylde Ave., Lancaster University, Bailrigg, Lancaster, LA1 4YR.

T-TAM was developed by the Trace Research and Development Centre in Madison, Wisconsin.

WiViK2, WiVOX and KeyREP are registered trademarks of the Hugh MacMillan Rehabilitation Centre and are supplied by Liberator Ltd.

WordWriter is copyrighted by McIntyre Computer Systems 22809 Shagbark, Birmingham, Michigan 48025 USA.

X-10 is a registered trademark of X-10, Inc. and is supplied in the UK by Quest Enabling Designs Ltd, Ability House, 242 Gosport Rd., Fareham, Hants PO16 0SS.

Bibliography

Abercrombie, D. (1967). *Elements of General Phonetics*. Edinburgh: Edinburgh University Press.

Adams, C., Bishop, D.V.M. (1989). Conversational characteristics of children with semantic–pragmatic disorder. I: Exchange structure, turntaking, repairs and cohesion. *British Journal of Disorders of Communication*, 24;3: 211-239.

Adams, S.G., Lang, A.E. (1992). Can the Lombard effect be used to improve voice intensity in Parkinson's Disease? *European Journal of Communication Disorders*, 27;2 121-128.

Aiken, L.R. (1985). *Psychological Testing and Assessment*. Massachusetts: Allyn and Bacon.

Ainsworth, M.D.S. (1979). Infant-Mother Attachment. *American Psychologist*, 34, 932-937.

Allerton, D.J. (1979). *Essentials of Grammatical Theory: A consensus of syntax and morphology*. London: Routledge and Kegan Paul.

Allum, D.J. (1996). *Cochlear Implant Rehabilitation in Children and Adults*. London: Whurr.

Argyle, M. (1994). *The Psychology of Interpersonal Behaviour*. London: Penguin.

Atkinson, R.L., Atkinson, R.C., Smith, E.E., Bem, D.J, Nolen-Hoeksema, S. (1993) (11th edn) *Introduction to Psychology*. New York: Harcourt Brace Jovanovich.

Atkinson, R.L., Atkinson, R.C., Smith, E.E., Bem, D.J, Nolen-Hoeksema, S. (1996) (12th ed) *Hilgard's Introduction to Psychology*. New York: Harcourt Brace Jovanovich.

Badman, A.L., Baker, B., Banajee, M., Cross, R., Lehr, J.S., Maro, J., Zucco, M. (1995). *Unity/128*. Wooster, Ohio: Prentke Romich Company.

Bailey, P., Jenkinson, J. (1982). The Application of Blissymbols. In M. Peter and R. Barnes (Eds), *Signs, Symbols and Schools: An introduction to the use of non-vocal communication systems and sign language in schools*. Chester: NCSE.

Baker B. (1982). Minspeak: A semantic compaction system that makes self-expression easier for communicatively disabled individuals. *Byte*, Sept.

Baker, B. (1989). Words Strategy. *Proceedings of 1st UK Minspeak Conference*, Sept. 1989.

Barker, P. (1981). *Basic Family Therapy*. London: Granada.

Barlow, D.H., Hersen, M. (1984). *Single Case Experimental Designs: Strategies for studying behaviour change*. Oxford: Pergamon Press.

Barr, M.L. (1979). *The Human Nervous System: An Anatomical Viewpoint*. Maryland: Harper and Row.

Basso, A. (1992). Prognostic factors in aphasia. *Aphasiology*, 6:4 337-348.

Beard, R.M. (1969). *An Outline of Piaget's Developmental Psychology*. London: Routledge and Kegan Paul.

Beech, J.R., Harding, L., Hilton-Jones, D. (1993). *Assessments in Speech and Language Therapy*. London: Routledge.

Bench, J. (1992). *Communication Skills in Hearing-Impaired Children*. London: Whurr.

Benson, D.F. (1979). Neurologic correlates of anomia. In H.A. Whitaker & H. Whitaker (Eds), *Studies in Neurolinguistics*, vol. 4. London: Academic Press.

Benson, D.F. and Geschwind, N. (1969). The Alexias. In P.J. Vinken and G.W. Bruyn (Eds), *Handbook of Clinical Neurology* vol 4, 112–140. Amsterdam: North Holland Publishing Company.

Berko, J., Brown, R. (1960) Psycholinguistic research in children's language. In P.H. Mussen (ed). *Handbook of Research Methods in Child Development*. New York: John Wiley & Sons.

Berry, P. (Ed.) (1976). *Language and Communication in the Mentally Handicapped*. London: Edward Arnold.

Beukelman, D.R., Mirenda, P. (1992). *Augmentative and Alternative Communication: Management of Severe Communication Disorders in Children and Adults*. Baltimore: Paul H. Brookes Publishing Co.

Bishop, D.V.M. (1979). Comprehension in developmental language disorders. *Developmental Medical Child Neurology,* **21**: 225-238.

Bishop, D.V.M. (1982). Comprehension of spoken, written and signed sentences in childhood language disorders. *Journal of Child Psychology Psychiatry,* **23**;1: 1-20.

Bishop, D.V.M. (1984). Automated LARSP: computer-assisted grammatical analysis. *British Journal of Disorders of Communication,* **19**;1: 78-87.

Bishop, D.V.M., Adams, C. (1989). Conversational characteristics of children with semantic-pragmatic disorders. II: What features lead to a judgement of innappropriacy? *British Journal of Disorders of Communication,* **24**;3: 241-263.

Bishop, D.V.M., Mogford, K. (1993). *Language Development in Exceptional Circumstances*. Hove: Lawrence Erlbaum Associates.

Bishop, P. (1985). *Comprehensive Computer Studies*. London: Hodder & Stoughton.

Blanken, G. (1991). The functional basis of speech automatisms (recurring utterances). *Aphasiology,* **5**;2: 103-128.

Bliss, C.K. (1965). *Semantography: Blissymbolics*. Sydney, Australia: Symantography Publications.

Boden, M.A. (1994). *Piaget*, 2nd edn. London: Fontana Press.

Bollinger, R.L., Musson, N.D., Holland, A.L. (1993). A study of group communication intervention with chronic aphasic persons. *Aphasiology,* **7**;3: 301-314.

Bolton, S.O., Dalshiell, S.E. (1984) *Interaction Checklist for Augmentative Communication*. California: Imaginative Communication Products.

Bornstein, H., Hamilton, L.B. (1978). *Signed English. Ways and Means*. Globe Education.

Bromley, D.B. (1988). *Human Ageing: An Introduction to Gerontology*. London: Penguin.

Brookshear, J. Glenn. (1991). *Computer Science: An Overview*. California: Benjamin Cummings.

Brosnahan, L.F., Malmberg, B. (1976). *Introduction to Phonetics*. Cambridge: Cambridge University Press.

Brown, K., Miller, J. (1991) *Syntax: A Linguistic Introduction to Sentence Structure,* 2nd edn. London: Routledge.

Brown, R. (1973). *A First Language: The Early Stages*. Cambridge, MA: Harvard University Press.

Bruno, J. (1989). Interaction, Education and Play. *Proceedings of 1st UK Minspeak Conference*. Swinstead: Liberator.

Bruno, J. (1992). *Topics to Learn Communication*. Wooster, Ohio: Prentke Romich company.

Butterworth B. (1984). Jargon Aphasia: processes and strategies. In S.K. Newman, & R. Epstein (Eds), *Current Perspectives in Dysphasia*. Edinburgh: Churchill Livingstone.

Byers Brown, B. (1976). Language vulnerability, speech delay and therapeutic intervention. *British Journal of Disorders of Communication*, **11**: 43-56.

Byers Brown, B. (1981). *Speech Therapy: Principles and Practice*. Edinburgh: Churchill Livingstone.

Byers Brown, B., Edwards, M. (1989). *Development Disorders of Language*. London: Whurr.

Byrne, K., Abbeduto, L., Brooks, P. (1990). The language of children with spina bifida and hydrocephalus meeting tasks demands and mastering syntax. *Journal of Speech and Hearing Disorders*, **55;1**: 118-123.

Canning, B.A., Rose, M.F. (1974). Clinical measurements of the speed of tongue and lip movements in British children with normal speech. *British Journal of Disorders of Communication*, **9;1**: 45-50.

Carr, P. (1993). *Phonology*. London: MacMillan.

Catford, J.C. (1977). *Fundamental Problems in Phonetics*. Edinburgh: Edinburgh University Press.

Catford, J.C. (1989). *Practical Introduction to Phonetics*. Oxford: Clarendon Press.

Chandor, A., Graham, J., Williamson, R. (1985). *The Penguin Dictionary of Computers*. London: Penguin.

Chomsky, N. (1957). *Syntactic Structures*. The Hague: Mouton.

Chomsky, N. (1965). *Aspects of the Theory of Syntax*. Cambridge, Mass.: M.I.T. Press.

Chomsky, N., Halle, M. (1968). *The Sound Pattern of English*. New York: Harper and Row.

Chomsky, N. (1972). *Language and Mind*. New York: Harcourt Brace Jovanovich.

Chomsky, N. (1982). *Some Concepts and Consequences of the Theory of Government and Binding*. Cambridge, Mass.: M.I.T. Press.

Clark, H.H., Clark E.V., (1977). *Psychology and Language*: An Introduction to *Psycholinguistics*. New York: Harcourt Brace Jovanovich.

Clarke, A.M., Clarke, A.D.B. (1974). *Readings in Mental Deficiency*: The changing outlook. London: Methuen.

Clarke, G.M., Cooke, D. (1992). *A Basic Course in Statistics*. London: Edward Arnold.

Code, C., Müller, D.J. (1989). *Aphasia Therapy*. London: Whurr.

Code, C., Müller, D.J. (1995). *Treatment of Aphasia: From Theory to Practice*. London: Whurr.

Code, C., Müller, D.J. (1996). *Forums in Clinical Aphasiology*. London: Whurr.

Coltheart, M. (1983). Aphasia therapy research: A single case study approach. In C. Code and D.J. Müller. *Aphasia Therapy*. London: Whurr.

Crockford, C., Lesser, R. (1994). Assessing functional communication in aphasia: clinical utility and time demands of three methods. *European Journal of Communication Disorders*, **29;2**: 165-182.

Cross, R.T. (1991). *Intro Talker IEP+*. Wooster, Ohio: Prentke Romich.

Crossley, R. (1988). Unexpected communication attainment by persons diagnosed as autistic and intellectually impaired. *Proceedings of 5th ISAAC Conference*, Anaheim, Calif.

Crossley, R., McDonald, A. (1984). *Annie's Coming Out*. New York: Viking Penguin.

Cruttenden, A. (1970). A phonetic study in babbling. *British Journal of Disorders of Communication*, **5**: 110-117.

Cruttenden, A. (1972). Phonological procedures for child language. *British Journal of Disorders of Communication*. 7;30–37.

Cruttenden, A. (1979). *Language in Infancy and Childhood*. Manchester: Manchester University Press.

Cruttenden, A. (1994). *Gimson's Pronunciation of English 5th Edition*. London: Edward Arnold.

Crystal, D. (1981). *Clinical Linguistics*. London: Whurr.

Crystal, D. (1992). *Profiling Linguistic Disability*. London: Whurr.

Crystal, D. (1993). *Introduction to Language Pathology*. London: Whurr.

Crystal, D. (1984). *Linguistic Encounters with Language Handicap*. London: Blackwell.

Crystal, D., Davy, D. (1969). *Investigating English Style*. London: Longman.

Crystal, D., Fletcher, P., Garman, M. (1989). *The Grammatical Analysis of Language Disability*. London: Whurr.

Culler, J. (1986). *Saussure, 2nd edn*. London: Fontana.

Cunningham, C. (1982). *Down's Syndrome: An Introduction for Parents*. London: Souvenir Press.

Dalton, P. (1983). *Approaches to the Treatment of Stuttering*. Beckenham, Kent: Croom Helm.

Dalton, P. (1994). *Counselling People with Communication Problems*. London: Sage Publications Ltd.

Dalton, P., Hardcastle, W.J. (1989). *Disorders of Fluency and their Effect on Communication*. London: Whurr.

Darley, F.L., Aranson, A.E., Brown, J.R. (1975). *Motor Speech Disorders*. Philadelphia: Saunders.

Davison, G.C., Neale, J.M. (1994). *Abnormal Psychology, 6th rev edn*. New York: Wiley.

De Meyer, W. (1972). Megalencephaly in Children. *Neurology*, **22**: 634-643.

Denes, P.B., Pinson, E.N. (1973). *The Speech Chain: The Physics and Biology of Spoken Language*. New York: Anchor.

Diagnostic and Statistical Manual of Mental Disorders, 4th edn (DSM-IV) (1991). Washington, DC: American Psychiatric Association.

Donaldson, Margaret (1987). *Children's Minds*. Glasgow: Fontana/Collins.

Draper, I.T. (1980). *Lecture Notes on Neurology*. Oxford: Blackwell.

Duckworth, M. (1990). A report on changes to the IPA symbols. *The Bulletin*, **462**: 5-7, Royal College of Speech and Language Therapy.

Edels, Y. (Ed.) (1983). *Laryngectomy: Diagnosis to Rehabilitation*. Beckenham, Kent: Croom Helm.

Edwards, A.D.N. (1990). *Speech Synthesis – Technology for Disabled People*. London: Paul Chapman.

Edwards, M., Watson, A.C.H. (Eds)(1980). *Advances in the Management of Cleft Palate*. Edinburgh: Churchill Livingstone.

Eisenson, J. (1984). *Adult Aphasia*. New Jersey: Prentice Hall.

Ellis, A. W. (1993). *Reading, Writing and Dyslexia: A Cognitive Analysis*. Hove: Lawrence Erlbaum Associates.

Ellis, A., Beattie, G. (1986). *The Psychology of Language and Communication*. Hove: Lawrence Erlbaum Associates.

Ellis, K. (Ed.) (1990). *Autism: Professional Perspectives and Practice*. London: Chapman & Hall.

Enderby, P. (1987). *Assistive Communication Aids for the Speech Impaired*. Edinburgh: Chuchill Livingstone.

Erikson, E. H. (1963). *Childhood and Society*. New York: Norton.

Fawcus, M. (1989). Group therapy: A learning situation. In C. Code & D.J. Müller (Eds) (1989), *Adult Aphasia*. London: Whurr.

Fawcus, M. (Ed.) (1991). *Voice Disorders and Their Management*. London: Chapman & Hall.

Fawcus, M. (Ed.) (1992). *Group Encounters in Speech and Language Therapy*. London: Whurr.

Fay, W.H. (1993). Infantile autism. In D. Bishop & K. Mogford (Eds), *Language Development in Exceptional Circumstances*. Hove: Lawrence Erlbaum Associates.

Fitch, J.L. (1986). *Clinical Applications of Microcomputers in Communication Disorders*. London: Academic Press.

Fransella, F. (1972). *Personal Change and Reconstruction*. London & New York: Academic Press.

Fromkin,V., Rodman, R. (1993). *An Introduction to Language, 5th edn*. New York: Holt-Saunders International Editions.

Fry, D.B. (1979). *The Physics of Speech*. Cambridge: Cambridge University Press.

Garnham, A. (1985). *Psycholinguistics: Central topics*. London: Routledge.

Garvey, C. (1977). *Play: The Developing Child*. Glasgow: J Fontana/Collins.

German, D.J. (1986) *Test of Word Finding*. DLM Teaching Resources.

Gillham, W. (1979). *The First Words Language Programme*. London: George Allen & Unwin and Beaconsfield Publishers.

Gilroy, J., Holliday, P.L. (1982). *Basic Neurology*. New York: Macmillan.

Ginsberg, I. A. and White, T. P. (1985). Otologic considerations in audiology. In J. Katz, *Handbook of Clinical Audiology*. Baltimore: Williams & Wilkins.

Goodglass, H., Kaplan, E. (1983). *The Assessment of Aphasia and Related Disorders*. Philadelphia: Lea & Febiger.

Goodman, R.M., Gorlin, R.J. (1983). *The Malformed Infant: An Illustrated Guide*. Oxford: Oxford University Press.

Gordon, N. and McKinley, I. (1980). *Helping Clumsy Children*. Edinburgh: Churchill Livingstone.

Green, D.S. (1978). Pure tone air conduction testing. In J. Katz (1985), *Handbook of Clinical Audiology*. Baltimore: Williams & Wilkins.

Green, G. (1984). Communication in therapy: some of the procedures and issues involved. *British Journal of Disorders of Communication, 19*: 35-46.

Green, J.H. (1978). *Basic Clinical Physiology*. Oxford: Oxford University Press.

Greenbaum, S., Quirk, R. (1990). *A Student's Grammar of the English Language*. (8th impression, 1995). Essex: Longman.

Greene, M.C.L., Mathieson, L. (1989). *The Voice and its Disorders*. London: Whurr.

Greven, A.J., Meijer, M.F., Tiwari, R.M. (1994). Articulation after total glossectomy: a clinical study of six patients. *European Journal of Disorders of Communication, 29;1*: 85-94.

Grove,N., Walker, M. (1990). The Makaton Vocabulary: Using manual signs and graphic symbols to develop interpersonal communication. *Alternative and Augmentative Communication, 6*: 15–28.

Grunwell, P. (1987). *Clinical Phonology*. Beckenham, Kent: Croom Helm.

Grunwell, P. (Ed.) (1993). *Analysing Cleft Palate Speech*. London: Whurr.

Haas, W. (1963). Phonological analysis of a case of dyslexia. *Journal of Speech and Hearing Disorders, 28;3*: 239–246.

Haines, R.W., Mohiuddin, A. (1972). *Handbook of Embryology*. Edinburgh: Churchill Livingstone.

Halliday, M. (1994). *An Introduction to Functional Grammar, 2nd edn*. London: Edward Arnold.

Hodgson, W.R. (1985). Testing infants and young children. In J. Katz (1985), *Handbook of Clinical Audiology*. Baltimore: Williams & Wilkins.

Hood, J.D. (1981). Speech audiometry. In H. A. Beagley, *Audiology and Audiological Medicine*. Vol. 1, chap. 7, Oxford: Oxford University Press.

Hopkins, H.L., Smith H.D. (1993) *Willard and Spackman's Occupational Therapy, 8th edn*. Philadelphia: Lippinott Co.

Hornsby, B. (1984). *Overcoming Dyslexia*. London: Dunitz.

Hornstein, N., Lightfoot, D. (Eds) (1981). *Explanation in Linguistics: The Logical Problem of Language Acquisition*. London: Longman.

Hosking, G. (1982). *An Introduction to Paediatric Neurology*. London: Faber & Faber.

Huddleston, R. (1976). *An Introduction to English Transformational Grammar*. London: Longman.

Hyman, L.M. (1975). *Phonology, Theory and Analysis*. London: Holt Rinehart and Winston.

Illingworth, R.S. (1987). *The Development of the Young Infant and Young Child: Normal and Abnormal*. Edinburgh: Churchill Livingstone.

Jacobson, J.T., Hyde M.L. (1985). An introduction to auditory evoked potentials. In J. Katz (1985), *Handbook of Clinical Audiology*. Baltimore: Williams & Wilkins.

Jakobson, R., Halle, M. (1956) *Fundamentals of Language*. The Hague: Mouton.

Jennings, A.A. (1984). What do I get for my money? *The Bulletin*, **382**: Royal College of Speech and Language Therapists.

Johns, D.F. (1981). *Clinical Management of Neurogenic Communicative Disorders*. Boston: Little, Brown & Company.

Jones, A.P. (1989). Language, Learning and Living. *Proceedings of 1st UK Minspeak Conference*, Sept. 1989, 70-91. Swinstead: Liberator.

Jones, A.P. (1991). *Language, Learning & Living*. Wooster, Ohio: Prentke Romich.

Jones, A.P. (1992). *Teaching Language, Learning & Living*. Swinstead: Liberator.

Jones, A.P. (1995a). *IMPACT: Implementing Augmentative Communication Training – A manual for staff training*. Swinstead: Liberator.

Jones, A.P. (1995b). *PATHWAYS: Language, Learning and Living for beginners*. Swinstead: Liberator.

Joseph, J. (1979). *Essential Anatomy*. Lancaster: MTP Press.

Josey, A.F. (1985). Auditory brainstem response in site of lesion testing. In J. Katz (1985), *Handbook of Clinical Audiology*. Baltimore: William & Wilkins.

Kallen, D., Marshall, R.C., Casey, D.E. (1986). Atypical dysarthria in Munchausen syndrome. *British Journal of Disorders of Communication*, **21;3**: 377-380.

Katz, J. (1985). *Handbook of Clinical Audiology*. Baltimore: Williams & Wilkins.

Katz, J. (1994) *Handbook of Clinical Audiology 4th edn*. Baltimore: Williams & Wilkins.

Katz, R.C. (1986). *Aphasia Treatment and Microcomputers*. London: Taylor and Francis.

Kaye, A. (1991). *Essential Neurosurgery*. Edinburgh: Churchill Livingstone.

Kazdin, A. (1981). The token economy. In G. Davey (Ed.) (1981), *Applications of Conditioning Theory*. London: Methuen.

Keller, E. (1994). *Fundamentals of Speech Synthesis and Speech Recognition*. New York: Wiley.

Kelly, G.A. (1955). *The Psychology of Personal Constructs*. New York: Norton.

Kempe, R.S., Kempe, C.H. (1978). *Child Abuse*. Suffolk: Fontana/Open Books.

Kennedy, M., Murdoch, B.E. (1994). Thalamic aphasia and striato-capsular aphasia as independent aphasic syndromes: a review. *Aphasiology*, **8;4**: 303-313.

Kenstowicz, M. (1994). *Phonology in Generative Grammar*. Massachusetts: Blackwell Publishers.

Kersner, M. (1992). *Tests of Voice, Speech and Language*. London: Whurr.

Kiernan, C., Reid, B., Jones, L. (1982). *Signs and Symbols*. London: Heinemann Educational Books.

Kleppe, S.A., Katayama, K.C., Shipley, K.G., Foushee, D.R. (1990). The speech and language characteristics of children with Prader-Willi syndrome. *Journal of Speech and Hearing Disorders*, 55;2: 300-309.

Kolb, B., Whishaw, I.Q. (1990). *Fundamentals of Human Neuropsychology*. New York: W.H. Freeman and Co.

Ladefoged, P. (1962). *Elements of Acoustic Phonetics*. Chicago: Chicago University Press.

Ladefoged, P. (1971). *Preliminaries to Lingistic Phonetics*. Chicago: Chicago University Press.

Ladefoged, P. (1993). *A Course in Phonetics*. New York: Harcourt Brace Jovanovich.

Langley, J. (1987). *Working with Swallowing Disorders*. London: Winslow Press.

Le Dorze, G., Dionne, L., Ryalls, J., Julien, Ouellet M. (1992). The effects of speech and language therapy for a case of dysarthria associated with Parkinson's disease. *European Journal of Communication Disorders*, 27: 313-324.

Lebrun, Y. (1988). Language and epilepsy. *British Journal of Disorders of Communication*, 23;2: 97-110.

Lees, J. (1993). *Children with Acquired Aphasias*. London: Whurr.

Leeson, T.S., Leeson, C.R., Papano, A.A. (1985). *Textbook of Histology*. Philadelphia: W.B. Saunders.

Lepschy, G.C. (1982). *A Survey of Structural Linguistics*. London: Andre Deutsch.

Lesser, R. (1989). *Linguistic Investigations of Asphasia*. London: Whurr.

Lewis, V., Boucher, J., Astell, A. (1992). The assessment of symbolic play in young children: A prototype test. *European Journal of Disorders of Communication*, 27: 231-245.

Locke, A. (1985). *Living Language*. Berks: NFER-Nelson.

Lyons, J. (1968). *Introduction to Theoretical Linguistics*. Cambridge: Cambridge University Press.

Lyons, J. (1981). *Language and Linguistics*. Cambridge: Cambridge University Press.

Lyons, J. (1991). *Chomsky, 3rd edn*. London: Fontana.

Lysons, K. (1978). *Your Hearing Loss and How to Cope with it*. Vancouver, BC: David & Charles.

MacKay, D. (1975). *Clinical Psychology: Theory and Therapy*. London: Methuen.

MacMahon, M.K.C. (1990). *Basic Phonetics*. Unpublished.

McNaughton, S. (1992). *Blissymbol Component Minspeak Words Strategy*. Woosten, OH: Prentke Romich Company.

McTear, M.F. (1985). Pragmatic disorders: a case of conversational disability? *British Journal of Disorders of Communication*, 20;2: 129-142.

Mark, V.W., Thomas, B.E., Berndt, R.S. (1992). Factors associated with improvement in global aphasia. *Aphasiology*, 6;2: 121-134.

Martin, M. (Ed.) (1996). *Speech Audiometry*. London: Whurr.

Martins, I.P., Ferro, J.M. (1992). Recovery of acquired aphasia in children. *Aphasiology*, 6;4: 431-438.

Matthews, P.H. (1974). *Morphology: An Introduction to the Theory of Word-Structure*. Cambridge: Cambridge University Press.

Meadow, K. (1980). *Deafness and Child Development*. London: Edward Arnold.

Miller, M.H. (1972). *Hearing Aids*. Indianapolis: Bobbs-Merrill.

Miller, N. (1986). *Dyspraxia and Its Management*. Beckenham: Croom-Helm.

Miller, N. (1990). Review of the Pragmatics Profile by Dewart and Summers. *Clinical Linguistics and Phonetics*, 4: 179-182.

Miller, S. (1975). *Experimental Design and Statistics*. London: Methuen.

Morris, D. W. H. (1994). Speech and language therapy in the United Kingdom in the 1990s. *Logopedie*, 7;4: 18–21.

Morris, D.W.H. (1995a). AAC & Aphasia: Does Minspeak have a role to play? *Communication Matters Journal* (ISAAC UK), 9;1: 5–7.

Morris, D.W.H. (1995b). AAC & Aphasia II: Treatment, Technology and Language. *Proceedings of 9th Annual Minspeak Conference*, July 1995. Wooster, Ohio: Prentke Romich Company.

Murdoch, B.E., Hudson-Tennent, L.J. (1994). Speech disorders in children treated for posterior fossa tumours: ataxic and developmental features. *European Journal of Disorders of Communication*, 29;4: 379-397.

Murphy, J. and Scott, J. (1995). Attitudes and Strategies towards AAC: A training package for AAC users and carers. Stirling: University of Stirling.

Nelson-Jones, R. (1982). *The Theory and Practice of Counselling Psychology*. London: Holt, Rinehart and Winston.

Nickels, L. (1995). Reading too little into reading?: Strategies in the rehabilitation of acquired dyslexia. *European Journal of Disorders of Communication*, 30;1: 37-50.

Northern, J., Downs, M. (1984). *Hearing in Children*. Baltimore: Williams & Wilkins.

Nowell, R.C., (1985). Psychology of Hearing Impairment. In J. Katz, (1985). *Handbook of Clinical Audiology*. Baltimore: Williams & Wilkins.

Obler, L.K., Albert, M.L. (1981) Language in the elderly aphasic and in the dementing Patient. In M. T. Sarno (Ed.) (1981), *Acquired Aphasia*. London: Academic Press.

Palmer, F.R. (1976). *Semantics: A New Outline*. Cambridge: Cambridge University Press.

Palmer, L.R. (1978). *Descriptive and Comparative Linguistics: A Critical Introduction*. London: Faber.

Patel, P.G., Satz, P. (1994). The language production system and senile dementia of Alzheimer's type: neuropathological implications. *Aphasiology*, 8;1: 1-18.

Patterson, K., Kay, J. (1982). Letter-by-letter reading: psychological descriptions of a neurological syndrome. *Quarterly Journal of Experimental Psychology*, 34A: 411-441.

Pennington, L., Jolleff, N., McConachie, H., Wisbeach, A., Price, K. (1993). *My Turn to Speak: A Team Approach to Augmentative Communication*. London: Hospitals for Sick Children and the Institute of Child Health.

Peter, M., Barnes, R. (1982). *Signs, Symbols and Schools: An introduction to the use of non-vocal communication systems and sign language in schools*. Chester: NSCE.

Pit Corder, S. (1973). *Introducing Applied Linguistics*. London: Penguin.

Plant, G. (1993). The speech of adults with acquired profound hearing losses I: a perceptual evaluation. *European Journal of Communication Disorders*, 273-288.

Porch, B. (1971). *The Porch Index of Communicative Ability in Children*. Palo Alto: Consulting Psychologists Press.

Porkess, R. (1988). *Dictionary of Statistics*. Glasgow: Collins.

Pracy, R., Siegler, J., Stell, P.M. (1974). *A Short Textbook of Ear, Nose and Throat*. London: Hodder & Stoughton.

Pulvermüller, F., Roth, V.M. (1991). Communicative aphasia treatment as a further development of PACE therapy. *Aphasiology*, 5;1: 39-50.

Purser, H. (1982). *Psychology for Speech Therapists*. London: Macmillan.

Quirk, R. and Greenbaum, S. (1979). *A University Grammar of English*. London: Longman.

Rachman, S.J., Wilson, G.T. (1980). *The Effects of Psychological Therapy*. Oxford: Pergamon Press.

Rapin, I., Allen, D.A. (1983). Developmental language disorders: nosological considerations. In U. Kirk, (Ed) *Neuropsychology of Language, Reading and Spelling*. New York: Academic Press.

Reber, A.S. (1985). *The Penguin Dictionary of Psychology*. London: Penguin.

Renfrew, C. E. (1966). Persistence of the open syllable in defective articulation. *Journal of Speech and Hearing Disorders*, **31**: 370–373.

Renfrew, C. E. (1991) *The Bus Story, 3rd edn*. Oxford: the author.

Riedel, K. (1981). Auditory comprehension in aphasia. In M.T.Sarno (Ed.) (1981), *Acquired Aphasia*. London: Academic Press.

Robertson, S.J., Thomson, F. (1986). *Working with Dysarthrics*. London: Winslow Press.

Robins, R.H. (1971). *General Linguistics: An Introductory Survey*. London: Longman.

Robins, R.H. (1979). *A Short History of Linguistics*. London: Longman.

Rosenbek, J.C., LaPointe, L.L., Wertz, R.T. (1989). *Aphasia: A Clinical Approach*. Texas: Pro-ed.

Rumble, G.D., Robertson, J. (1995). *Lesson Plans for Minspeak Application Programmes*. Swinstead: Liberator.

Rutter, M. (1975). *Helping Troubled Children*. London: Penguin.

Ryan, B. P. and van Kirk, B. (1978). *Monterey Fluency Program*. Palo Alto, California: Monterey Learning Systems.

Salkie, R. (1990). *The Chomsky Update: Linguistics and Politics*. London: Routledge.

Salmon, M.A. (1978). *Developmental Defects and Syndromes*. Chichester: HM+M Publishers.

Sanders, D.A. (1977). *Auditory Perception of Speech*. London & New York: Prentice-Hall.

Sarno, M.T. (1969). The Functional Communication Profile: Manual of Directions. In *Rehabilitation Monograph*, **42**: New York: Institute of Rehabilitation Medicine.

Sarno. M.T. (Ed.) (1991). *Acquired Aphasia, 2nd edn*. London: Academic Press.

Satz, P., Bullard-Bates, C. (1981). Acquired aphasia in children. In M.T.Sarno (Ed.) (1981), *Acquired Aphasia*. London: Academic Press.

Sauber, G.R., L'Abate, L., Weeks, G.R., Buchanan, W.L. (1993). *The Dictionary of Family Psychology and Family, 2nd edn*. California: Sage Publications.

Saussure, F. de (1916). *Cours de Linguistique Générale*. Paris: Payot.

Scott, S., Caird, F. I. and Williams, B. O. (1985). *Communication in Parkinson's Disease*. London: Croom-Helm.

Searle, J.R. (1969). *Speech Acts: An Essay in the Philosophy of Language*. Cambridge: Cambridge University Press.

Sell, D., Grunwell, P. (1994). Speech studies and the unoperated cleft palate subject. *European Journal of Communication Disorders*, **29;2**: 151-164.

Sell, D., Harding, A., Grunwell, P. (1994). A screening assessment of cleft palate speech (Great Ormond Street Speech Assessment). *European Journal of Communication Disorders*, **29;1**: 1-16.

Shakespeare, R. (1975). *The Psychology of Handicap*. London: Methuen.

Shearer, D.E., Shearer, M.S. (1974). The Portage Project. A paper presented at the *Conference on Early Intervention for High Risk Infants and Young Children*, N. Carolina.

Silver, L.B. (1992). *The Misunderstood Child: A Guide for Parents of Children with*

Learning Disabilities. Florida: McGraw Hill.

Silverman, E.H., Elfant, I.L., (1979). An evaluation and treatment program for the adult. *American Journal of Occupational Therapy*, **33**;6: 382-392.

Simmons, N.N., Buckingham Jr, H.W. (1992). Recovery in jargon aphasia. *Aphasiology*, **6**;4: 403-414.

Skelly, M. (1979). *Amerind Gestural Code Based on Universal American Hand Talk*. New York: Elsevier.

Smith, D.W. (1985). *Recognizable Patterns of Human Malformation*. Volume VII in the series *Major Problems of Clinical Pediatrics*.

Sparks, R.W., Holland, A.L. (1976). Method: Melodic intonation therapy for aphasia. *Journal of Speech and Hearing Disorders*, **41**, 287–297.

Sparks, R., Helm, N., Albert, M. (1974). Aphasia rehabilitation resulting from melodic intonation therapy. *Cortex*, **10**: 303.

Stackhouse, J. (1992). Developmental verbal dyspraxia I: A review and critique. *European Journal of Disorders of Communication*, **27**;1: 19-34.

Stackhouse, J., Snowling, M. (1992). Developmental verbal dyspraxia II: A developmental perspective on two case studies. *European Journal of Disorders of Communication*, **27**;1: 35-54.

Stackhouse, J., Wells, B. (1993). Psycholinguistic assessment of developmental speech disorders. *European Journal of Disorders of Communication*, **28**;4: 331-348.

Stafford-Clark, D., Smith, A.C. (1983). *Psychiatry for Students*. London: George Allen & Unwin.

Sternberg, D.D. (1982). *Psycholinguistics: Language, Mind and World*. London: Longman.

Sternberg, D.D (1993). *An Introduction to Psychology*. London: Longman

Stevens, S.J. (1992). Differentiating the language disorder in dementia from dysphasia – the potential of a screening test. *European Journal of Disorders of Communication*, **27**;4: 275-288.

Stockwell, R.P. (1977). *Foundations of Syntactic Theory*. New Jersey: Prentice-Hall.

Strang, M.H. (1968). *Modern English Structure*. London: Edward Arnold.

Stuart-Smith, V.G., Wilks, V. (1979). Gesture program: A supplement to verbal communication for severely aphasic individuals. *Australian Journal of Human Communication Disorders*, **7**;2.

Swiffin, A.L., Arnott, J.L., Pickering, A., Newell, A.F. (1987). Adaptive and predictive techniques in a communication prosthesis. *Augmentative Alternative Communication*, 181-191.

Taverner, D. (1983). *Taverner's Physiology*. London: Hodder & Stoughton.

Taylor, A., Sluckin, W., Davies, D.R., Reason, J.T., Thomson, R., Colman, A.M. (1982). *Introducing Psychology*. London: Penguin.

Tortora, G.J., Grabowski, S.R. (1993). *Principles of Anatomy and Physiology, 7th edn*. New York: Harper & Row.

Travis, L.E. (Ed.) (1971). *Handbook of Speech Pathology and Audiology*. New York: Appleton-Century-Crofts.

Trower, P., Bryant, B., Argyle, M. (1978). *Social Skills and Mental Health*. London: Methuen.

Trudgill, P. (1974). *Sociolinguistics: An Introduction*. London: Penguin.

Tudor, C., Selley, W. G. (1974). A palatal training appliance and visual aid for use in the treatment of hypernasal speech. *British Journal of Disorders of Communication*, **9**: 117–122.

Valot, L. (1995). BUILLD: *Bringing Unity Into Language and Learning Development*.

Wooster, Ohio: Prentke Romich Company.

van der Gaag, A., Dormandy, K. (1993). *Communication and Adults with Learning Disabilities*. London: Whurr.

van Dijk, T.A. (1980). *Text and Context: Exploration in the Semantics and Pragmatics of Discourse*. London: Longman.

van Mourik, M., Verschaeve, M., Boon, P., Paquier, P., van Harskamp, F. (1992). Cognition in global aphasia: indicators for therapy. *Aphasiology*, **6;5**: 491-500.

van Tatenhove, G. (1989). Power in Play. *Proceedings of 1st UK Minspeak Conference*. Sept. 1989.

Vance, M. (1991). Education and therapeutic approaches used with a child presenting with aquired aphasia with convulsive disorder (Landau-Kleffner Syndrome). *Child Language Teaching and Therapy*, **7**: 1.

Walker, M. Armfield, A (1982). What is the Makatan Vocubulary? In M. Peter, R. Barnes (Eds) *Signs, Symbols and Schools: An Introduction to the Use of Non-vocal communicative Systems and Sign Language in Schools*. Stratford-on-Avon: NCSE.

Warner, J. (1981). *Helping the Handicapped Child with Early Feeding: A Checklist and Manual for Parents and Professionals*. Oxon: PTM Winslow.

Wells, G. (1985). *Language Development in the Pre-school Years*. Cambridge: Cambridge University Press.

Wells, J.C. (1982). *Accents of English 1: An Introduction*. Cambridge: Cambridge University Press.

Wertz, R.T. (1981). Neuropathologies of Speech and Language: an Introduction to patient management. In D.F. Johns (1981), *Clinical Management of Neurogenic Communicative Disorders*. Boston: Little, Brown and Company.

Wheldall, K. (1987). Assessing young children's receptive language development: A revised edition of the sentence comprehension test. *Child Language Teaching and Therapy*, **3;1**: 72-85.

White, M. (1985). *Good Basic Programming with the BBC Microcomputer*. London: Macmillan.

Whitton, M., Zloch, R. (1995). *Talking Lifestyles*. Lancaster: Mardis.

Williamson, I., Sheridan, C. (1994). The development of a test of speech reception disability for use in 5 to 8-year-old children with otitis media with effusion. *European Journal of Communication Disorders*, **29;1**: 27-37.

Wilson, D.K. (1979). *Voice Problems in Children*. Baltimore: Williams & Wilkins.

Wing, L. (1980). *Autistic Children: A Guide for Parents*. New York: Constable.

Wolff, S. (1981). *Children under Stress*. London: Penguin.

Wood, M.E. (1981). *The Development of Personality and Behaviour in Children*. London: Harrap.

World Health Organization (1967). *Manual of the International Statistical Classification of Diseases, Injuries and Causes of Death*, revised edn. Geneva: WHO.

Wyke, M. (Ed.) (1978). *Developmental Dysphasia*. London: Academic Press.